Intrinsically Disordered Proteins and Chronic Diseases

Intrinsically Disordered Proteins and Chronic Diseases

Editors

Prakash Kulkarni
Vladimir N. Uversky

MDPI • Basel • Beijing • Wuhan • Barcelona • Belgrade • Manchester • Tokyo • Cluj • Tianjin

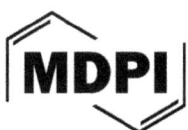

Editors
Prakash Kulkarni
Department of Medical Oncology
USA

Vladimir N. Uversky
University of South Florida
USA

Editorial Office
MDPI
St. Alban-Anlage 66
4052 Basel, Switzerland

This is a reprint of articles from the Special Issue published online in the open access journal *Biomolecules* (ISSN 2218-273X) (available at: https://www.mdpi.com/journal/biomolecules/special_issues/IDPs_Chronic_Diseases).

For citation purposes, cite each article independently as indicated on the article page online and as indicated below:

LastName, A.A.; LastName, B.B.; LastName, C.C. Article Title. *Journal Name* **Year**, *Volume Number*, Page Range.

ISBN 978-3-0365-1262-4 (Hbk)
ISBN 978-3-0365-1263-1 (PDF)

© 2021 by the authors. Articles in this book are Open Access and distributed under the Creative Commons Attribution (CC BY) license, which allows users to download, copy and build upon published articles, as long as the author and publisher are properly credited, which ensures maximum dissemination and a wider impact of our publications.

The book as a whole is distributed by MDPI under the terms and conditions of the Creative Commons license CC BY-NC-ND.

Contents

About the Editors vii

Prakash Kulkarni and Vladimir N. Uversky
Intrinsically Disordered Proteins in Chronic Diseases
Reprinted from: *Biomolecules* **2019**, *9*, 147, doi:10.3390/biom9040147 1

Christophe Bignon, Francesca Troilo, Stefano Gianni and Sonia Longhi
Modulation of Measles Virus N_{TAIL} Interactions through Fuzziness and Sequence Features of Disordered Binding Sites
Reprinted from: *Biomolecules* **2019**, *9*, 8, doi:10.3390/biom9010008 7

Taranpreet Kaur, Ibraheem Alshareedah, Wei Wang, Jason Ngo, Mahdi Muhammad Moosa and Priya R. Banerjee
Molecular Crowding Tunes Material States of Ribonucleoprotein Condensates
Reprinted from: *Biomolecules* **2019**, *9*, 71, doi:10.3390/biom9020071 21

Xingcheng Lin, Prakash Kulkarni, Federico Bocci, Nicholas P. Schafer, Susmita Roy, Min-Yeh Tsai, Yanan He, Yihong Chen, Krithika Rajagopalan, Steven M. Mooney, Yu Zeng, Keith Weninger, Alex Grishaev, José N. Onuchic, Herbert Levine, Peter G. Wolynes, Ravi Salgia, Govindan Rangarajan, Vladimir Uversky, John Orban and Mohit Kumar Jolly
Structural and Dynamical Order of a Disordered Protein: Molecular Insights into Conformational Switching of PAGE4 at the Systems Level
Reprinted from: *Biomolecules* **2019**, *9*, 77, doi:10.3390/biom9020077 39

Wenning Wang and Dongdong Wang
Extreme Fuzziness: Direct Interactions between Two IDPs
Reprinted from: *Biomolecules* **2019**, *9*, 81, doi:10.3390/biom9030081 57

Oluwakemi T. Sowemimo, Patrick Knox-Brown, Wade Borcherds, Tobias Rindfleisch, Anja Thalhammer and Gary W. Daughdrill
Conserved Glycines Control Disorder and Function in the Cold-Regulated Protein, COR15A
Reprinted from: *Biomolecules* **2019**, *9*, 84, doi:10.3390/biom9030084 69

Robin Levy, Emily Gregory, Wade Borcherds and Gary Daughdrill
p53 Phosphomimetics Preserve Transient Secondary Structure but Reduce Binding to Mdm2 and MdmX
Reprinted from: *Biomolecules* **2019**, *9*, 83, doi:10.3390/biom9030083 87

Hiroto Anbo, Masaya Sato, Atsushi Okoshi and Satoshi Fukuchi
Functional Segments on Intrinsically Disordered Regions in Disease-Related Proteins
Reprinted from: *Biomolecules* **2019**, *9*, 88, doi:10.3390/biom9030088 101

Raj Kumar and E. Brad Thompson
Role of Phosphorylation in the Modulation of the Glucocorticoid Receptor's Intrinsically Disordered Domain
Reprinted from: *Biomolecules* **2019**, *9*, 95, doi:10.3390/biom9030095 119

Kateřina Melková, Vojtěch Zapletal, Subhash Narasimhan, Séverine Jansen, Jozef Hritz, Rostislav Škrabana, Markus Zweckstetter, Malene Ringkjøbing Jensen, Martin Blackledge and Lukáš Žídek
Structure and Functions of Microtubule Associated Proteins Tau and MAP2c: Similarities and Differences
Reprinted from: *Biomolecules* **2019**, *9*, 105, doi:10.3390/biom9030105 129

Ucheor B. Choi, Hugo Sanabria, Tatyana Smirnova, Mark E. Bowen and Keith R. Weninger
Spontaneous Switching among Conformational Ensembles in Intrinsically Disordered Proteins
Reprinted from: *Biomolecules* **2019**, *9*, 114, doi:10.3390/biom9030114 . . . . **161**

Tarsila G. Castro, Florentina-Daniela Munteanu and Artur Cavaco-Paulo
Electrostatics of Tau Protein by Molecular Dynamics
Reprinted from: *Biomolecules* **2019**, *9*, 116, doi:10.3390/biom9030116 . . . . **177**

Supriyo Bhattacharya and Xingcheng Lin
Recent Advances in Computational Protocols Addressing Intrinsically Disordered Proteins
Reprinted from: *Biomolecules* **2019**, *9*, 146, doi:10.3390/biom9040146 . . . . **193**

About the Editors

Prakash Kulkarni obtained his PhD in biochemistry in India and did postdoctoral training in cell biology at New York University School of Medicine. Subsequently, he held Staff Scientist positions in the Division of Chemistry and Chemical Engineering, as well as in the Division of Biology and Biological Engineering at the California Institute of Technology, and later, in the Department of Genetics at Yale University School of Medicine. Dr. Kulkarni began his independent academic career as an Assistant Professor of Urology and Oncology in the Brady Urological Institute at Johns Hopkins University. He then moved as Research Associate Professor to the W. M. Keck Laboratory for Structural Biology at the Institute of Bioscience & Biotechnology Research, University of Maryland, before he moved to City of Hope, where he is currently a Research Professor and the Director of Translational Research. His main research interests are in intrinsically disordered proteins (IDPs), cancer biology, translational mathematical oncology and cancer systems biology, and are focused on answering fundamental questions concerning phenotypic switching, self-organization, synchronization, and evolution, that have important biological and biomedical implications. His long-term goals are to understand how a normal cell is transformed into a malignant one by factors from within, as is seen in sporadic cancers, and how a cancer cell progresses to colonize distant locations, acquire stem cell-like properties, and develop drug resistance, and whether these phenotypic changes can be reversed so that ultimately, this knowledge can be used to develop new and effective cancer therapeutics. Dr. Kulkarni has authored ~100 peer-reviewed publications and is co-editor of a book, "Phenotypic Switching: Implications in Biology and Medicine", published by Academic Press, 2020. He is a Fellow of the Royal Society of Biology, UK.

Vladimir N. Uversky is a Professor in the Department of Molecular Medicine at the University of South Florida (USF). He obtained his PhD from Moscow Institute of Physics and Technology and DSc from Institute of Experimental and Theoretical Biophysics, Russia. He is the discoverer of intrinsically disordered proteins (IDPs). He has authored over 850 scientific publications and edited several books and book series on protein structure, function, folding and misfolding. He is also an editor of several scientific journals. Dr. Uversky's research is focused on protein physics, including protein structure, stability, dynamics, function, folding, misfolding, and non-folding, and tries to establish relationships between the protein sequence and function in light of pharmaceutical biophysics. His laboratory uses a combination of experimental and bioinformatics approaches to describe the structural properties, functions, dynamics, and conformational stability of different proteins; to characterize their partially folded states; to analyze the molecular mechanisms of their folding and misfolding; to quantify structural consequences of protein interaction with various binding partners; to evaluate structural consequences of protein posttranslational modifications; to understand the effect of various environmental factors on protein folding, misfolding and conformational stability; to uncover the relationship between protein structure, stability and pathogenesis of various protein conformation-based diseases.

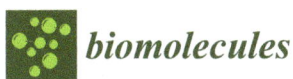

Editorial

Intrinsically Disordered Proteins in Chronic Diseases

Prakash Kulkarni [1],* and Vladimir N. Uversky [2,3],*

1 Department of Medical Oncology and Therapeutics Research, City of Hope National Medical Center, Duarte, CA 91010, USA
2 Department of Molecular Medicine, Morsani College of Medicine, University of South Florida, Tampa, FL 33612, USA
3 Laboratory of New Methods in Biology, Institute for Biological Instrumentation, Russian Academy of Sciences, 142290 Pushchino, Moscow Region, Russia
* Correspondence: pkulkarni@coh.org (P.K.); vuversky@health.usf.edu (V.N.U.)

Received: 3 April 2019; Accepted: 3 April 2019; Published: 11 April 2019

It is now increasingly evident that a large fraction of the human proteome comprises proteins that, under physiological conditions, lack fixed, ordered 3D structures as a whole or have segments that are not likely to form a defined 3D structure [1–7]. These proteins and regions are referred to as intrinsically disordered proteins (IDPs) and intrinsically disordered protein regions (IDPRs), respectively. Despite their lack of a stable structure, IDPs/IDPRs are involved in a multitude of crucial biological functions related to regulation, recognition, signaling, and control, where binding to multiple partners and high-specificity/low-affinity interactions plays a crucial role [8–14]. Furthermore, intrinsic disorder is a unique structural feature that enables IDPs/IDPRs to participate in both one-to-many and many-to-one signaling [9,10]. Since they serve as general regulators of various cellular processes, IDPs/IDPRs themselves are tightly controlled [15,16]. However, when misexpressed, misprocessed, mismodified, or dysregulated, IDPs/IDPRs are prone to engage in promiscuous, often unwanted interactions and, thus, are associated with the development of various pathological states. In fact, the majority of human cancer-related proteins [8], as well as many proteins associated with neurodegeneration [17,18], diabetes [19], cardiovascular disease [20], amyloidosis [21], and genetic diseases [22], are either intrinsically disordered or contain long IDPRs. This broad involvement of misbehaving IDPs/IDPRs in human diseases is known as "disorder in disorders" (or D^2) concept [23,24].

It is generally believed that IDPs/IDPRs stochastically sample all possible configurations driven by thermal fluctuations. While this may be true for many extended IDPs, which behave as "random" coils, it is likely that due to the variability in interaction energy between different amino acid sequences, some configurations may be strongly preferred while others are forbidden. Furthermore, unlike folded proteins that exhibit a high degree of structural order and undergo collective motions, albeit fairly constrained, IDPs/IDPRs also exhibit some structural and dynamical ordering, being much less constrained in their motions than folded proteins. Thus, the larger structural plasticity of IDPs emphasizes the importance of entropically driven motions. Because of their simplified spatial organization and globally reduced structural content, IDPs/IDPRs are characterized by the exceptional spatiotemporal heterogeneity, where different parts of a protein are ordered (or disordered) to a different degree, and this distribution is constantly changing over time [25,26]. Therefore, IDPs/IDPRs are not homogeneous, but have a very complex mosaic architecture reflecting their highly heterogeneous spatiotemporal structural organization that includes foldons (independently foldable units of a protein), inducible foldons (disordered regions that can fold at least in part due to their interaction with binding partners), non-foldons (non-foldable protein regions), semi-foldons (regions that are always in a semi-folded form), and unfoldons (ordered regions that have to undergo an order-to-disorder transition to become functional) [25,26]. Since these differently (dis)ordered structural elements might have well-defined and specific functions, an IDP/IDPR can be multifunctional, being involved in interaction with, regulation of, and be controlled by a multitude of structurally unrelated partners [27].

Although high-specificity/low-affinity interactions are considered a functional hallmark of IDPs/IDPRs, these proteins can also interact with ultrahigh (picomolar) affinity, but fully retain their structural disorder, long-range flexibility, and highly dynamic character [28]. Such structures, wherein bound IDPs/IDPRs retain structural plasticity, have been defined as fuzzy complexes [29,30]. While a large number of fuzzy complexes have been characterized, many of such interactions are between an IDP/IDPR and a structured protein. There are also examples of direct interactions between IDPs/IDPRs leading to the formation of a fuzzy complex without disorder-to-order transition [31–33]. With recent advances in experimental techniques and better integration with computational simulations, the picture that is emerging suggests that the modest structural ordering and large amplitude collective motions of IDPs/IDPRs enable them to mediate multiple interactions with different partners in the cell.

This Special Issue of *Biomolecules* is dedicated to elucidating how conformational dynamics affects interactions of IDP/IDPR with partner proteins, especially in those IDPs that are implicated in chronic diseases. Because of the unique properties they possess, and also because they are not amenable to classical tools and methods used to study ordered proteins, the IDPs/IDPRs have attracted attention across disciplines and scales. In fact, increasing curiosity in understanding how these fascinating molecules that lack unique structure but carry out the myriad functions resulted in an explosive expansion of the disorder-related literature, and scientists from various backgrounds as diverse as protein biochemists, classical physics, polymer physics, biophysics, theoretical physics, bioengineering, and computational and information science have begun to unravel many mysteries of IDPs/IDPRs. Technological advances, and the availability of more and more sophisticated computational tools, have further contributed to a deeper understanding of how IDPs are able carry out their functions. Therefore, it is not surprising that the various contributions to this Special Issue are from experts in biology, bioinformatics, biochemistry, biophysics, structural biology, and computational physics.

The contributions by Bignon et al. 'Modulation of measles virus NTAIL interactions through fuzziness and sequence features of disordered binding sites' [34], and by Kumar and Thompson 'Role of phosphorylation in the modulation of glucocorticoid receptor's intrinsically disordered domain' [35] provide an overview of the disorder-based functionality mostly from a biochemical perspective. Bignon et al. review recent findings on the different interaction mechanisms of the C-terminal domain of the intrinsically disordered nucleoprotein (N) of measles virus (MeV) N_{TAIL}, with two of its known binding partners, namely, the C-terminal X domain of the phosphoprotein of MeV XD (a globular viral protein) and the heat-shock protein 70 (hsp70, a globular cellular protein). Kumar and Thompson, on the other hand, delve in the important role of phosphorylation in gene regulation by glucocorticoid receptor (GR) [34]. The GR N-terminal domain is highly disordered and undergoes disorder-to-order transition following site-specific phosphorylation. And this transition from disorder to order is critical for AF1's efficient interaction with several coregulatory proteins and subsequent AF1-mediated GR activity [35].

Three articles comprise the structural biology section. Of course, protein NMR remains the work horse for gaining insight into IDP/IDPR (un)structure/function relationships. Levy et al., in their article 'p53 phosphomimetics preserve transient secondary structure but reduce binding to Mdm2 and MdmX' [36], examined the disordered p53 transactivation domain (p53TAD) using a combination of biophysical techniques including NMR. The p53TAD contains transient helical structures that are necessary for its binding to the negative regulators, mouse double minute 2 (Mdm2) and MdmX. The second paper in this section, 'Conserved glycines control disorder and function in the Cold-Regulated Protein, COR15A' by Sowemimo et al. [37], analyzes the plant cold-regulated protein COR15A from *Arabidopsis* that is important for freeze tolerance. During freezing-induced cellular dehydration, COR15A transitions from a disordered to mostly α-helical structure. The authors tested whether mutations that increase the helicity of COR15A also increase its protective function using a combination of NMR, circular dichroism, and fluorescence spectroscopy. The results of these experiments showed that the mutants with higher content of α-helical structure were characterized by an increased membrane stabilization potential during freezing [37]. Finally, the paper by Melková et al. 'Structure and functions of microtubule associated proteins tau and MAP2c: similarities and differences' [38] used a combination of NMR and cryo-electron microscopy to examine the propensities of MAPs, tau40 and MAP2, to form transient local structures and long-range contacts in the free state, and conformations adopted by these proteins in complexes with microtubules and filamentous actin, as well as in pathological aggregates. For both molecules, the authors identified transient structural motifs by conformational analysis of the experimental data and observed that many of the short sequence motifs that exhibit transient structural features are linked to functional properties, manifested by specific interactions. Therefore, this detailed structure–function analysis may help in explaining the observed differences between biological activities of tau40 and MAP2c [38].

Single-molecule fluorescence resonance energy transfer (or smFRET) is yet another powerful tool used to study IDPs/IDPRs. It is one of the few approaches that are sensitive to transient populations of substrates within molecular ensembles, and therefore, is ideally suited to discern conformational preferences of IDP/IDPR ensembles. The first paper in the section, 'Spontaneous switching among conformational ensembles in intrinsically disordered proteins', by Choi et al. [39] describes a growing number of proteins that appear intrinsically disordered by biochemical and bioinformatics characterization but switch between restricted regions of conformational space. Such switching between disparate corners of conformational space could bias ligand binding and regulate the volume of IDPs acting as structural or entropic elements. Therefore, mapping the accessible energy landscape and capturing dynamics across a wide range of timescales are essential for recognition of when an IDP/IDPR is acting as such a switch [39]. In the paper entitled 'Extreme fuzziness: Direct interactions between two IDPs', Wang and Wang [40] examined whether two IDPs can interact directly to form a fuzzy complex without disorder-to-order transition. Using a combination of smFRET, NMR, and molecular dynamics (MD) simulation, the authors demonstrate that direct interactions between the two pairs of IDPs, 4.1G-CTD/NuMA and H1/ProTα, do form fuzzy complexes while retaining high conformational dynamics of the isolated proteins, which they name as the extremely fuzzy complexes. Therefore, extreme fuzziness completes the full spectrum of protein–protein interaction modes, suggesting that a more generalized model beyond existing binding mechanisms is required [40].

Using a different biophysical approach, confocal fluorescence microscopy, Kaur et al. [41] in their paper entitled 'Molecular crowding tunes material states of ribonucleoprotein condensates', study how molecular crowding impacts ribonucleoprotein (RNP) liquid condensation using an archetypal disordered RNP, called fused in sarcoma (FUS), as an example. RNP condensation is largely governed by promiscuous attractive inter-chain interactions mediated by low-complexity domains (LCDs). The authors demonstrate that the liquid–liquid coexistence boundary of FUS is lowered by polymer crowders, consistent with an excluded volume model. With increasing bulk crowder concentration, the RNP partition increases and the diffusion rate decreases in the condensed phase. These results reveal that the impact of crowding is largely independent of LCD charge and sequence patterns. These results are consistent with a thermodynamic model of crowder-mediated depletion interaction, which suggests that inter-RNP attraction is enhanced by molecular crowding [41].

Characterizing the structure–function relationship of IDPs/IDPRs is no doubt an essential but daunting task as they can adapt transient structure. Molecular dynamics simulations (MDS) has emerged as a natural complement to various experimental approaches for atomic-level characterizations and mechanistic investigations of this intriguing class of proteins. This SI includes three interesting papers that have exploited this computational technique in conjunction with experimental data to gain new insight into the IDP/IDPR structure/function paradigm. In the first article in this section, 'Electrostatics of Tau protein by molecular dynamics', Castro et al. [42] employed MDS to study the structure of a microtubule associated protein Tau that promotes microtubule assembly and stability. To date, the 3D structure of Tau has not been fully solved, experimentally. This is the first MDS study of full-length Tau in conjunction with a region from the microtubule tubulin with which it interacts. The results bring a new insight into Tau and tubulin proteins, their characteristics and structure-function relationship, and highlights the fact that Tau is a disordered protein with discrete portions of well-defined secondary structure mostly at the microtubule binding region [42].

The second paper, 'Structural and dynamical order of a disordered protein: Molecular insights into conformational switching of PAGE4 at the systems level', describes another MDS study by Lin et al. [43]. Using prostate-associated gene 4 (PAGE4), an IDP implicated in prostate cancer (PCa), as an example, the authors describe the quantitative reproduction of experimental observations and reveal how structural and dynamic ordering are encoded in the sequence of PAGE4, and how these features can be modulated by different extents of phosphorylation by different kinases. This ordering is reflected in changing populations of certain secondary structural elements, as well as in the regularity of its collective motions, and correlate with the functional interactions of the different conformational ensembles of PAGE4 to give rise to repeated transitions between cellular phenotypes with important physiological consequences [43].

The third paper in this section on MDS and biophysical computation, 'Recent advances in computational protocols addressing intrinsically disordered proteins' by Bhattacharya and Lin [44], argues that to understand the conformational dynamics of IDPs/IDPRs and how their structural ensembles recognize multiple binding partners and small molecule inhibitors, knowledge-based and physics-based sampling techniques, guided by the experimental structural data, can be utilized for the comprehensive and focused in silico analyses. However, efficient sampling of the IDP/IDPR conformational ensemble requires traversing the numerous degrees of freedom in the IDP/IDPR energy landscape, as well as force-fields that accurately model the protein and solvent interactions. Therefore, these authors provide an overview of the current state of computational methods for studying IDP/IDPR structure and dynamics and discuss the major challenges in this field.

Finally, the paper 'Functional segments on intrinsically disordered regions in disease-related proteins' by Anbo et al. [45] describes a bioinformatics approach to study IDPs/IDPRs. IDPRs, which are often found in the ordered proteins, are known to play important roles in signaling pathways and transcriptional regulation. Therefore, the authors performed a bioinformatics analysis and found more than a thousand potential functional IDPR segments in disease-related proteins, which are found in cancers, congenital disorders, digestive system diseases, and reproductive system diseases. A detailed analysis of some of these regions showed that the functional segments are located on experimentally verified IDPRs. Since IDPs involved in disease pathology tend to have numerous protein–protein interactors, these data suggest that, by occupying hub positions in the protein–protein interaction networks, IDPs can have huge impacts on human diseases. This study highlights the utility of bioinformatics approaches in conjunction with experimental data to in casting new light on the IDPs/IDPRs [45].

In summary, we trust these articles on the IDPs/IDPRs will not only serve as excellent references, but will also stimulate a flurry of activity toward gaining a deeper insight into these fascinating molecules that constitute a large fraction of the proteomes across all three kingdoms of life and engage in myriad biological activities in ways that seem to challenge conventional wisdom. With new advances in experimental techniques, theoretical concepts, and computational capabilities that permit observations across spatiotemporal scales, it is likely that we may have a better understanding of the IDPs and be able to design strategies to target them for therapeutic purposes.

References

1. Peng, Z.; Yan, J.; Fan, X.; Mizianty, M.J.; Xue, B.; Wang, K.; Hu, G.; Uversky, V.N.; Kurgan, L. Exceptionally abundant exceptions: Comprehensive characterization of intrinsic disorder in all domains of life. *Cell Mol. Life Sci.* **2015**, *72*, 137–151.
2. Colak, R.; Kim, T.; Michaut, M.; Sun, M.; Irimia, M.; Bellay, J.; Myers, C.L.; Blencowe, B.J.; Kim, P.M. Distinct types of disorder in the human proteome: Functional implications for alternative splicing. *PLoS Comput. Biol.* **2013**, *9*, e1003030. [CrossRef]

3. Xue, B.; Dunker, A.K.; Uversky, V.N. Orderly order in protein intrinsic disorder distribution: Disorder in 3500 proteomes from viruses and the three domains of life. *J. Biomol. Struct. Dyn.* **2012**, *30*, 137–149. [CrossRef] [PubMed]
4. Uversky, V.N. The mysterious unfoldome: Structureless, underappreciated, yet vital part of any given proteome. *J. Biomed. Biotechnol.* **2010**, *2010*, 568068. [CrossRef] [PubMed]
5. Shimizu, K.; Toh, H. Interaction between intrinsically disordered proteins frequently occurs in a human protein-protein interaction network. *J. Mol. Biol.* **2009**, *392*, 1253–1265. [CrossRef]
6. Ward, J.J.; Sodhi, J.S.; McGuffin, L.J.; Buxton, B.F.; Jones, D.T. Prediction and functional analysis of native disorder in proteins from the three kingdoms of life. *J. Mol. Biol.* **2004**, *337*, 635–645. [CrossRef] [PubMed]
7. Dunker, A.K.; Obradovic, Z.; Romero, P.; Garner, E.C.; Brown, C.J. Intrinsic protein disorder in complete genomes. *Genome Inform. Ser. Workshop Genome Inform.* **2000**, *11*, 161–171.
8. Iakoucheva, L.M.; Brown, C.J.; Lawson, J.D.; Obradovic, Z.; Dunker, A.K. Intrinsic disorder in cell-signaling and cancer-associated proteins. *J. Mol. Biol.* **2002**, *323*, 573–584. [CrossRef]
9. Dunker, A.K.; Cortese, M.S.; Romero, P.; Iakoucheva, L.M.; Uversky, V.N. Flexible nets: The roles of intrinsic disorder in protein interaction networks. *FEBS Journal* **2005**, *272*, 5129–5148. [CrossRef] [PubMed]
10. Uversky, V.N.; Oldfield, C.J.; Dunker, A.K. Showing your id: Intrinsic disorder as an id for recognition, regulation and cell signaling. *J. Mol. Recognit.* **2005**, *18*, 343–384. [CrossRef] [PubMed]
11. Radivojac, P.; Iakoucheva, L.M.; Oldfield, C.J.; Obradovic, Z.; Uversky, V.N.; Dunker, A.K. Intrinsic disorder and functional proteomics. *Biophys. J.* **2007**. [CrossRef]
12. Vucetic, S.; Xie, H.; Iakoucheva, L.M.; Oldfield, C.J.; Dunker, A.K.; Obradovic, Z.; Uversky, V.N. Functional anthology of intrinsic disorder. 2. Cellular components, domains, technical terms, developmental processes, and coding sequence diversities correlated with long disordered regions. *J. Proteome Res.* **2007**, *6*, 1899–1916. [CrossRef]
13. Xie, H.; Vucetic, S.; Iakoucheva, L.M.; Oldfield, C.J.; Dunker, A.K.; Obradovic, Z.; Uversky, V.N. Functional anthology of intrinsic disorder. 3. Ligands, post-translational modifications, and diseases associated with intrinsically disordered proteins. *J. Proteome Res.* **2007**, *6*, 1917–1932. [CrossRef] [PubMed]
14. Xie, H.; Vucetic, S.; Iakoucheva, L.M.; Oldfield, C.J.; Dunker, A.K.; Uversky, V.N.; Obradovic, Z. Functional anthology of intrinsic disorder. 1. Biological processes and functions of proteins with long disordered regions. *J. Proteome Res.* **2007**, *6*, 1882–1898. [CrossRef] [PubMed]
15. Gsponer, J.; Futschik, M.E.; Teichmann, S.A.; Babu, M.M. Tight regulation of unstructured proteins: From transcript synthesis to protein degradation. *Science* **2008**, *322*, 1365–1368. [CrossRef] [PubMed]
16. Uversky, V.N.; Dunker, A.K. Biochemistry. Controlled chaos. *Science* **2008**, *322*, 1340–1341. [CrossRef]
17. Uversky, V.N. The triple power of d(3): Protein intrinsic disorder in degenerative diseases. *Front. Biosci. (Landmark Ed.)* **2014**, *19*, 181–258. [CrossRef]
18. Uversky, V.N. Intrinsic disorder in proteins associated with neurodegenerative diseases. *Front. Biosci. (Landmark Ed.)* **2009**, *14*, 5188–5238. [CrossRef] [PubMed]
19. Du, Z.; Uversky, V.N. A comprehensive survey of the roles of highly disordered proteins in type 2 diabetes. *Int. J. Mol. Sci.* **2017**, *18*, 10. [CrossRef]
20. Cheng, Y.; LeGall, T.; Oldfield, C.J.; Dunker, A.K.; Uversky, V.N. Abundance of intrinsic disorder in protein associated with cardiovascular disease. *Biochemistry* **2006**, *45*, 10448–10460. [CrossRef] [PubMed]
21. Uversky, V.N. Amyloidogenesis of natively unfolded proteins. *Curr. Alzheimer. Res.* **2008**, *5*, 260–287. [CrossRef] [PubMed]
22. Midic, U.; Oldfield, C.J.; Dunker, A.K.; Obradovic, Z.; Uversky, V.N. Protein disorder in the human diseasome: Unfoldomics of human genetic diseases. *BMC Genomics* **2009**, *10* 1, S12. [CrossRef]
23. Uversky, V.N.; Oldfield, C.J.; Dunker, A.K. Intrinsically disordered proteins in human diseases: Introducing the d2 concept. *Annu. Rev. Biophys.* **2008**, *37*, 215–246. [CrossRef] [PubMed]
24. Uversky, V.N.; Dave, V.; Iakoucheva, L.M.; Malaney, P.; Metallo, S.J.; Pathak, R.R.; Joerger, A.C. Pathological unfoldomics of uncontrolled chaos: Intrinsically disordered proteins and human diseases. *Chem. Rev.* **2014**, *114*, 6844–6879. [CrossRef]
25. Uversky, V.N. Unusual biophysics of intrinsically disordered proteins. *Biochim. Biophys. Acta* **2013**, *1834*, 932–951. [CrossRef]
26. Uversky, V.N. Paradoxes and wonders of intrinsic disorder: Complexity of simplicity. *Intrinsically Disord. Proteins* **2016**, *4*, e1135015. [CrossRef]

27. Uversky, V.N. Functional roles of transiently and intrinsically disordered regions within proteins. *FEBS J.* **2015**, *282*, 1182–1189. [CrossRef]
28. Borgia, A.; Borgia, M.B.; Bugge, K.; Kissling, V.M.; Heidarsson, P.O.; Fernandes, C.B.; Sottini, A.; Soranno, A.; Buholzer, K.J.; Nettels, D.; et al. Extreme disorder in an ultrahigh-affinity protein complex. *Nature* **2018**, *555*, 61–66. [CrossRef] [PubMed]
29. Fuxreiter, M. Fold or not to fold upon binding - Does it really matter? *Curr. Opin. Struct. Biol.* **2018**, *54*, 19–25. [CrossRef] [PubMed]
30. Tompa, P.; Fuxreiter, M. Fuzzy complexes: Polymorphism and structural disorder in protein-protein interactions. *Trends Biochem. Sci.* **2008**, *33*, 2–8. [CrossRef]
31. Shen, Q.; Shi, J.; Zeng, D.; Zhao, B.; Li, P.; Hwang, W.; Cho, J.H. Molecular mechanisms of tight binding through fuzzy interactions. *Biophys. J.* **2018**, *114*, 1313–1320. [CrossRef] [PubMed]
32. Teixeira, J.M.C.; Fuentes, H.; Bielskute, S.; Gairi, M.; Zerko, S.; Kozminski, W.; Pons, M. The two isoforms of lyn display different intramolecular fuzzy complexes with the sh3 domain. *Molecules* **2018**, *23*, 2731. [CrossRef] [PubMed]
33. Sigalov, A.B.; Zhuravleva, A.V.; Orekhov, V.Y. Binding of intrinsically disordered proteins is not necessarily accompanied by a structural transition to a folded form. *Biochimie* **2007**, *89*, 419–421. [CrossRef] [PubMed]
34. Bignon, C.; Troilo, F.; Gianni, S.; Longhi, S. Modulation of measles virus ntail interactions through fuzziness and sequence features of disordered binding sites. *Biomolecules* **2018**, *9*, 8. [CrossRef] [PubMed]
35. Kumar, R.; Thompson, E.B. Role of phosphorylation in the modulation of the glucocorticoid receptor's intrinsically disordered domain. *Biomolecules* **2019**, *9*, 77. [CrossRef] [PubMed]
36. Levy, R.; Gregory, E.; Borcherds, W.; Daughdrill, G. P53 phosphomimetics preserve transient secondary structure but reduce binding to mdm2 and mdmx. *Biomolecules* **2019**, *9*, 83. [CrossRef]
37. Sowemimo, O.T.; Knox-Brown, P.; Borcherds, W.; Rindfleisch, T.; Thalhammer, A.; Daughdrill, G.W. Conserved glycines control disorder and function in the cold-regulated protein, cor15a. *Biomolecules* **2019**, *9*, 84. [CrossRef]
38. Melkova, K.; Zapletal, V.; Narasimhan, S.; Jansen, S.; Hritz, J.; Skrabana, R.; Zweckstetter, M.; Ringkjobing Jensen, M.; Blackledge, M.; Zidek, L. Structure and functions of microtubule associated proteins tau and map2c: Similarities and differences. *Biomolecules* **2019**, *9*, 105. [CrossRef]
39. Choi, U.B.; Sanabria, H.; Smirnova, T.; Bowen, M.E.; Weninger, K.R. Spontaneous switching among conformational ensembles in intrinsically disordered proteins. *Biomolecules* **2019**, *9*, 114. [CrossRef]
40. Wang, W.; Wang, D. Extreme fuzziness: Direct interactions between two idps. *Biomolecules* **2019**, *9*, 81. [CrossRef]
41. Kaur, T.; Alshareedah, I.; Wang, W.; Ngo, J.; Moosa, M.M.; Banerjee, P.R. Molecular crowding tunes material states of ribonucleoprotein condensates. *Biomolecules* **2019**, *9*, 71. [CrossRef]
42. Castro, T.G.; Munteanu, F.D.; Cavaco-Paulo, A. Electrostatics of tau protein by molecular dynamics. *Biomolecules* **2019**, *9*, 116. [CrossRef]
43. Lin, X.; Kulkarni, P.; Bocci, F.; Schafer, N.P.; Roy, S.; Tsai, M.Y.; He, Y.; Chen, Y.; Rajagopalan, K.; Mooney, S.M; et al. Structural and dynamical order of a disordered protein: Molecular insights into conformational switching of page4 at the systems level. *Biomolecules* **2019**, *9*, 77. [CrossRef]
44. Bhattacharya, S.; Lin, X. Recent advances in computational protocols addressing intrinsically disordered proteins. *Biomolecules* **2019**, *9*, 146. [CrossRef]
45. Anbo, H.; Sato, M.; Okoshi, A.; Fukuchi, S. Functional segments on intrinsically disordered regions in disease-related proteins. *Biomolecules* **2019**, *9*, 88. [CrossRef]

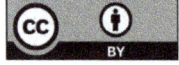 © 2019 by the authors. Licensee MDPI, Basel, Switzerland. This article is an open access article distributed under the terms and conditions of the Creative Commons Attribution (CC BY) license (http://creativecommons.org/licenses/by/4.0/).

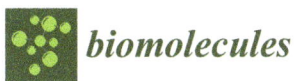

Review

Modulation of Measles Virus N_{TAIL} Interactions through Fuzziness and Sequence Features of Disordered Binding Sites

Christophe Bignon [1,*], Francesca Troilo [1,2], Stefano Gianni [2] and Sonia Longhi [1,*]

[1] CNRS and Aix-Marseille Univ Laboratoire Architecture et Fonction des Macromolecules Biologiques (AFMB), UMR 7257 Marseille, France; francesca.troilo@uniroma1.it
[2] Istituto Pasteur—Fondazione Cenci Bolognetti, Dipartimento di Scienze Biochimiche 'A. Rossi Fanelli' and Istituto di Biologia e Patologia Molecolari del Consiglio Nazionale delle Ricerche, Sapienza Università di Roma, 00185 Rome, Italy; stefano.gianni@uniroma1.it
* Correspondence: christophe.bignon@afmb.univ-mrs.fr (C.B.); sonia.longhi@afmb.univ-mrs.fr (S.L.)

Received: 22 November 2018; Accepted: 18 December 2018; Published: 27 December 2018

Abstract: In this paper we review our recent findings on the different interaction mechanisms of the C-terminal domain of the nucleoprotein (N) of measles virus (MeV) N_{TAIL}, a model viral intrinsically disordered protein (IDP), with two of its known binding partners, i.e., the C-terminal X domain of the phosphoprotein of MeV XD (a globular viral protein) and the heat-shock protein 70 hsp70 (a globular cellular protein). The N_{TAIL} binds both XD and hsp70 via a molecular recognition element (MoRE) that is flanked by two fuzzy regions. The long (85 residues) N-terminal fuzzy region is a natural dampener of the interaction with both XD and hsp70. In the case of binding to XD, the N-terminal fuzzy appendage of N_{TAIL} reduces the rate of α-helical folding of the MoRE. The dampening effect of the fuzzy appendage on XD and hsp70 binding depends on the length and fuzziness of the N-terminal region. Despite this similarity, N_{TAIL} binding to XD and hsp70 appears to rely on completely different requirements. Almost any mutation within the MoRE decreases XD binding, whereas many of them increase the binding to hsp70. In addition, XD binding is very sensitive to the α-helical state of the MoRE, whereas hsp70 is not. Thus, contrary to hsp70, XD binding appears to be strictly dependent on the wild-type primary and secondary structure of the MoRE.

Keywords: IDP; fuzzy interactions; protein complementation assays; split-GFP reassembly; kinetics

1. Structural Properties and Molecular Partnership of N_{TAIL}

The nucleoprotein (N) of measles virus (MeV) consists in a large structured moiety (N_{CORE}, aa 1 to 400) and in a C-terminal domain (N_{TAIL}, aa 401 to 525 of N) that is intrinsically disordered [1] (Figure 1A). The N_{TAIL} protrudes from the globular core of N and is exposed at the surface of the viral nucleocapsid [2–6]. The latter is made of a regular array of N monomers wrapping the RNA genome into a helicoidal arrangement. The exposure of N_{TAIL} at the surface of the nucleocapsid allows recruitment of the phosphoprotein (P) via interaction with the C-terminal X domain (XD) of the latter [7–10]. The phosphoprotein (P) is required for both transcription and replication, as it tethers the viral Large protein (L), which possesses all the enzymatic activities required for RNA synthesis, onto the nucleocapsid template (for a review see [11]).

Structural disorder is known to be a determinant of protein interactivity: the enhanced plasticity of intrinsically disordered proteins (IDPs) and regions (IDRs) allows for the enlargement of their molecular partnership [12–14]. In line with this, MeV N$_{TAIL}$ binds to numerous partners. Beyond the X domain of the P protein, N$_{TAIL}$ also interacts with the viral matrix protein [15]. In addition, it also interacts with host proteins, such as the major inducible heat shock protein 70 (hsp70) [16–18], a nuclear export protein [19], the interferon regulatory factor 3 [20,21], a cell receptor involved in MeV-induced immunosuppression [22,23], peroxiredoxin 1 [24], and proteins of the cell cytoskeleton [25,26].

The N$_{TAIL}$ and XD proteins interact with each other forming a 1:1 stoichiometric complex with an equilibrium dissociation constant (K_D) in the µM range [27,28]. The crystal structure of MeV XD has revealed that this domain consists of a bundle of three antiparallel α-helices [9,10,29] (Figure 1B). In solution however, two distinct structural forms differing in their degree of compactness coexist [30,31].

The structural arrangement of XD in a triple α-helical bundle, as well as the disordered nature of N$_{TAIL}$ [32], are also conserved in the related Nipah and Hendra viruses, whose N$_{TAIL}$-XD complexes are similar to that of MeV [27,33]. Binding to XD triggers α-helical folding of a short N$_{TAIL}$ region (Box2, aa 486 to 504 of MeV N, and Box3, aa 473 to 493 of *Henipavirus* N), referred to as a Molecular Recognition Element or MoRE [7,9,10,27] (Figure 1A). The MoREs are short, transiently populated secondary structures within IDRs that are often structurally biased towards their bound state [34]. The crystal structure of a MeV chimeric construct in which XD is covalently attached to the MoRE of N$_{TAIL}$ (aa 486 to 504) was solved at 1.8 Å [10]. The structure consists of a pseudo-four helix complex in which the MoRE of N$_{TAIL}$ adopts a parallel orientation with respect to XD and is embedded in a large hydrophobic cleft delimited by XD helices α2 and α3 [10] (Figure 1C).

The MoRE is partly preconfigured as an α-helix in the absence of XD in both MeV and henipaviruses [5,29,33,35–38]. This partial pre-configuration facilitates the folding-upon-binding process by rendering the structural transition to the (partially) folded conformation energetically less demanding [34]. In spite of this pre-configuration, N$_{TAIL}$ was shown to fold according to a folding-after-binding mechanism [28,33,39,40].

Mutational studies coupled to Φ-value analysis led to a detailed structural description of the folding and binding events occurring in the recognition between MeV N$_{TAIL}$ and XD [41]. Analysis of the impact of single-amino acid substitutions in N$_{TAIL}$ on the reaction mechanism allowed the identification of key residues involved in the initial recognition between N$_{TAIL}$ and XD, and enabled unraveling of the general features of the folding pathway of N$_{TAIL}$. In addition, analysis of the changes in stability of all the variants revealed that a few substitutions favor the folding step, which highlighted the inherent poor folding efficiency of N$_{TAIL}$, a property that we proposed that could arise from the weakly funneled nature of the energy landscape of IDPs in their unbound state that might dictate a considerable structural heterogeneity (or structural frustration) of the bound state [41].

In both MeV and henipaviruses, following binding to XD, most of N$_{TAIL}$ remains disordered and does not establish stable contacts with XD [8,27,29,33,35–38,42–44]. These N$_{TAIL}$-XD complexes are therefore illustrative examples of fuzziness [45]. Fuzziness may confer various functional advantages, such as the ability to interact with alternative partners and/or to establish simultaneous interactions with different partners. Fuzziness also provides a way to reduce the entropic penalty that accompanies the disorder-to-order transition, thereby leading to enhanced affinity. Tuning fuzziness therefore constitutes an additional manner by which IDPs can modulate the interaction strength with their partners. Furthermore, disordered appendages can harbor regulatory post-translational modification sites, can serve for partner fishing via non-specific, transient contacts, and can accommodate binding sites for additional partners [46–48].

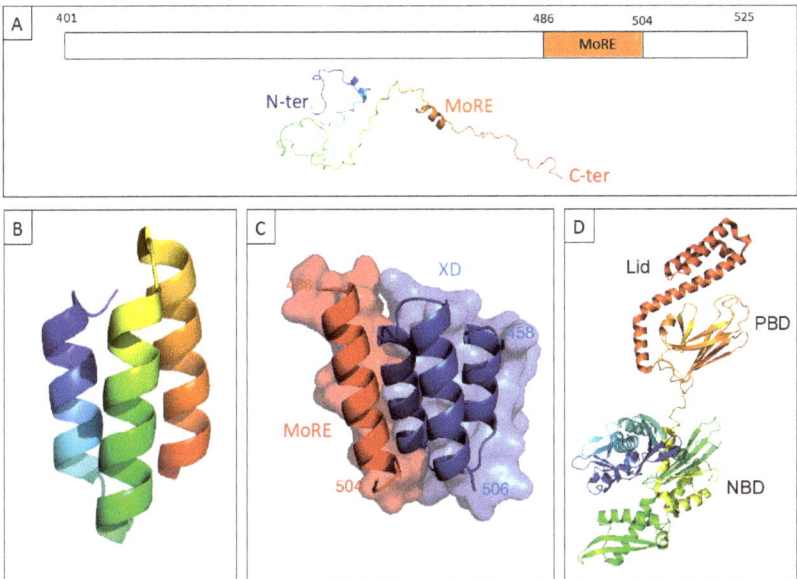

Figure 1. (**A**) Schematic representation of the C-terminal domain of the nucleoprotein (N) of measles virus (MeV) N_{TAIL} (upper panel) and cartoon representation of an N_{TAIL} conformer generated using Flexible-Mecano [49]. (**B**) Ribbon representation of the crystal structure of the C-terminal X domain of the phosphoprotein of MeV XD (PDB code 1OKS). (**C**) The structure of the chimeric construct made of MeV XD (blue) and of the molecular recognition element MoRE of N_{TAIL} (red) (PDB code 1T6O). (**D**) Cartoon representation of the crystal structure of hsp70 based on PDB codes 1HJO and 4JNF. The relative orientation of the two hsp70 domains (i.e., amino acids 3 to 382 and amino acids 389 to 610) is based on the structure of a form encompassing residues 1 to 554 (PDB code 1YUW). The three constituent domains of hsp70, i.e., nucleotide binding domain (NBD, aa 1 to 384), peptide binding domain (PBD, aa 384 to 543) and "lid" (aa 543 to 641) (see [18] and references therein cited) are highlighted.

In line with these abilities, the C-terminal fuzzy region of MeV N_{TAIL} encompassing residues 517 to 525 was shown to serve as a low-affinity binding site for hsp70 [17,18], a large cellular protein with a markedly different structural organization (Figure 1D) with respect to XD. The heat shock protein 70 (hsp 70) was shown to stimulate both viral transcription and replication, with this ability relying on interaction with N_{TAIL} [16,17,50–55]. Binding experiments showed that the major hsp70-binding site is however located within Box2 [56]. Since hsp70 was found to competitively inhibit the binding of XD to N_{TAIL} [17], it has been proposed that hsp70 could enhance viral transcription and replication by destabilizing the P–N_{TAIL} interaction, thereby promoting successive cycles of binding and release that are essential for the polymerase to progress along the nucleocapsid template [8,17]. The hsp70-dependent reduction of the stability of P–N_{TAIL} complexes would thus rely on competition between hsp70 and XD for binding to the α-MoRE of N_{TAIL}, with recruitment of hsp70 being ensured by both Box2 and Box3 [17]. Although the hsp70-binding site(s) within N_{TAIL} have been mapped, no structural information on the complex is available.

In the following sections we summarize available data pertaining to the impact of the long, N-terminal fuzzy appendage of N_{TAIL} on binding to both XD and hsp70. We also summarize the available molecular information on the sequence and secondary structure requirements for N_{TAIL}-XD and N_{TAIL}-hsp70 binding. Altogether, these studies contribute to enlarge our knowledge of the molecular determinants underlying the ability of hsp70 to interact with N_{TAIL} and, more generally, add "another brick to the wall" towards the ambitious goal of building up a comprehensive understanding of the mechanisms by which IDPs recognize their partners.

2. The N-Terminal Fuzzy Region of N$_{TAIL}$ down Regulates the Binding of the MoRE to Both XD and Hsp70

As recalled in the introduction, the MoRE of N$_{TAIL}$ (aa 486 to 504) is responsible for XD binding and is preceded by a long, N-terminal fuzzy region (aa 401 to 488). We have investigated the role of this region by shortening it by ten residue intervals from aa 401 to aa 481 (Figure 2A), and then assessing the binding ability of each truncation variant using a split-green fluorescent protein (GFP) complementation assay [57,58]. In this assay, two proteins (X and Y) known to interact with each other are respectively fused to the C-terminal end of the first seven N-terminal moiety of GFP (NGFP) and the N-terminal end of the last four β-strands C-terminal moiety of GFP (CGFP) of GFP. Separately, NGFP-X and Y-CGFP are unable to fluoresce. However, when NGFP-X and Y-CGFP are co-expressed in E. coli, X and Y bind to each other within the cell, allowing NGFP and CGFP to reconstitute the full-length fluorescent GFP. Since the fluorescence is proportional to the affinity between X and Y [59,60], the interaction between different combinations of NGFP-X and Y-CGFP can be compared by simply measuring the fluorescence of the bacteria co-expressing NGFP-X and Y-CGFP. In our case, X was N$_{TAIL}$ or its truncation variants and Y was either XD or hsp70.

Results show a non-monotonic fluorescence increase with the truncation, with both XD (Figure 2B) and hsp70 (Figure 2C). In agreement with the known higher affinity of N$_{TAIL}$ for XD (3 µM) [28] compared to that for hsp70 (70 µM) [18], the overall fluorescence was found to be higher for XD than for hsp70 (see the different Y-axis scales between Figure 2B,C). Thus, the fuzzy N-terminal region of N$_{TAIL}$ negatively regulates the binding of N$_{TAIL}$ to two partners that differ in both size and affinity. We have obtained similar results when N$_{TAIL}$ and XD from NiV and HeV were used [61] or when another protein complementation assay based on split-luciferase [62] was used. Thus, the negative effect of the fuzzy N-terminal region of N$_{TAIL}$ on XD binding is shared by at least three paramyxoviruses and is maintained irrespective of whether the assay generates reversible (luciferase) or irreversible (GFP) complexes [61].

We sought possible reasons for this negative effect. The importance of the primary structure of N$_{TAIL}$ N-terminal region was first assessed. Since this region remains disordered after binding, a possible reason for its observed negative effect on binding could be its mere fuzziness. If this were the case, then swapping the wild-type sequence with another unrelated sequence would be expected to elicit similar effects provided that it is similarly disordered. To test this hypothesis, we replaced the wild-type N-terminal fuzzy region of N$_{TAIL}$ (aa 401 to 480) with another non-natural sequence. Compared to its wild-type counterpart, this artificial sequence (i) has the same number of residues, (ii) is predicted to be slightly more disordered (Figure 2D), (iii) shares only 6% identity. This artificial sequence was fused to the remaining part (aa 481 to 525) of wild-type N$_{TAIL}$ to reconstitute an artificial full-length N$_{TAIL}$ (aa 401 to 525) (artN$_{TAIL}$). We then generated the same series of truncation variants as those previously generated from the wild-type sequence (wtN$_{TAIL}$) (Figure 2A) and compared their effect on the binding to XD. As shown in Figure 2E, wtN$_{TAIL}$ and artN$_{TAIL}$ truncation variants yielded similar binding patterns, with the binding strength increasing non-monotonically with the truncation. However, results were not identical. Compared to wtN$_{TAIL}$, the profile obtained with artN$_{TAIL}$ was more linear, and each artN$_{TAIL}$ variant displayed a slightly lower interaction strength towards XD than its wild-type counterpart, a property that could be related to the higher disorder probability of full-length artN$_{TAIL}$ (Figure 2D). Thus, the negative effect of N$_{TAIL}$ N-terminal fuzzy region (aa 401 to 485) on XD binding was not due to its specific sequence but to a combination of length and fuzziness. The sequence-independent nature of the effect exerted by the disordered appendage is not unique to N$_{TAIL}$, having also been observed in the case of human UDP-α-D-glucose-6-dehydrogenase. This enzyme possesses a C-terminal disordered region that entropically rectifies the dynamics and structure of the enzyme to favor binding of an allosteric inhibitor, with this effect being independent from both primary structure and chemical composition [63].

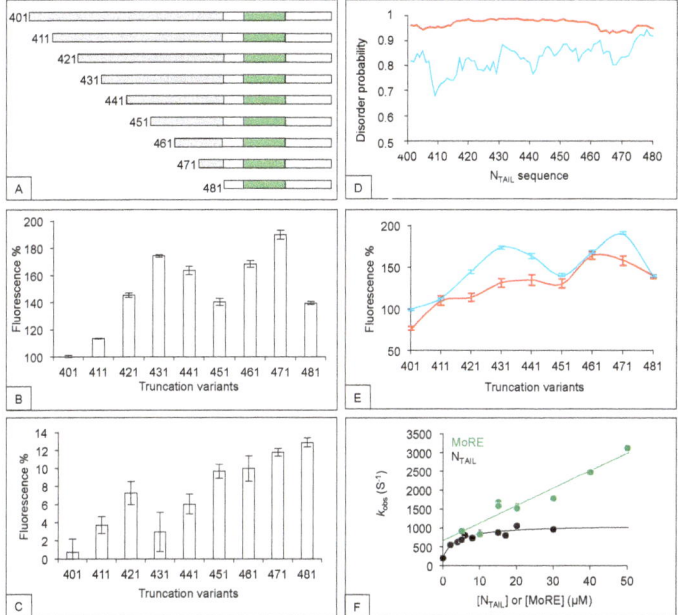

Figure 2. Effect of the N-terminal fuzzy region of N_{TAIL} on XD and hsp70 binding. (**A**) N_{TAIL} deletion variants were generated as described [60]. The N-terminal residue is indicated. The N-terminal fuzzy region subjected to truncation is shown in grey and the MoRE is shown in green. (**B,C**) Split-green fluorescent protein (GFP) complementation assay using XD (**B**) and hsp70 (**C**). Shown are the mean values and standard deviation (SD) of an experiment performed in triplicate. Results are expressed as percentage with 100% being the fluorescence value provided by full-length N_{TAIL} (401). For a detailed description of the procedure see Supplementary Information. (**D**) IUPred [64] disorder prediction of wtN_{TAIL} (blue) and artN_{TAIL} (red) from residue 401 to residue 480. (**E**) Fluorescence values obtained by split-GFP complementation assays using wild type (wt) (blue line) and art (red line) N_{TAIL} truncation variants and XD. Shown are the mean values and SD of an experiment performed in triplicate. Results are expressed as percentage with 100% being the fluorescence value provided by full-length wtN_{TAIL} (401). (**F**) Binding kinetics of XD (at a constant concentration of 2 µM) with excess concentrations of either wtNTAIL (black circles) or a peptide mimicking the MoRE (green circles) in 10 mM sodium phosphate buffer and 150 mM NaCl at pH 7.0. Under all conditions, there was an at least fivefold difference in concentration between the two proteins to ensure pseudo-first order conditions. Experiments were carried out using a PTJ-64 capacitor-discharge T-jump apparatus (Hi-Tech, Salisbury, UK). The temperature was rapidly changed with a jump size of 9 °C, from 11 °C to 20 °C. Data were taken from [60].

We tried to perform the same experiments using hsp70, but got results suffering from low reproducibility for unknown reasons (not illustrated). We further investigated the molecular mechanisms by which the fuzzy appendage of MeV N_{TAIL} influences the interaction with XD by analyzing binding kinetics (Figure 2F). In the case of full-length N_{TAIL} (aa 401–525), a hyperbolic dependence of k_{obs} (the macroscopic observed rate constant) on ligand concentration was observed, which accounts for the folding of N_{TAIL} becoming rate-limiting at high reactant concentrations [28]. Conversely, when a MoRE-mimicking peptide (aa 485 to 506) was used, linear kinetics was observed. Kinetic experiments could not be performed using hsp70 because of the low affinity of the interaction, and due to the presence of numerous tryptophan residues that could jeopardize the analysis. In conclusion, the N_{TAIL} N-terminal region could dampen the N_{TAIL}/XD interaction, at least in part, by lowering the rate of folding of the MoRE, although the subtle mechanisms underlying this ability remain elusive and await future studies to be unraveled.

3. The Bindings of XD and Hsp70 to N_{TAIL} MoRE Rely on Different Primary and Secondary Structure Requirements

We have seen that MeV N_{TAIL} N-terminal region (401 to 485) has comparable negative effects on the binding of two different N_{TAIL} partners: XD, a small viral protein [9] with a relatively high affinity (3 μM) [28] and hsp70, a large cellular protein with a lower affinity (70 μM) for N_{TAIL} [18]. Although the MoRE has been shown to be the major hsp70-binding site [17,18], the structure of N_{TAIL}-hsp70 complex has not been solved yet contrary to the N_{TAIL}-XD complex [10]. As a consequence, we do not know whether the MoRE folds into an α-helix upon binding to hsp70 as it does upon XD binding and whether the interaction relies on the same MoRE residues. The relevance of investigating the molecular mechanisms governing the N_{TAIL}/hsp70 interaction lies in its well-documented impact on viral transcription and replication [16,17] and on the innate immune response [65].

3.1. Sequence Requirements of N_{TAIL} Molecular Recognition Element for XD and Hsp70 Binding

To gain insights into this biologically relevant question, we first alanine scanned the MoRE, and assessed the effect of these substitutions by monitoring the binding of each individual variant to XD and hsp70 using the split-GFP complementation assay [64]. We used N_{TAIL} truncation variant 471 (aa 471 to 525) as backbone to derive single-site variants because it binds XD better than full-length N_{TAIL} (Figure 2B) [61], and therefore provides higher fluorescence signals in split-GFP complementation assay that are more appropriate than weak signals to study subtle modulation effects. In the case of XD binding (Figure 3A), most alanine variants exhibited a decreased binding compared to that of the wild-type sequence and, in a few cases (residues Ser491, Ala494, Leu495, Met501), the single alanine (or glycine) substitution essentially abrogates binding [66]. These latter residues can therefore be defined as critical for XD binding, a conclusion in agreement with the 3D structure of the MeV MoRE-XD complex in which all these residues point toward XD and not to the solvent [10]. Very different results were obtained with hsp70 (Figure 3B) [64]. First, several variants exhibited an increased binding compared to the wild-type sequence. Secondly, no single residue proved to be mandatory for binding to hsp70. Thus, although N_{TAIL} binding to both XD and hsp70 was down-regulated by the N_{TAIL} N-terminal fuzzy region (Figure 2), these two proteins bind the MoRE using different residues thereof, and hence through different mechanisms.

Based on the results provided by the alanine-scanning mutagenesis, we conceived an hsp70 "super binder" (hsb) that was obtained by collectively introducing all the substitutions that individually increased the binding to hsp70 (see Figure 4A) in the context of truncated variant 471 (hsb471). This rationally designed variant displayed a much higher binding strength (2.35 times) towards full-length hsp70 than wt471 in a split-GFP complementation assay (compare wt471 to hsb471 and wtMoRE to hsbMoRE in Figure 4B). Because of the dampening effect of the N-terminal fuzzy appendage (Figure 2C), this enhancement in affinity was even more pronounced when hsbMoRE was used alone rather than in the context of truncated variant 471 (compare hsb471 and hsbMoRE bindings in Figure 4B).

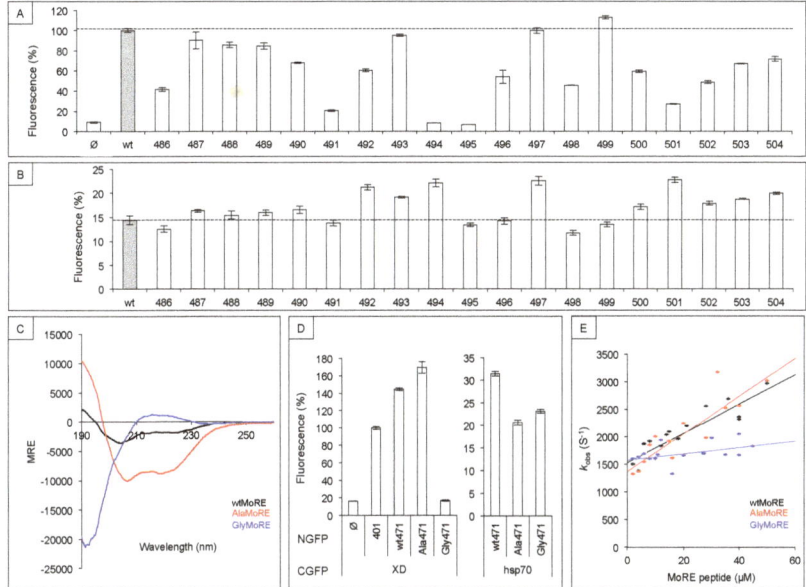

Figure 3. Effect of primary and secondary structures of the MoRE on XD and hsp70 binding. (**A**,**B**) Alanine scanning mutagenesis of N_{TAIL} MoRE. MoRE residues (aa 486 to 504) of MeV N_{TAIL} truncation variant 471 were individually mutated into an alanine (or a glycine when the wild-type residue was an alanine). The binding ability of each single N_{TAIL} variant was then compared to that of wild-type N_{TAIL} by split-GFP complementation assay using either XD (**A**) or hsp70 (**B**). Ø, negative control (fluorescence background obtained using an empty vector encoding NGFP alone); wt, positive control (i.e., wild-type truncation variant 471). Results are expressed as percentage with 100% being the fluorescence value provided by wt truncation variant 471. The horizontal dotted line indicates the binding of the positive control. (**C**) Far-UV circular dichroism spectra of wtMoRE, AlaMoRE, and GlyMoRE peptides. (**D**) Fluorescence values obtained by split-GFP complementation assays using N_{TAIL} MoRE variants with different α-helicities. See A for details; 401, full-length wtN_{TAIL}; wt471, 471 truncated variant with a wtMoRE; Ala471, 471 truncated variant with AlaMoRE; Gly471, 471 truncated variant with GlyMoRE. (**E**) Binding kinetics of MoRE peptides to XD. Data shown in panels A, B, and D are the mean values and SD of an experiment performed in triplicate. Data were taken from [66].

The three-fold increase in binding strength towards hsp70 upon replacement of as many as 13 residues out of 19 (i.e., almost 70%) of the sequence of the wtMoRE with alanine or glycine (Figure 4A) is puzzling. How can N_{TAIL} binding to hsp70 be specific of the MoRE while being relatively independent of the sequence of the latter? Conceivably, hsp70 may recognize not a precise amino acid sequence or motif, but rather a set of few residues with specific chemical features and no strict positional conservation. While hydrophobicity on its own cannot explain the increased binding strength of hsbMoRE [64], the enrichment in Ala, Gly, and Leu residues (in this order) and the depletion in Asp residues of hsbMoRE (Figure 4A) might provide a rational explanation: indeed, previous studies identified these features as favoring binding of peptides to hsp33, a redox-regulated chaperone [67].

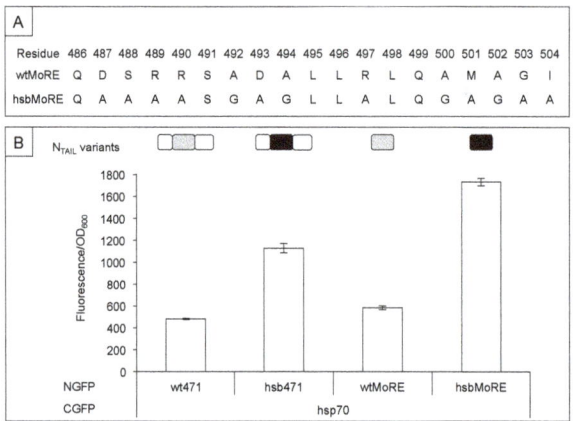

Figure 4. Binding abilities of hsb towards hsp70. (**A**) Amino acid sequence of wt and hsbMore. In the latter, all the residues individually shown to lead to increased N_{TAIL}-hsp70 binding strength by the alanine scanning mutagenesis were collectively replaced with alanine, or with glycine when the wild-type residue was alanine. (**B**) Binding abilities of N_{TAIL} variants as obtained by split-GFP complementation assays. Y-axis: fluorescence values of each culture divided by the optical density at 600 nm. X-axis: N_{TAIL} variants-hsp70 pairs. Shown are the mean values and SD of an experiment performed in triplicate. The scheme of the N_{TAIL} constructs is shown above the graph, with wt and hsb MoREs being represented in grey and black, respectively, and fuzzy regions in white. Orientation is from left (N-terminal end) to right (C-terminal end). Data were taken from [66].

3.2. Secondary Structure Requirements of N_{TAIL} Molecular Recognition Element for XD and Hsp70 Binding

Single residue substitutions of the alanine scanning aimed at providing information on the sequence requirement of XD and hsp70 binding but not at changing the secondary structure of the MoRE. The latter is known to fold into an α-helix upon XD binding. However, nothing is known about the conformation it takes upon binding to hsp70. To address this question, we constructed two MoRE variants with opposite folding properties [66]. Both MoRE variants were generated using truncation variant 471 as backbone for the reason given above. In the first one (Ala471), all residues the alanine scanning identified as non-critical for XD binding were replaced with alanine. In the second one (Gly471), those residues were replaced with glycine. Since alanine promotes α-helix formation whereas glycine has the opposite effect [68], Ala471 and Gly471 were expected to be more and less α-helical than wtMoRE, respectively. This assumption, strengthened by disorder prediction and modeling [66], was experimentally confirmed by circular dichroism (CD) analysis of MoRE peptides (Figure 3C).

The wt471, Ala471, and Gly471 variants were then tested for their ability to bind XD or hsp70 by split-GFP complementation assay. Results (Figure 3D, left panel), indicated that increasing the α-helicity (Ala471) slightly increased binding to XD compared to wt471, whereas the lack of α-helicity (Gly471) resulted in a complete loss of binding in spite of the presence of the residues revealed to be critical for XD binding by alanine scanning [64]. Conversely, Ala471 and Gly471 behaved similarly when assessed for their binding to hsp70: they both exhibited a moderately decreased binding compared to wt471 (Figure 3D, right panel) [66]. The lower XD binding ability of Gly471 compared to that of wt471 and Ala471 was also confirmed by kinetics experiments (Figure 3E). While AlaMoRE and wtMoRE behaved similarly, there was a detectable destabilization of the complex in the case of GlyMoRE as judged from the lower slope of its binding kinetics [64]. These results definitely indicate that XD and hsp70 did not rely on the same structural requirements to bind to the MoRE of N_{TAIL}. More specifically, increasing the α-helicity of the MoRE increased XD binding but decreased hsp70 binding suggesting that the latter did not trigger α-helical folding of the MoRE, a conclusion strengthened by the ability of hsp70 to bind a MoRE that is unable to fold into an α-helix.

In conclusion, in addition to using a different set of N_{TAIL} residues, XD and hsp70 did not induce the same folding within the MoRE, therefore indicating that they likely interacted with N_{TAIL} through completely different mechanisms.

4. Conclusions

Deletion studies have shown that the long, N-terminal fuzzy region of N_{TAIL} inhibits the interaction with XD and hsp70. This raises the question of what could be the possible functional role of this auto-inhibition. According to the so-called cartwheeling mechanism, the N_{TAIL}-XD interaction needs to be dynamically made and broken to ensure progression of the polymerase complex onto the nucleocapsid to allow transcription and replication [69]. A too strong interaction between N_{TAIL} and XD is therefore predicted to hinder the polymerase processivity. The discovery that the fuzzy appendage acts as a natural dampener of the interaction provides a conceptual framework to understand why the MoRE is preceded by such a long arm. It is tempting to speculate that in the course of evolution, the length of this region has been under selective pressure so as to ensure an optimal affinity towards XD. This speculation is in agreement with recent studies by the group of Plemper that showed that a mutated measles virus in which the region preceding the MoRE has been shortened suffers from an imbalance between transcription and replication [70].

Alanine-scanning mutagenesis of the MoRE unveiled that XD is very sensitive to substitutions, in line with experimental evidence showing that the MoRE of N_{TAIL} is poorly evolvable in terms of XD binding [58]. This implies that the sequence of the MoRE has been shaped during evolution to achieve maximal binding to XD, a finding in striking contrast with the postulated positive selection of a long fuzzy appendage dampening the interaction. Although apparently contradictory, these effects of natural selection have in fact resulted in a finely tuned system in which the strongest possible MoRE-XD interaction is "entropically rectified" [63] by the N-terminal fuzzy region of N_{TAIL} to achieve a precise N_{TAIL}-XD interaction strength. The latter is in fact required to ensure dynamic anchoring of the L–P polymerase complex [71] and efficient transcription re-initiation at each intergenic junction of the MeV genome [72].

By contrast, hsp70 is much more tolerant to substitutions within the MoRE, and the MoRE-hsp70 interaction appears to be highly evolvable. The high evolvability of the N_{TAIL}-hsp70 interaction might arise from the fact that the two binding partners have not been subjected to an as tight co-evolution as that of the N_{TAIL}-XD pair due to the multiple functional roles that hsp70 plays in the cell and that are not exclusively related to MeV infection. In addition, a high affinity between N_{TAIL} and hsp70 might not be required for the interaction to take place and elicit the known effects on viral transcription and replication [17,73] and on the innate immune response [65] given the very high intracellular concentrations of both hsp70 and N in MeV infected cells [53]. A high affinity could even be deleterious for the viral replication since hsp70 could then fully out compete XD for N_{TAIL} binding [17].

The discovery that the N_{TAIL}-hsp70 interaction does not rely on the same residues mediating the N_{TAIL}-XD interaction, and does not imply α-helical folding emphasizes the plasticity and polymorphism of this IDP. The structure adopted in the bound form seems therefore to be "sculpted" by the partner, thereby providing an additional example of "templated folding" [41]. This high extent of malleability with respect to the partner challenges the role of preconfiguration of MoREs in the recognition process. N_{TAIL} seems indeed to be relatively insensitive to the structure of its pre-recognition motif, being able to adopt a non α-helical conformation upon binding to hsp70 in spite of the partial α-helical preconfiguration of its MoRE.

Finally, and from a more applied perspective, the much higher affinity of hsb compared to wt MoRE towards hsp70 holds promise for future potential therapeutic applications. Since the N_{TAIL}-hsp70 interaction stimulates viral transcription and replication [16,17], and since hsbMoRE binds hsp70 three times better than wtMoRE, over-expressing hsbMoRE in MeV-infected cells might expectedly inhibit MeV replication (provided that hsbMoRE is non-toxic for eukaryotic cells).

Incidentally, hsbMoRE could also be used as an anti-cancer drug, based on previous studies that have described the anti-viral [74] and anti-cancer [75,76] effect of 2-phenylethynesulfonamide, a specific hsp70 inhibitor. Experiments are ongoing in our lab to assess the therapeutic potential of hsbMoRE.

Supplementary Materials: The following are available online at http://www.mdpi.com/2218-273X/9/1/8/s1.

Author Contributions: C.B. and S.L. wrote the manuscript. All authors approved the final version of the manuscript.

Funding: The studies herein reviewed were carried out with the financial support of the CNRS, of the Direction Générale de l'Armement (DGA), and of the Agence Nationale de la Recherche, specific programs "Physico-Chimie du Vivant", ANR-08-PCVI-0020-01, and "ASTRID", ANR-11-ASTR-003-01 to S.L. They were also partly supported by the European program H2020 under the EVAg Research Infrastructure (grant agreement Nb. 653316 to C.B.), and by the Italian Ministero dell'Istruzione dell'Università e della Ricerca (Progetto di Interesse 'Invecchiamento' to S.G.) and by Sapienza University of Rome (C26A155S48 to S.G.). F.T. is a recipient of a Ph.D. fellowship from the Italo-French University.

Acknowledgments: S.L. wishes to thank former members of her lab who contributed to these studies: D. Blocquel (The Scripps Institute, La Jolla, CA, USA), A. Gruet (Memorial Sloan Kettering Cancer Center, New York, USA) and M. Dosnon. The authors also thank D. Gerlier (CIRI, INSERM U758, Lyon, FR), R. Das (Dept. of Biomedical Engineering and Center for Biological Systems Engineering, Washington University in St. Louis, St. Louis, MO, USA) and M. Fuxreiter (Hungarian Academy of Sciences, Momentum Laboratory of Protein Dynamics, Department of Biochemistry and Molecular Biology, University of Debrecen, Hungary).

Conflicts of Interest: The authors declare no conflict of interest. The funders had no role in study design, data collection and analysis, decision to publish, or preparation of the manuscript.

References

1. Longhi, S.; Receveur-Brechot, V.; Karlin, D.; Johansson, K.; Darbon, H.; Bhella, D.; Yeo, R.; Finet, S.; Canard, B. The C-terminal domain of the measles virus nucleoprotein is intrinsically disordered and folds upon binding to the C-terminal moiety of the phosphoprotein. *J. Biol. Chem.* **2003**, *278*, 18638–18648. [CrossRef] [PubMed]
2. Heggeness, M.H.; Scheid, A.; Choppin, P.W. Conformation of the helical nucleocapsids of paramyxoviruses and vesicular stomatitis virus: Reversible coiling and uncoiling induced by changes in salt concentration. *Proc. Natl. Acad. Sci. USA* **1980**, *77*, 2631–2635. [CrossRef] [PubMed]
3. Heggeness, M.H.; Scheid, A.; Choppin, P.W. The relationship of conformational changes in the Sendai virus nucleocapsid to proteolytic cleavage of the NP polypeptide. *Virology* **1981**, *114*, 555–562. [CrossRef]
4. Karlin, D.; Longhi, S.; Canard, B. Substitution of two residues in the measles virus nucleoprotein results in an impaired self-association. *Virology* **2002**, *302*, 420–432. [CrossRef] [PubMed]
5. Ringkjøbing Jensen, M.; Communie, G.; Ribeiro, E.D., Jr.; Martinez, N.; Desfosses, A.; Salmon, L.; Mollica, L.; Gabel, F.; Jamin, M.; Longhi, S.; et al. Intrinsic disorder in measles virus nucleocapsids. *Proc. Natl. Acad. Sci. USA* **2011**, *108*, 9839–9844. [CrossRef] [PubMed]
6. Gutsche, I.; Desfosses, A.; Effantin, G.; Ling, W.L.; Haupt, M.; Ruigrok, R.W.; Sachse, C.; Schoehn, G. Near-atomic cryo-EM structure of the helical measles virus nucleocapsid. *Science* **2015**, *348*, 704–707. [CrossRef] [PubMed]
7. Bourhis, J.; Johansson, K.; Receveur-Bréchot, V.; Oldfield, C.J.; Dunker, A.K.; Canard, B.; Longhi, S. The C-terminal domain of measles virus nucleoprotein belongs to the class of intrinsically disordered proteins that fold upon binding to their physiological partner. *Virus Res.* **2004**, *99*, 157–167. [CrossRef] [PubMed]
8. Bourhis, J.M.; Receveur-Bréchot, V.; Oglesbee, M.; Zhang, X.; Buccellato, M.; Darbon, H.; Canard, B.; Finet, S.; Longhi, S. The intrinsically disordered C-terminal domain of the measles virus nucleoprotein interacts with the C-terminal domain of the phosphoprotein via two distinct sites and remains predominantly unfolded. *Protein Sci.* **2005**, *14*, 1975–1992. [CrossRef]
9. Johansson, K.; Bourhis, J.M.; Campanacci, V.; Cambillau, C.; Canard, B.; Longhi, S. Crystal structure of the measles virus phosphoprotein domain responsible for the induced folding of the C-terminal domain of the nucleoprotein. *J. Biol. Chem.* **2003**, *278*, 44567–44573. [CrossRef]
10. Kingston, R.L.; Hamel, D.J.; Gay, L.S.; Dahlquist, F.W.; Matthews, B.W. Structural basis for the attachment of a paramyxoviral polymerase to its template. *Proc. Natl. Acad. Sci. USA* **2004**, *101*, 8301–8306. [CrossRef]

11. Longhi, S.; Bloyet, L.M.; Gianni, S.; Gerlier, D. How order and disorder within paramyxoviral nucleoproteins and phosphoproteins orchestrate the molecular interplay of transcription and replication. *Cell. Mol. Life Sci.* **2017**, *74*, 3091–3118. [CrossRef] [PubMed]
12. Dunker, A.K.; Cortese, M.S.; Romero, P.; Iakoucheva, L.M.; Uversky, V.N. Flexible nets. *FEBS J.* **2005**, *272*, 5129–5148. [CrossRef] [PubMed]
13. Uversky, V.N.; Oldfield, C.J.; Dunker, A.K. Showing your ID: Intrinsic disorder as an ID for recognition, regulation and cell signaling. *J. Mol. Recognit.* **2005**, *18*, 343–384. [CrossRef] [PubMed]
14. Haynes, C.; Oldfield, C.J.; Ji, F.; Klitgord, N.; Cusick, M.E.; Radivojac, P.; Uversky, V.N.; Vidal, M.; Iakoucheva, L.M. Intrinsic disorder is a common feature of hub proteins from four eukaryotic interactomes. *PLoS Comput. Biol.* **2006**, *2*, e100. [CrossRef] [PubMed]
15. Iwasaki, M.; Takeda, M.; Shirogane, Y.; Nakatsu, Y.; Nakamura, T.; Yanagi, Y. The matrix protein of measles virus regulates viral RNA synthesis and assembly by interacting with the nucleocapsid protein. *J. Virol.* **2009**, *83*, 10374–10383. [CrossRef] [PubMed]
16. Zhang, X.; Glendening, C.; Linke, H.; Parks, C.L.; Brooks, C.; Udem, S.A.; Oglesbee, M. Identification and characterization of a regulatory domain on the carboxyl terminus of the measles virus nucleocapsid protein. *J. Virol.* **2002**, *76*, 8737–8746. [CrossRef] [PubMed]
17. Zhang, X.; Bourhis, J.M.; Longhi, S.; Carsillo, T.; Buccellato, M.; Morin, B.; Canard, B.; Oglesbee, M. Hsp72 recognizes a P binding motif in the measles virus N protein C-terminus. *Virology* **2005**, *337*, 162–174. [CrossRef]
18. Couturier, M.; Buccellato, M.; Costanzo, S.; Bourhis, J.M.; Shu, Y.; Nicaise, M.; Desmadril, M.; Flaudrops, C.; Longhi, S.; Oglesbee, M. High Affinity Binding between Hsp70 and the C-Terminal Domain of the Measles Virus Nucleoprotein Requires an Hsp40 Co-Chaperone. *J. Mol. Recognit.* **2010**, *23*, 301–315. [CrossRef]
19. Sato, H.; Masuda, M.; Miura, R.; Yoneda, M.; Kai, C. Morbillivirus nucleoprotein possesses a novel nuclear localization signal and a CRM1-independent nuclear export signal. *Virology* **2006**, *352*, 121–130. [CrossRef]
20. TenOever, B.R.; Servant, M.J.; Grandvaux, N.; Lin, R.; Hiscott, J. Recognition of the Measles Virus Nucleocapsid as a Mechanism of IRF-3 Activation. *J. Virol.* **2002**, *76*, 3659–3669. [CrossRef]
21. Colombo, M.; Bourhis, J.M.; Chamontin, C.; Soriano, C.; Villet, S.; Costanzo, S.; Couturier, M.; Belle, V.; Fournel, A.; Darbon, H.; et al. The interaction between the measles virus nucleoprotein and the Interferon Regulator Factor 3 relies on a specific cellular environment. *Virol. J.* **2009**, *6*, 59. [CrossRef] [PubMed]
22. Laine, D.; Bourhis, J.; Longhi, S.; Flacher, M.; Cassard, L.; Canard, B.; Sautès-Fridman, C.; Rabourdin-Combe, C.; Valentin, H. Measles virus nucleoprotein induces cell proliferation arrest and apoptosis through NTAIL/NR and NCORE/FcgRIIB1 interactions, respectively. *J. Gen. Virol.* **2005**, *86*, 1771–1784. [CrossRef] [PubMed]
23. Laine, D.; Trescol-Biémont, M.; Longhi, S.; Libeau, G.; Marie, J.; Vidalain, P.; Azocar, O.; Diallo, A.; Canard, B.; Rabourdin-Combe, C.; et al. Measles virus nucleoprotein binds to a novel cell surface receptor distinct from FcgRII via its C-terminal domain: Role in MV-induced immunosuppression. *J. Virol.* **2003**, *77*, 11332–11346. [CrossRef] [PubMed]
24. Watanabe, A.; Yoneda, M.; Ikeda, F.; Sugai, A.; Sato, H.; Kai, C. Peroxiredoxin 1 is required for efficient transcription and replication of measles virus. *J. Virol.* **2011**, *85*, 2247–2253. [CrossRef] [PubMed]
25. De, B.P.; Banerjee, A.K. Involvement of actin microfilaments in the transcription/replication of human parainfluenza virus type 3: Possible role of actin in other viruses. *Microsc. Res. Tech.* **1999**, *47*, 114–123. [CrossRef]
26. Moyer, S.A.; Baker, S.C.; Horikami, S.M. Host cell proteins required for measles virus reproduction. *J. Gen. Virol.* **1990**, *71*, 775–783. [CrossRef] [PubMed]
27. Habchi, J.; Blangy, S.; Mamelli, L.; Ringkjobing Jensen, M.; Blackledge, M.; Darbon, H.; Oglesbee, M.; Shu, Y.; Longhi, S. Characterization of the interactions between the nucleoprotein and the phosphoprotein of Henipaviruses. *J. Biol. Chem.* **2011**, *286*, 13583–13602. [CrossRef] [PubMed]
28. Dosnon, M.; Bonetti, D.; Morrone, A.; Erales, J.; di Silvio, E.; Longhi, S.; Gianni, S. Demonstration of a folding after binding mechanism in the recognition between the measles virus NTAIL and X domains. *ACS Chem. Biol.* **2015**, *10*, 795–802. [CrossRef]

29. Gely, S.; Lowry, D.F.; Bernard, C.; Ringkjobing-Jensen, M.; Blackledge, M.; Costanzo, S.; Darbon, H.; Daughdrill, G.W.; Longhi, S. Solution structure of the C-terminal X domain of the measles virus phosphoprotein and interaction with the intrinsically disordered C-terminal domain of the nucleoprotein. *J. Mol. Recognit.* **2010**, *23*, 435–447. [CrossRef]
30. D'Urzo, A.; Konijnenberg, A.; Rossetti, G.; Habchi, J.; Li, J.; Carloni, P.; Sobott, F.; Longhi, S.; Grandori, R. Molecular Basis for Structural Heterogeneity of an Intrinsically Disordered Protein Bound to a Partner by Combined ESI-IM-MS and Modeling. *J. Am. Soc. Mass Spectrom.* **2015**, *26*, 472–481. [CrossRef]
31. Bonetti, D.; Camilloni, C.; Visconti, L.; Longhi, S.; Brunori, M.; Vendruscolo, M.; Gianni, S. Identification and Structural Characterization of an Intermediate in the Folding of the Measles Virus X Domain. *J. Biol. Chem.* **2016**, *291*, 10886–10892. [CrossRef]
32. Habchi, J.; Mamelli, L.; Darbon, H.; Longhi, S. Structural Disorder within Henipavirus Nucleoprotein and Phosphoprotein: From Predictions to Experimental Assessment. *PLoS ONE* **2010**, *5*, e11684. [CrossRef] [PubMed]
33. Communie, G.; Habchi, J.; Yabukarski, F.; Blocquel, D.; Schneider, R.; Tarbouriech, N.; Papageorgiou, N.; Ruigrok, R.W.; Jamin, M.; Ringkjøbing-Jensen, M.; et al. Atomic resolution description of the interaction between the nucleoprotein and phosphoprotein of Hendra virus. *PLoS Pathog.* **2013**, *9*, e1003631. [CrossRef] [PubMed]
34. Fuxreiter, M.; Simon, I.; Friedrich, P.; Tompa, P. Preformed structural elements feature in partner recognition by intrinsically unstructured proteins. *J. Mol. Biol.* **2004**, *338*, 1015–1026. [CrossRef] [PubMed]
35. Morin, B.; Bourhis, J.M.; Belle, V.; Woudstra, M.; Carrière, F.; Guigliarelli, B.; Fournel, A.; Longhi, S. Assessing induced folding of an intrinsically disordered protein by site-directed spin-labeling EPR spectroscopy. *J. Phys. Chem. B* **2006**, *110*, 20596–20608. [CrossRef]
36. Belle, V.; Rouger, S.; Costanzo, S.; Liquiere, E.; Strancar, J.; Guigliarelli, B.; Fournel, A.; Longhi, S. Mapping alpha-helical induced folding within the intrinsically disordered C-terminal domain of the measles virus nucleoprotein by site-directed spin-labeling EPR spectroscopy. *Proteins Struct. Funct. Bioinform.* **2008**, *73*, 973–988. [CrossRef] [PubMed]
37. Martinho, M.; Habchi, J.; El Habre, Z.; Nesme, L.; Guigliarelli, B.; Belle, V.; Longhi, S. Assessing induced folding within the intrinsically disordered C-terminal domain of the Henipavirus nucleoproteins by site directed spin labeling EPR spectroscopy. *J. Biomol. Struct. Dyn.* **2013**, *31*, 453–471. [CrossRef] [PubMed]
38. Baronti, L.; Erales, J.; Habchi, J.; Felli, I.C.; Pierattelli, R.; Longhi, S. Dynamics of the intrinsically disordered C-terminal domain of the Nipah virus nucleoprotein and interaction with the X domain of the phosphoprotein as unveiled by NMR spectroscopy. *ChemBioChem* **2015**, *16*, 268–276. [CrossRef]
39. Wang, Y.; Chu, X.; Longhi, S.; Roche, P.; Han, W.; Wang, E.; Wang, J. Multiscaled exploration of coupled folding and binding of an intrinsically disordered molecular recognition element in measles virus nucleoprotein. *Proc. Natl. Acad. Sci. USA* **2013**, *110*, e3743–e3752. [CrossRef]
40. Shang, X.; Chu, W.; Chu, X.; Xu, L.; Longhi, S.; Wang, J. Exploration of nucleoprotein alpha-MoRE and XD interactions of Nipah and Hendra viruses. *J. Mol. Model.* **2018**, *24*, 113. [CrossRef]
41. Bonetti, D.; Troilo, F.; Toto, A.; Brunori, M.; Longhi, S.; Gianni, S. Analyzing the folding and binding steps of an intrinsically disordered protein by protein engineering. *Biochemistry* **2017**, *56*, 3780–3786. [CrossRef] [PubMed]
42. Belle, V.; Rouger, S.; Costanzo, S.; Longhi, S.; Fournel, A. Site-directed spin labeling EPR spectroscopy. In *Instrumental Analysis of Intrinsically Disordered Proteins: Assessing Structure and Conformation*; Uversky, V.N., Longhi, S., Eds.; John Wiley and Sons: Hoboken, NJ, USA, 2010.
43. Blocquel, D.; Habchi, J.; Gruet, A.; Blangy, S.; Longhi, S. Compaction and binding properties of the intrinsically disordered C-terminal domain of Henipavirus nucleoprotein as unveiled by deletion studies. *Mol. Biosyst.* **2012**, *8*, 392–410. [CrossRef] [PubMed]
44. Troilo, F.; Bignon, C.; Gianni, S.; Fuxreiter, M.; Longhi, S. Experimental characterization of fuzzy protein assemblies: Interactions of paramyxoviral NTAIL domains with their functional partners. *Methods Enzymol.* **2018**, *611*, 137–192. [PubMed]
45. Tompa, P.; Fuxreiter, M. Fuzzy complexes: Polymorphism and structural disorder in protein-protein interactions. *Trends Biochem. Sci.* **2008**, *33*, 2–8. [CrossRef] [PubMed]
46. Fuxreiter, M. Fuzziness: Linking regulation to protein dynamics. *Mol. Biosyst.* **2012**, *8*, 168–177. [CrossRef] [PubMed]

47. Fuxreiter, M. Fuzziness in protein interactions—A historical perspective. *J. Mol. Biol.* **2018**, *430*, 2278–2287. [CrossRef]
48. Fuxreiter, M. Fold or not to fold upon binding—Does it really matter? *Curr. Opin. Struct. Biol.* **2018**, *54*, 19–25. [CrossRef]
49. Ozenne, V.; Bauer, F.; Salmon, L.; Huang, J.R.; Jensen, M.R.; Segard, S.; Bernado, P.; Charavay, C.; Blackledge, M. Flexible-meccano: A tool for the generation of explicit ensemble descriptions of intrinsically disordered proteins and their associated experimental observables. *Bioinformatics* **2012**, *28*, 1463–1470. [CrossRef]
50. Carsillo, T.; Zhang, X.; Vasconcelos, D.; Niewiesk, S.; Oglesbee, M. A single codon in the nucleocapsid protein C terminus contributes to in vitro and in vivo fitness of Edmonston measles virus. *J. Virol.* **2006**, *80*, 2904–2912. [CrossRef]
51. Oglesbee, M. Nucleocapsid protein interactions with the major inducible heat shock protein. In *Measles Virus Nucleoprotein*; Longhi, S., Ed.; Nova Publishers Inc.: Hauppage, NY, USA, 2007; pp. 53–98.
52. Oglesbee, M.J.; Kenney, H.; Kenney, T.; Krakowka, S. Enhanced production of morbillivirus gene-specific RNAs following induction of the cellular stress response in stable persistent infection. *Virology* **1993**, *192*, 556–567. [CrossRef]
53. Oglesbee, M.J.; Liu, Z.; Kenney, H.; Brooks, C.L. The highly inducible member of the 70 kDa family of heat shock proteins increases canine distemper virus polymerase activity. *J. Gen. Virol.* **1996**, *77*, 2125–2135. [CrossRef] [PubMed]
54. Vasconcelos, D.; Norrby, E.; Oglesbee, M. The cellular stress response increases measles virus-induced cytopathic effect. *J. Gen. Virol.* **1998**, *79*, 1769–1773. [CrossRef] [PubMed]
55. Vasconcelos, D.Y.; Cai, X.H.; Oglesbee, M.J. Constitutive overexpression of the major inducible 70 kDa heat shock protein mediates large plaque formation by measles virus. *J. Gen. Virol.* **1998**, *79*, 2239–2247. [CrossRef]
56. Longhi, S.; Oglesbee, M. Structural disorder within the measles virus nucleoprotein and phosphoprotein. *Protein Peptide Lett.* **2010**, *17*, 961–978. [CrossRef]
57. Wilson, C.G.; Magliery, T.J.; Regan, L. Detecting protein-protein interactions with GFP-fragment reassembly. *Nat. Methods* **2004**, *1*, 255–262. [CrossRef] [PubMed]
58. Gruet, A.; Dosnon, M.; Vassena, A.; Lombard, V.; Gerlier, D.; Bignon, C.; Longhi, S. Dissecting partner recognition by an intrinsically disordered protein using descriptive random mutagenesis. *J. Mol. Biol.* **2013**, *425*, 3495–3509. [CrossRef]
59. Jackrel, M.E.; Cortajarena, A.L.; Liu, T.Y.; Regan, L. Screening libraries to identify proteins with desired binding activities using a split-GFP reassembly assay. *ACS Chem. Biol.* **2010**, *5*, 553–562. [CrossRef]
60. Magliery, T.J.; Wilson, C.G.; Pan, W.; Mishler, D.; Ghosh, I.; Hamilton, A.D.; Regan, L. Detecting protein-protein interactions with a green fluorescent protein fragment reassembly trap: Scope and mechanism. *J. Am. Chem. Soc.* **2005**, *127*, 146–157. [CrossRef]
61. Gruet, A.; Dosnon, M.; Blocquel, D.; Brunel, J.; Gerlier, D.; Das, R.K.; Bonetti, D.; Gianni, S.; Fuxreiter, M.; Longhi, S.; et al. Fuzzy regions in an intrinsically disordered protein impair protein-protein interactions. *FEBS J.* **2016**, *283*, 576–594. [CrossRef]
62. Cassonnet, P.; Rolloy, C.; Neveu, G.; Vidalain, P.O.; Chantier, T.; Pellet, J.; Jones, L.; Muller, M.; Demeret, C.; Gaud, G.; et al. Benchmarking a luciferase complementation assay for detecting protein complexes. *Nat. Methods* **2011**, *8*, 990–992. [CrossRef]
63. Keul, N.D.; Oruganty, K.; Schaper Bergman, E.T.; Beattie, N.R.; McDonald, W.E.; Kadirvelraj, R.; Gross, M.L.; Phillips, R.S.; Harvey, S.C.; Wood, Z.A. The entropic force generated by intrinsically disordered segments tunes protein function. *Nature* **2018**. [CrossRef] [PubMed]
64. Dosztanyi, Z.; Csizmok, V.; Tompa, P.; Simon, I. IUPred: Web server for the prediction of intrinsically unstructured regions of proteins based on estimated energy content. *Bioinformatics* **2005**, *21*, 3433–3434. [CrossRef]
65. Kim, M.Y.; Shu, Y.; Carsillo, T.; Zhang, J.; Yu, L.; Peterson, C.; Longhi, S.; Girod, S.; Niewiesk, S.; Oglesbee, M. Hsp70 and a novel axis of type I interferon-dependent antiviral immunity in the measles virus-infected brain. *J. Virol.* **2013**, *87*, 998–1009. [CrossRef] [PubMed]
66. Bignon, C.; Troilo, F.; Gianni, S.; Longhi, S. Partner-mediated polymorphism of an intrinsically disordered protein. *J. Mol. Biol.* **2018**, *430*, 2493–2507. [CrossRef] [PubMed]

67. Reichmann, D.; Xu, Y.; Cremers, C.M.; Ilbert, M.; Mittelman, R.; Fitzgerald, M.C.; Jakob, U. Order out of disorder: Working cycle of an intrinsically unfolded chaperone. *Cell* **2012**, *148*, 947–957. [CrossRef] [PubMed]
68. O'Neil, K.T.; DeGrado, W.F. A thermodynamic scale for the helix-forming tendencies of the commonly occurring amino acids. *Science* **1990**, *250*, 646–651. [CrossRef] [PubMed]
69. Kolakofsky, D.; Le Mercier, P.; Iseni, F.; Garcin, D. Viral DNA polymerase scanning and the gymnastics of Sendai virus RNA synthesis. *Virology* **2004**, *318*, 463–473. [CrossRef]
70. Thakkar, V.D.; Cox, R.M.; Sawatsky, B.; da Fontoura Budaszewski, R.; Sourimant, J.; Wabbel, K.; Makhsous, N.; Greninger, A.L.; von Messling, V.; Plemper, R.K. The Unstructured Paramyxovirus Nucleocapsid Protein Tail Domain Modulates Viral Pathogenesis through Regulation of Transcriptase Activity. *J. Virol.* **2018**, *92*. [CrossRef]
71. Brunel, J.; Chopy, D.; Dosnon, M.; Bloyet, L.M.; Devaux, P.; Urzua, E.; Cattaneo, R.; Longhi, S.; Gerlier, D. Sequence of events in measles virus replication: Role of phosphoprotein-nucleocapsid interactions. *J. Virol.* **2014**, *88*, 10851–10863. [CrossRef]
72. Bloyet, L.; Brunel, J.; Dosnon, M.; Hamon, V.; Erales, J.; Gruet, A.; Lazert, C.; Bignon, C.; Roche, P.; Longhi, S.; et al. Modulation of re-initiation of measles virus transcription at intergenic regions by PXD to NTAIL binding strength. *PLoS Pathog.* **2016**, *12*, e1006058. [CrossRef]
73. Shu, Y.; Habchi, J.; Costanzo, S.; Padilla, A.; Brunel, J.; Gerlier, D.; Oglesbee, M.; Longhi, S. Plasticity in structural and functional interactions between the phosphoprotein and nucleoprotein of measles virus. *J. Biol. Chem.* **2012**, *287*, 11951–11967. [CrossRef] [PubMed]
74. Wang, H.; Bu, L.; Wang, C.; Zhang, Y.; Zhou, H.; Zhang, X.; Guo, W.; Long, C.; Guo, D.; Sun, X. The Hsp70 inhibitor 2-phenylethynesulfonamide inhibits replication and carcinogenicity of Epstein-Barr virus by inhibiting the molecular chaperone function of Hsp70. *Cell Death Dis.* **2018**, *9*, 734. [CrossRef] [PubMed]
75. Leu, J.I.; Pimkina, J.; Frank, A.; Murphy, M.E.; George, D.L. A small molecule inhibitor of inducible heat shock protein 70. *Mol. Cell* **2009**, *36*, 15–27. [CrossRef] [PubMed]
76. Granato, M.; Lacconi, V.; Peddis, M.; Lotti, L.V.; Di Renzo, L.; Gonnella, R.; Santarelli, R.; Trivedi, P.; Frati, L.; D'Orazi, G.; et al. HSP70 inhibition by 2-phenylethynesulfonamide induces lysosomal cathepsin D release and immunogenic cell death in primary effusion lymphoma. *Cell Death Dis.* **2013**, *4*, e730. [CrossRef] [PubMed]

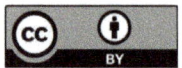

© 2018 by the authors. Licensee MDPI, Basel, Switzerland. This article is an open access article distributed under the terms and conditions of the Creative Commons Attribution (CC BY) license (http://creativecommons.org/licenses/by/4.0/).

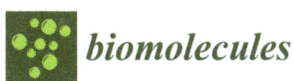

Article

Molecular Crowding Tunes Material States of Ribonucleoprotein Condensates

Taranpreet Kaur [1], Ibraheem Alshareedah [1], Wei Wang [1], Jason Ngo [1], Mahdi Muhammad Moosa [2] and Priya R. Banerjee [1,*]

[1] Department of Physics, University at Buffalo, SUNY, NY 14260, USA; tkaur2@buffalo.edu (T.K.); ialshare@buffalo.edu (I.A.); wwang23@buffalo.edu (W.W.); jasonngo@buffalo.edu (J.N.)
[2] Department of Pharmacology and Chemical Biology, Baylor College of Medicine, Houston, TX 77030, USA; mahdi.moosa@gmail.com
* Correspondence: prbanerj@buffalo.edu

Received: 31 December 2018; Accepted: 5 February 2019; Published: 19 February 2019

Abstract: Ribonucleoprotein (RNP) granules are membraneless liquid condensates that dynamically form, dissolve, and mature into a gel-like state in response to a changing cellular environment. RNP condensation is largely governed by promiscuous attractive inter-chain interactions mediated by low-complexity domains (LCDs). Using an archetypal disordered RNP, fused in sarcoma (FUS), here we study how molecular crowding impacts the RNP liquid condensation. We observe that the liquid–liquid coexistence boundary of FUS is lowered by polymer crowders, consistent with an excluded volume model. With increasing bulk crowder concentration, the RNP partition increases and the diffusion rate decreases in the condensed phase. Furthermore, we show that RNP condensates undergo substantial hardening wherein protein-dense droplets transition from viscous fluid to viscoelastic gel-like states in a crowder concentration-dependent manner. Utilizing two distinct LCDs that broadly represent commonly occurring sequence motifs driving RNP phase transitions, we reveal that the impact of crowding is largely independent of LCD charge and sequence patterns. These results are consistent with a thermodynamic model of crowder-mediated depletion interaction, which suggests that inter-RNP attraction is enhanced by molecular crowding. The depletion force is likely to play a key role in tuning the physical properties of RNP condensates within the crowded cellular space.

Keywords: membraneless organelles; optical tweezer; liquid–liquid phase separation; protein diffusion; depletion interaction; entropic force; low-complexity sequences; intrinsically disordered proteins

---

1. Introduction

Ribonucleoprotein (RNP) granules or particles are a diverse group of subcellular compartments that are utilized by eukaryotic cells to spatiotemporally organize various biomolecular processes. These non-membranous assemblies, also termed as membraneless organelles (MLOs), dynamically form, dissolve, and tune their physicochemical microenvironment in response to changing cellular cues [1–3]. RNP granules are enriched in proteins with low-complexity domains (LCDs) that are structurally disordered [4–6], and are assumed to be formed by RNP liquid–liquid phase separation (LLPS) [7]. LLPS is a spontaneous physical process that results in the formation of co-existing liquid phases of varying densities from a homogeneous solution [2,8]. At the molecular level, low-affinity multivalent interactions amongst different LCDs and their partner nucleic acids provide the necessary energetic input to drive the LLPS of RNPs [9]. Furthermore, LCD-mediated promiscuous interactions can act synergistically with sequence-specific interactions in many RNPs, thereby shaping their global phase behavior [10]. Experimentally, it was observed that these promiscuous interactions are tuned by several cellular physicochemical perturbations (e.g., pH, salt concentration, and non-specific interactions with biomacromolecules) [10–14].

Unlike in typically utilized in vitro experimental conditions, in cellulo environments are crowded by a plethora of macromolecules that are ubiquitous within the cellular milieu [15]. To effectively capture biomolecular dynamics in a crowded cellular environment, in vitro studies utilizing recombinant proteins employ buffer systems containing inert biocompatible polymers as crowding agents. One of the most widely used crowders is polyethylene glycol (PEG), a neutral hydrophilic polymer with numerous applications in crystallography, biotechnology, and medicine [16–19]. Macromolecular crowding by PEG and similar polymer agents imparts a significant excluded volume effect (i.e., a space occupied by one molecule cannot be accessed by another) and results in alterations of molecular and mesoscale properties of biomolecules. For example, molecular crowding was shown to affect protein conformation [20–23], RNA folding [24], conformational dynamics of intrinsically disordered proteins [25], energetics of protein self-association [26–28], molecular recognition [29], and LLPS of globular proteins [30–33]. However, how macromolecular crowding alters disordered RNP condensation remains underexplored.

The well-established excluded-volume model of colloid–polymer mixtures predicts that the addition of a polymer chain to a neutral colloidal suspension will trigger inter-colloid attraction [34]. The underlying driving force, known as the depletion interaction, is originated due to a net entropy gain by the system via maximizing the free volume available to the polymer chains. For globular protein–crowder mixtures, this depletion interaction can induce various phase transition processes, including protein crystallization [35]. In a similar vein, for RNP systems containing low-complexity "sticky" domains, a considerable impact of macromolecular crowding on their phase transition is expected [36]. This idea is supported by multiple recent observations such as (i) crowding induces homotypic LLPS of the nucleolar phosphoprotein Npm1 in vitro [37], (ii) PEG induces a robust liquid phase transition of the Alzheimer's disease-linked protein Tau [38], and (iii) macromolecular crowding results in a substantial decrease in protein concentration required for inducing hnRNPA1 phase separation [39,40]. However, it remains unknown whether molecular crowding impacts the fluid dynamics of RNP condensates.

The material properties of intracellular RNP granules are important determinants of their function in intracellular storage and signaling [1,41]. Notably, many RNP condensates are competent to mature into a fiber-like state, which is implicated in several neurological diseases [11,42–45]. While the roles of LCD sequence compositions and charge patterns in controlling mesoscale dynamics of the RNP condensates have been the subject of some recent investigations [46,47], little is known regarding the effect of generalized thermodynamic forces such as crowding on RNP condensation. Here we conduct an experimental study to evaluate the impact of macromolecular crowding on the RNP liquid–liquid coexistence boundary, condensate fluidity in the micron-scale, and transport property by RNP diffusion in the nano-scale. Utilizing an archetypal RNP, fused in sarcoma (FUS), as well as representatives of the two commonly occurring LCD sequences in eukaryotic RNPs, we demonstrate an important role of crowding in modulating the mesoscale fluid dynamics of RNP condensates.

2. Results

2.1. Macromolecular Crowding Facilitates FUS Condensation and Alters Droplet Fluid Properties

Initially, we chose to study the effects of molecular crowding on the phase behavior of FUS using PEG8000 at concentrations that mimic cellular macromolecular density ($\geq$150 mg/mL) [48]. FUS is a stress-granule-associated RNP that undergoes LLPS in vitro and in cellulo via attractive inter-protein interactions [49,50]. Persistent FUS condensates also mature into a solid-like state during aging that is augmented by amyotrophic lateral sclerosis (ALS)-linked mutations [42,51]. Therefore, FUS serves as an ideal model system for this study. Firstly, we tested the impact of crowding on the liquid–liquid coexistence boundary of the full-length FUS (FUS^{FL}) in a physiologically-relevant buffer (25 mM Tris, 150 mM NaCl; pH 7.5) with variable PEG8000 concentrations. We used solution turbidity measurements in conjunction with optical microscopy to construct a phase diagram of FUS^{FL}–PEG8000 mixtures, which is presented in Figure 1a. We observed that FUS^{FL} formed micron-scale phase-separated droplets in vitro at protein concentrations ≥2 µM without any crowding agents (Figure 1), consistent with the protein's ability to undergo LLPS at physiologically relevant concentrations [47,51]. Increasing PEG8000 concentration in the buffer solution from 0 to 150 mg/mL decreased FUS^{FL} phase separation concentration to <1 µM (Figure 1a). These results suggest that crowding by PEG8000 facilitates FUS^{FL} condensation.

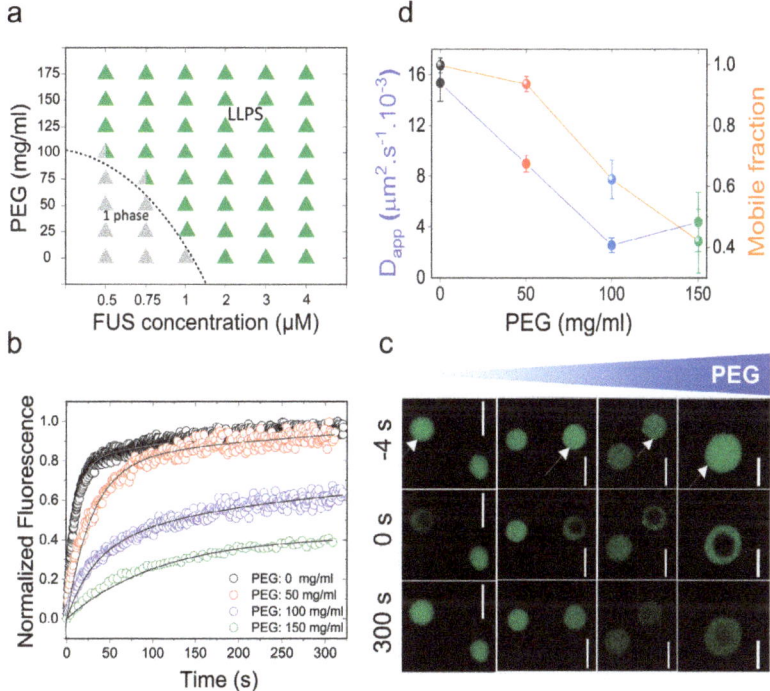

Figure 1. Molecular crowding facilitates full-length fused in sarcoma (FUS^{FL}) liquid–liquid phase separation (LLPS) and tunes protein droplet viscoelastic properties. (**a**) Isothermal phase diagram of FUS-polyethylene glycol (PEG) 8000 mixtures. The dotted line indicates the liquid–liquid phase boundary. (**b**) Fluorescence recovery after photobleaching (FRAP) plots of FUS (10 µM) condensates at various concentrations of PEG8000. (**c**) Confocal fluorescence microscopy images corresponding to the data in Figure 1b are shown. Scale bar = 4 µm. Negative time implies droplets before bleaching. (**d**) An analysis of these FRAP results on the basis of a diffusion model reveals a scaling of apparent diffusion coefficients (D_{app}; left axis, blue line) and the fraction of the mobile phase (right axis, orange line) with increasing concentration of PEG8000.

The observed effect of PEG on lowering the RNP liquid–liquid coexistence boundary can be explained by a crowder-mediated depletion force that effectively increases the net inter-RNP attractive interaction with increasing concentrations of the crowder [52] (also see Note S1). If that is the case, we expect that the fluidity of RNP droplets will decrease with increasing macromolecular crowding due to the enhanced inter-molecular network strength within the condensed phase [41]. A similar phenomenon is known to drive colloidal gel formation in polymer–colloid mixtures [53]. In the case of the RNP condensates, we expected a considerable alteration in the mesoscale dynamics, such as the biomolecular diffusion rate, with increasing PEG. Therefore, we next investigated the physical properties of the FUS^{FL} condensates as a function of PEG8000 concentration at a fixed protein concentration (10 µM; Figure 1b–d). We used two complementary methods to probe FUS^{FL} condensate material states: (a) Fluorescence recovery after photobleaching (FRAP), and (b) controlled fusion of suspended droplets using a dual-trap optical tweezer. Using FRAP, we measured the half-time of fluorescence recovery ($\tau_{\frac{1}{2}}^{FRAP}$) of the fluorescently-tagged RNP (Alexa488-FUS) after photobleaching a circular region at the center of the droplet (Figure 1b,c and Figure S1). Analysis of the $\tau_{\frac{1}{2}}^{FRAP}$ and effective bleach radius (r_e) allowed us to estimate an apparent diffusion coefficient (D_{app}) of a fluorescently tagged RNP within the protein-dense phase (see SI methods and Figure S1). The fraction of the mobile phase was also estimated from FRAP data and was used as a relative measure of the viscoelastic properties of FUS^{FL} droplets [8]. With increasing PEG8000, our FRAP data revealed two distinct trends (Figure 1b–d): (i) An increase in the fluorescence recovery half-time and, hence, a concomitant decrease in molecular diffusivity dynamics; and (ii) a decrease in the fraction of the mobile phase. The observed molecular diffusion rate decreased nearly fourfold upon increasing the PEG8000 concentration from 0 to 150 mg/mL. Concurrently, total fluorescence recovery after bleaching decreased from 100% to ~40% for FUS^{FL} droplets. These data suggest that macromolecular crowding mediates a progressive transition of FUS^{FL} droplets from a viscous fluid state to a viscoelastic state, resulting in substantially arrested protein diffusion.

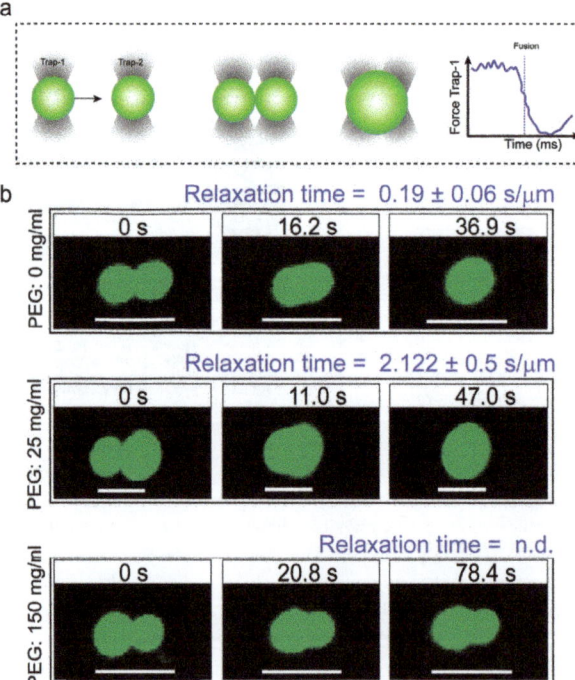

Figure 2. Coalescence dynamics of suspended condensates provide insight into FUS^{FL} droplet material states. (**a**) Experimental scheme of RNP condensate fusion using a dual-trap optical tweezer. (**b**) Controlled fusion of suspended FUS^{FL} droplets by the optical tweezer in the presence of 0 (top), 25 (middle), and 150 (bottom) mg/mL of PEG8000. The normalized relaxation times are indicated in each case. For 150 mg/mL PEG samples, droplets did not completely fuse. Scale bar = 5 µm. n.d.: not determined. Additionally, see Movies S1–3.

To gain further insight into the altered physical properties of FUS^{FL} droplets in the presence of macromolecular crowders, we performed quantitative droplet fusion experiments using a dual-trap optical tweezer. In these experiments, we used one laser beam to hold one RNP droplet at a fixed position while another RNP droplet, trapped by a second laser, was moved towards the first droplet at a constant velocity (Figure 2a and Figure S2) [47]. As these droplets were brought into proximity, liquid FUS^{FL} droplets coalesced rapidly in the absence of any crowders with a timescale of ~200 ms/μm (Figure 2, top panel; movie S1). In the presence of 150 mg/mL PEG8000, the fusion events of FUS^{FL} droplets were almost arrested (incomplete fusion in Figure 2, bottom panel; movie S3). Instead, we observed that FUS^{FL} droplets clustered at the optical trap under this condition (Figure S3). These observations are consistent with our FRAP results (Figure 1b–d). Taken together, our experimental data suggest that macromolecular crowding by PEG leads to a substantial hardening of FUS^{FL} droplets. We note that the observed alteration in the material properties of FUS^{FL} condensates occurred in the presence of crowding without any conclusive evidence for fiber formation (Figure S4).

2.2. The Effect of Macromolecular Crowding on RNP Condensation is Largely Independent of the LCD Sequence

The phase separation of the FUS family of RNPs is assumed to be driven by enthalpy, that is, attractive protein–protein interactions, and, therefore, is sensitive to LCD sequence features that encode essential intermolecular interactions [7]. As such, recent studies focused on elucidating the sequence determinants of LLPS in RNPs, which revealed two major classes of LCDs [46,47]. These are (i) prion-like LCD (PrD), characterized by an overabundance in polar (S/G/Q) and aromatic (Y/F) residues but largely devoid of charged amino acids [1,2,7,8,41,54–56]; and (ii) arginine-rich polycationic LCD (R-rich LCD) [57], such as the disordered RGG-box sequences present in the RNA-binding domains of many RNPs [58]. In the ribonucleoprotein FUS, both of these LCD types (FUS^{PrD} and FUS^{RGG}) are present as individual domains in the N- and C-termini of the protein, respectively (Figure 3a; Supplementary Table S1). To gain a mechanistic understanding of the impact of crowding on the physical properties of RNP droplets formed by these distinct LCDs, we next studied the phase behavior and physical properties of FUS^{PrD} and FUS^{RGG} condensates independently. FUS^{PrD} is intrinsically disordered, as predicted bioinformatically [59] (Figure 3a) and verified experimentally [49]. FUS^{PrD} is also known to form amyloids in vitro that contain dynamic β-sheet-rich structures [60,61], the formation of which is assumed to facilitate the droplet aging process [42]. While FUS^{PrD} has been implicated as the major driver of FUS LLPS [62], the role of FUS^{RGG} in RNP condensation is only beginning to be explored [47]. Similar disordered RGG-box regions have previously been shown to form homotypic condensates [63]. Here, to study the effect of crowding, we first constructed phase diagrams of PEG–LCD mixtures for these two distinct LCDs separately. Both LCD types underwent concentration-dependent reversible phase separation upon lowering the solution temperature (Figure S5), suggesting that there exists an upper critical solution temperature (UCST) for these two disordered domains, above which a homogeneous phase is energetically favored. The UCST phase behavior for the two LCDs also indicates that their phase separation is driven predominantly by favorable free energy change during self-association via attractive protein–protein interactions [7]. In presence of PEG8000, we observed that the phase separation of both FUS LCDs are facilitated. The isothermal phase diagram (at 22 ± 1 °C) analyses for FUS^{PrD} and FUS^{RGG} as a function of PEG8000 are presented in Figure 3. We observed that PEG decreased the protein condensation critical concentration by approximately fivefold for FUS^{PrD} in response to an increase in the PEG concentration from 0 to 100 mg/mL. A similar trend was also observed for FUS^{RGG}, where the concentration required for the protein to undergo LLPS was decreased by approximately sevenfold in the presence of 100 mg/mL PEG. These results are consistent with the hypothesis that the crowder-mediated depletion force acts synergistically with the homotypic LCD–LCD interactions (see Note S1).

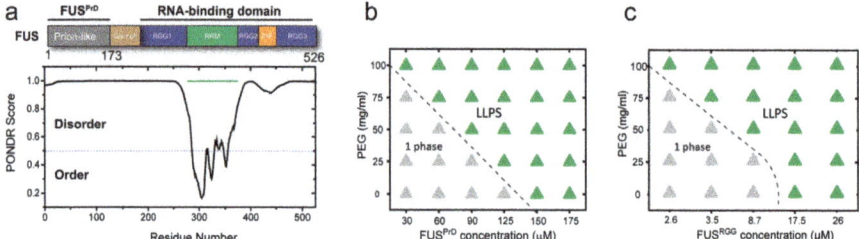

Figure 3. FUS^{FL} harbors distinct low-complexity disordered domains (LCDs) that individually undergo crowding-mediated liquid–liquid phase separation (LLPS). (**a**) Domain architecture of FUS; two distinct disordered domains are highlighted. The N-terminal FUS LCD has prion-like sequence features (FUS^{PrD}) and C-terminal LCD is enriched in RGG-repeats (FUS^{RGG}). The disorder prediction scores (using VSL2 algorithm [60]) are also shown in the bottom panel. (**b**,**c**) Effect of PEG on the LLPS of prion-like LCD and arginine-rich polycationic LCD (R-rich LCD). Shown here are the phase diagrams of FUS^{PrD} and FUS^{RGG} with PEG8000, respectively. The dotted lines indicate the liquid–liquid coexistence boundaries.

During the visualization of FUS^{PrD} and FUS^{RGG} condensates using a confocal fluorescence microscope, we noted that the well-dispersed LCD droplets underwent clustering at higher PEG concentrations (Figure S6). This observation indicates a crowding-dependent change of condensate physical properties. Therefore, we next investigated LCD droplet material properties in the presence of macromolecular crowders. Using Alexa488-labeled LCDs, we quantitatively analyzed fluorescence recovery after photobleaching in a well-defined region within FUS^{PrD}/FUS^{RGG} droplets (Figure 4). The recovery of fluorescence was modelled based on the diffusion of LCDs within the respective condensed phases (Figure S1). For FUS^{PrD} droplets, FRAP analyses revealed that the diffusion rate decreased significantly with an increase in the PEG8000 from 0 to 175 mg/mL. Only ~20% fluorescence recovery was observed at ≥150 mg/mL PEG8000 in a timescale of 300 s after bleaching (Figure 4a–c). The FUS^{RGG} droplets showed a similar arrest in protein mobility at a high concentration of PEG8000 (Figure 4d–f), although the changes were observed to be more gradual compared to FUS^{PrD}. We speculate that the differences observed in the FRAP trend between FUS^{PrD} and FUS^{RGG} as a function of crowder concentration is a manifestation of sequence-encoded distinct molecular interactions and polypeptide chain dynamics in respective LCDs. We also note that FUS^{FL} FRAP data (Figure 1b) showed a gradual change with increasing crowder concentration, similar to FUS^{RGG}. Overall, these data suggest that both FUS^{PrD} and FUS^{RGG} droplets undergo progressive hardening with increasing PEG, despite their diverse sequence features and charge patterning.

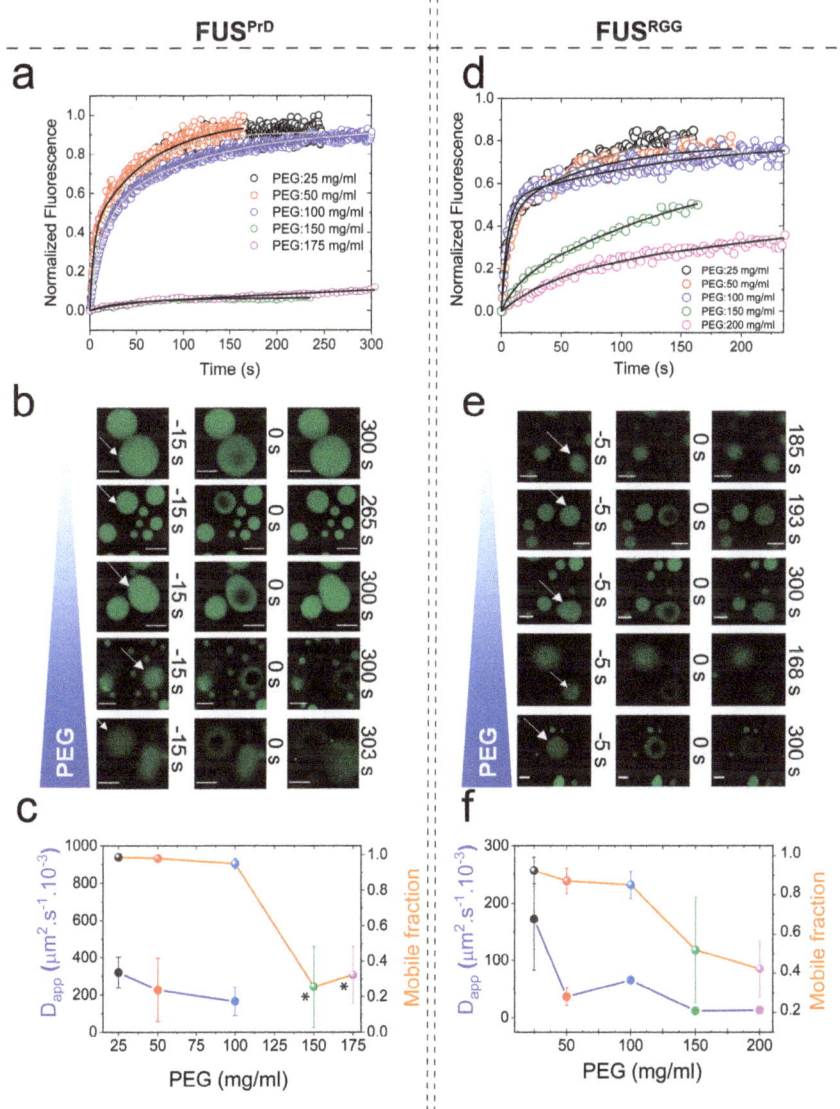

Figure 4. Macromolecular crowding tunes viscoelastic properties of both prion-like and R-rich LCDs. (**a,b,d,e**) Representative FRAP plots and images of FUS^{PrD}/FUS^{RGG} droplets at variable concentrations of PEG8000, respectively. Scale bar = 8 μm in (**b**) and = 4 μm in (**e**). Negative time implies droplets in pre-bleaching state in (**b,e**). (**c,f**) Analyses of the FRAP data estimating apparent diffusion coefficients (D_{app}) of respective LCDs within the condensed phase (left axis, blue) and the mobile phase fraction (right axis, orange) in respective cases. Due to a very low fraction of recovery, D_{app} estimation from the FRAP data for FUS^{PrD} droplets at 150 and 175 mg/mL PEG was omitted (indicated by the asterisks in (**c**)).

2.3. Crowding Impact on the Material Properties of FUS Condensates Is Observed for a Broad Range of Crowders

Macromolecular crowding in a cell arises from biopolymers with a plethora of sizes and shapes. In order to evaluate the excluded volume effect on RNP LLPS, it is necessary to use polymer crowders with variable chain lengths [25,64]. Therefore, we next considered the impact of crowders with different molecular weights on the FUS^{FL} condensation. To this end, we employed PEG polymers with molecular weights ranging from 300 to 35,000 gm/mol. FRAP experiments revealed that FUS^{FL} droplets were viscoelastic in the presence of all the crowders tested (crowder concentration = 150 mg/mL), with a significant degree of arrest in the dynamic exchange of the fluorescently tagged RNPs (Figure 5a and Figure S7b). Dextran, another widely utilized molecular crowder with a different chemical identity, also showed similar effects on FUS^{FL} condensates (Figure 5c and Figure S7d). These data collectively suggest that our observed viscoelastic tuning of FUS condensates is generally applicable to a broad range of polymer crowders and, therefore, represents a common effect of depletion interaction as induced by macromolecular crowding.

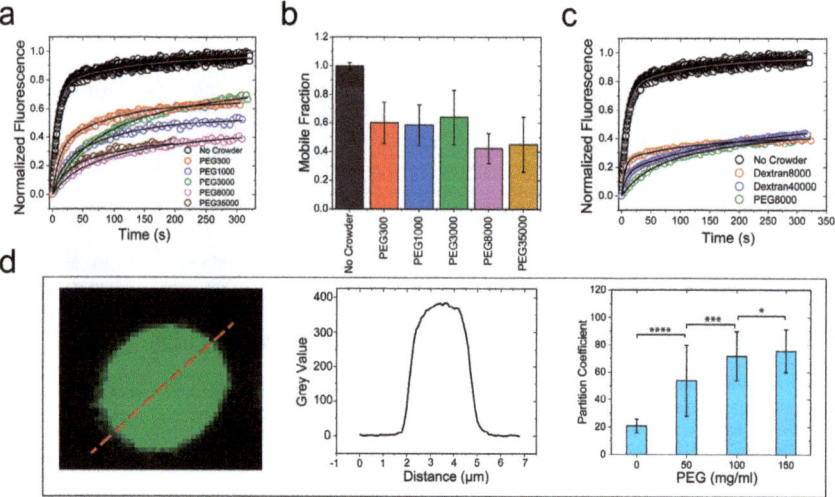

Figure 5. PEG and dextran produce similar effects on FUS^{FL} droplet physical properties. (a,c) Representative FRAP traces at 150 mg/mL PEG/dextran with a wide range of molecular weights, as indicated. The corresponding FRAP images and diffusion analyses are shown in Figure S7. (b) The fraction of the mobile phase decreased with increasing PEG molecular weight. (d) Increased ribonucleoprotein (RNP) partitioning within the FUS^{FL} droplets with increasing concentration of PEG8000, as probed by confocal image analysis. * p-value: 0.1–0.01, ** p-value: 0.01–0.001, *** p-value: 0.001–0.0001, **** p-value < 0.0001.

3. Discussion

Intracellular RNP granules are phase-separated bodies that display characteristic dynamics of complex fluids [2,65]. The mesoscale physical properties of RNP condensates are important modulators of their functions [3]. Aberrant alterations of the droplet material states, such as age onset loss of granule fluidity and formation of solid-like assemblies, are implicated in various neurological disorders, including ALS and frontotemporal dementia (FTD) [42,46,50]. Over the past two years, considerable efforts have been dedicated to characterizing RNP sequence-encoded molecular interactions that control the material properties of the RNP condensates [47]. In this study, we considered the role of molecular crowding—a ubiquitous thermodynamic force in the cellular environment—on the RNP condensate dynamics. We experimentally showed that crowding, as mimicked by biocompatible "inert" polymers, not only lowered the LLPS boundary, but also substantially altered the exchange dynamics of the RNP within the condensed phase. We observed that the aforementioned effects of crowding on LCD-driven LLPS, namely facilitating liquid condensation and droplet hardening, were largely independent of respective disordered domain sequences. In other words, while the saturation concentration and the condensate physical properties are governed by polypeptide sequence composition and patterning, their alterations by molecular crowding were observed to be a common effect in both types of LCDs. To provide a mechanistic picture of the observed effect of crowding on the RNP condensation, we consider a thermodynamic model that describes the perturbation of protein–protein interactions by a crowder in light of the well-established excluded volume effect [30,33]. According to this model, the introduction of a polymer crowder in the RNP–buffer solution leads to an isotropic inter-protein attraction by the depletion force (see Note S1), which acts in tandem with the intrinsic LCD–LCD homotypic attraction. The physical origin of the depletion attraction is the exclusion of the center of mass of a crowder molecule from a region surrounding an RNP molecule, which is typically called the depletion layer (Figure 6). The depletion layer thickness is directly proportional to the hydrodynamic radius of the polymer crowder [34]. This simple thermodynamic model predicts that increasing crowder concentration in the solution will increase the overlap of the RNP depletion layers in order to produce excess free volume available to the polymer crowders (Figure 6). This implies that the net attractive LCD–LCD attraction is enhanced by macromolecular crowding, which lowers the critical concentration of RNP LLPS and results in hardening of RNP condensates. Mathematically speaking, as the concentration of PEG increases, the chemical-potential derivative, $\left(\frac{\partial \mu_{protein}}{\partial c_{protein}}\right)_T$, which provides a thermodynamic basis of inter-protein attraction, decreases monotonically (see Equation (4) in Note S1). This quantity defines the spinodal curve, which is the boundary between the stable and unstable regions of the protein–crowder–buffer system (Figure S8). When $\left(\frac{\partial \mu_{protein}}{\partial c_{protein}}\right)_{T,c_{pol}} > 0$, the system is stable as a homogeneous solution, whereas it phase-separates into two coexisting liquids if $\left(\frac{\partial \mu_{protein}}{\partial c_{protein}}\right)_{T,c_{pol}} < 0$. Therefore, the net effect of the crowder may be physically interpreted as an effective increase in FUS–FUS attraction, manifested by depletion interactions. One key prediction of this model is that RNP partitioning in the dense phase should increase with increasing crowding (Figure S8). An increase in partitioning theoretically means a longer tie line that causes the volume fraction of the RNP in the dense phase to increase with a simultaneous decrease in the RNP volume fraction in the dilute phase. This is directly related to the strength of the inter-protein interaction parameter which increases the curvature of the free energy surface, pushing the coexisting states further apart (Figure S8). This was indeed experimentally verified for FUS^{FL} condensates using confocal fluorescence image analysis, which indicated that the RNP partition increased by about fourfold in response to an increase in the PEG8000 concentration from 0 to 150 mg/mL (Figure 5d). This observed increase in partition coefficient suggests that FUS^{FL} droplets become more dense with increasing crowder concentration. Such an increase in partitioning may also influence the rate at which FUS^{FL} condensates mature into a solid phase, which has been previously shown to accelerate with increasing FUS^{FL} concentration [42].

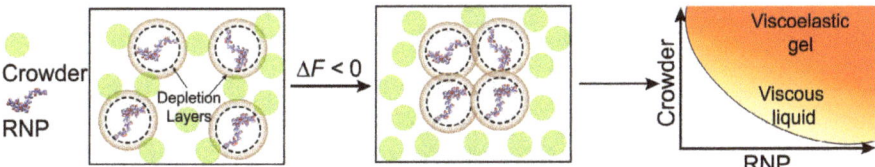

Figure 6. Schematic representation of depletion attraction: Proposed model showing crowder-mediated overlap of depletion layers as a driving force underlying RNP droplet formation and maturation into a gel-like phase in a crowded medium.

In summary, we demonstrated that depletion interaction, as induced by macromolecular crowding, continuously tunes the physical properties of RNP condensates ranging from purely viscous fluids to viscoelastic gel-like states. Alteration in the material properties of phase-separated membraneless compartments inside cells has been previously observed both in normal physiology and pathology [42,66,67]. Our results suggest that the hardening of RNP condensate is considerably influenced by the entropic forces in the crowded cellular environment. Several recent reports focused on identifying key RNP sequence features, post-translational protein modifications, and the role of RNA/protein partner binding that contribute to the gelation of RNP droplets [11,46,47]. Based on the data presented here, we postulate that generalized thermodynamic forces that can tune effective RNP homotypic interactions are likely to influence the rate at which physiological condensates mature into a viscoelastic gel.

4. Materials and Methods

4.1. Protein Samples

Codon optimized wild-type full-length FUS (FUS^{FL}), prion-like domain of FUS (FUS^{PrD}; AA: 1-173), and the RNA-binding domain of FUS without the zinc-finger domain (FUS^{RGG}:211-526Δ422-453) were gene synthesized by GenScript USA Inc. (Piscataway, NJ, USA) and cloned into (cloning site: SspI-BamHI) pET His6 MBP N10 TEV LIC cloning vector (2C-T). The plasmid vector was a gift from Scott Gradia (Addgene plasmid # 29706). TEV-cleaved proteins contained three exogenous amino acids (SNI) at its N-termini. *E. coli* cells (BL21(DE3)) were transformed with the plasmids containing FUS^{FL} and its variants in respective cases. Transformed cells were induced with IPTG (0.5 mM final concentration) at OD = 0.6–0.8 and further grown for an additional 3–5 h at 30 °C. Protein extraction was performed using a french press in lysis buffer (50 mM Tris-HCl, 10 mM imidazole, 1 M KCl, pH 8.0) containing protease inhibitor cocktail (Roche). Cell debris were removed by centrifugation. His-tag proteins were purified from the crude cell lysate using Ni-NTA agarose matrix (Qiagen Inc, Valencia, CA, USA) by gravity-flow chromatography following the manufacturer's protocol with the following modifications: the wash buffer included 1.5 M KCl to disrupt nucleic acid binding to the recombinant protein [68,69], which was eluted with elution buffer containing 250 mM imidazole and 150 mM NaCl. The purity of the eluted protein samples was checked using A_{280}/A_{260} measurements (to rule out presence of nucleic acids), and by polyacrylamide gel electrophoresis (PAGE) and Coomassie blue staining. The eluates (individual or pooled) were dialyzed against 25 mM Tris-HCl, pH 7.5 buffer containing 10% glycerol. The concentration of the protein samples were determined by absorbance at 280 nm using the following extinction coefficients: 103,600 M^{-1}·cm^{-1} for FUS^{PrD}-MBP, 86,750 M^{-1}·cm^{-1} for FUS^{RGG}-MBP, and 138,000 M^{-1}·cm^{-1} for FUS^{FL}-MBP (https://web.expasy.org/protparam). The protein samples were flash frozen in small aliquotes and stored in −80 °C.

4.2. Fluorescence Labeling

The S86C variant of FUS^{PrD} and A313C variant of the FUS^{RGG} were expressed and purified using an identical protocol as described above for the WT protein, except one modification: all buffers contained 2 mM DTT. The protein samples were fluorescently labeled with Alexa488 dye (C5-maleimide derivative, Molecular Probes) using Cys-maleimide chemistry as described in our earlier work [23]. The labeling efficiency for all samples were observed to be ≥ 90% (UV-Vis absorption measurements), and no additional attempt was made to purifiy them further, given that only labeled protein is observed in the fluorescence experiments.

4.3. Sample Preparation for Phase Separation Measurements

All of the protein samples were buffer exchanged into the phase separation buffer (25 mM Tris-HCl, pH 7.5) containing 150 mM NaCl unless otherwise noted. Prior to performing phase separation measurements, the His$_6$-MBP-N10 tag was removed by the action of TEV protease (1:25 ratio) (GenScript USA Inc.) for 1 h at 30 °C. The completion of the cleavage reaction was judged by polyacrylamide gel electrophoresis (PAGE) and Coomassie blue staining.

4.4. Phase Diagram Analysis

Phase diagrams were constructed by turbidity measurements at 350 nm using a NanoDrop oneC UV-Vis spectrophotometer at room temperature (22 ± 1 °C). Desired amounts of PEG solutions were added to the protein solutions from a 35% (w/v) stock in nuclease-free water with appropriate salt concentrations. Each sample was incubated ~120 s prior to turbidity measurements using a 1 mm optical path length. Simultaneously, visualization of protein droplets (or lack thereof) was performed using a Primo-vert inverted iLED microscope (Zeiss), equipped with a Zeiss Axiocam 503 monochrome camera. A global analysis of the turbidity and microscopy data was performed to construct phase diagrams in respective cases based on a simple binary criterion that identifies if droplets were present at a given protein/PEG concentration.

4.5. Confocal Fluorescence Microscopy

The fluorescence and DIC imaging were performed using a Zeiss LSM 710 laser scanning confocal microscope, equipped with a 63× oil immersion objective (Plan-Apochromat 63×/1.4 oil DIC M27) and a Zeiss Primovert inverted microscope. Samples were prepared and imaged using tween-coated (20% v/v) Nunc Lab-Tek Chambered Coverglass (ThermoFisher Scientific Inc.) at room temperature (22 ± 1 °C) unless otherwise noted, with ~ 1% labeled protein samples within the mixture of unlabeled proteins. All the samples were allowed to equilibrate in the chambered coverglass for ~30–45 min before imaging. For Alexa488-labeled samples, the excitation and emission wavelengths were 488 nm/503–549 nm; for Alexa594-labeled samples, the excitation and emission wavelengths were 595 nm/602–632 nm. Fluorescence recovery after photobleaching (FRAP) experiments were performed using the same confocal set up. The images and data were analyzed using Fiji software [70] and the FRAP curves were plotted and analyzed using origin software (OriginPro 2018).

4.6. Fluorescence Recovery after Photobleaching

FRAP experiments were performed using Zeiss LSM 710 laser scanning confocal microscope as described above. A circular region of interest (ROI) was bleached with 2–5 iterations of scanning using 100% laser power for a total time of 2–18 s. Fluorescence intensity changes with time were recorded for three different ROIs (bleached droplet, reference droplet, and background) for approximately 300 s or until the bleached ROI recovered and reached an equilibrium state. Data analyses were performed using Fiji software and MATLAB.

The fluorescence intensities from bleached ROI were corrected for photofading by multiplying with a correction factor obtained from reference ROI as follows:

$$C_f = \frac{R_i}{R(t)}$$

$$I_{corrected} = C_f \times I_{bleached}(t)$$

R_i: Initial intensity of reference droplet; $R(t)$: Intensity of reference ROI at time t; C_f: Correction factor; $I_{bleached}(t)$: Intensity of bleached ROI at time t; $I_{corrected}(t)$: Intensity of bleached ROI (corrected for photofading) at time t.

The corrected itensities were shifted to set the immediate post-bleach point to zero.

$$I_{shifted}(t) = I_{corrected} - \text{min. value of } I(t)$$

which were then normalized.

$$I_{Normalized}(t) = \frac{I_{shifted}(t)}{\text{max. value of } I_{shifted}(t)}$$

This normalized intensity post-bleach was plotted vs. time and fitted with a single exponential $y = A(1 - \exp(-t/\tau))$ using MATLAB. Half time of recovery ($\tau_{1/2}$) was obtained from the fitting parameter. To improve the goodness of the fit, two-exponential fit $y = A(1 - \exp(-t/\tau_A)) + B(1 - \exp(-t/\tau_B))$ was also used [71]. Half time of recovery ($\tau_{1/2}$) was obtained graphically for the latter (Figure S1c,d).

To account for diffusion during bleaching, instead of simply using user defined bleach radius (r_n) for diffusion coefficient calculations, an effective radius (r_e) from the immediate post bleach frame was calculated by taking a profile across bleached ROI in Fiji. The normalized fluorescence intensities were plotted with distance and fitted with an exponential of a Gaussian laser profile using MATLAB, as previously described [72,73].

$$f(x) = \exp\left(-K\exp\left(\frac{-2(x-b)^2}{r_e^2}\right)\right) \qquad (1)$$

r_e obtained from the fitting is the effective radius which corresponds to half width at 86 % of bleach depth K (Figure S1a,b).

The apparent diffusion coefficient [72] was calculated using the following equation:

$$D = \frac{r_e^2 + r_n^2}{8\tau_{1/2}} \qquad (2)$$

The mobile fraction [72,73] was calculated using the following formula:

$$M_f = \frac{I_\infty - I_0}{I_i - I_0} \qquad (3)$$

I_∞: Fluorescence intensity after recovery; I_0: Fluorescence intensity immediately after bleach; I_i: Fluorescence intensity before the bleach.

4.7. Coalescence of Suspended Droplets by Dual-Trap Optical Tweezer

Controlled fusion assays were conducted to investigate changes in the material properties of the FUS[FL] condensates as a function of crowder concentration. The samples were injected into a 25 mm × 75 mm × 0.1 mm single chamber custom-made flow cell. Samples at 10 µM protein concentration were prepared with different PEG8000 concentrations and equlibrated for ~30 min at room temperature. The trap-induced fusion was done using a dual-trap optical tweezer system coupled with laser scanning confocal fluorescence microscope (LUMICKS™ C-trap). In a typical fusion experiment, two droplets were trapped with a 1064 nm laser with minimum power to reduce heating effect. The trapping of droplets was acheived due to a difference in the refractive index between the condensate and the dilute phase. After trapping, one droplet is brought into contact with the other droplet at a constant velocity of 40 nm/s. The trap remains traveling at that velocity until the fusion is completed and the final droplet relaxes to a spherical shape. The force on the moving trap was recorded at 78.4 kHz sampling frequency and analyzed using a fusion relaxation model [45]. The following equation was used to fit the force-time curve:

$$F = ae^{(-t/\tau)} + bt + c \qquad (4)$$

where the parameter τ is the fusion relaxation time. We scaled the fusion time by the average of the radii of the two droplets for every event. The linear term in the model is added to account for the constant trap velocity. First, we did a control experiment on a slow fusion sample and the relaxation times were obtained both from force curves as well as from aspect ratio analysis using fluorescence images [74]. The results were in good quantitative agreement (data not shown). For FUS^{FL} samples, at least 15 droplet fusion events were collected for each PEG concentration and the scaled relaxation times were averaged. An example of a typical normalized force curve with the fitted model is shown in Figure S2.

4.8. Partition Analysis

Phase separated samples containing appropriate amount of fluorescently tagged protein were placed in a single-chambered custom-made flow cell (see Section 4.7). Droplets were imaged at the surface using laser scanning confocal fluorescence microscope using 60× water-immersion objective (LUMICKS^{TM}, C-trap). Images were analyzed using Fiji software. To calculate the partition coefficient, the mean intensity of the entire droplet was divided by mean background intensity for several droplets per sample for statistical accuracy using Excel. Statistical analysis were carried out using MATLAB.

4.9. Thioflavin T Assay

To probe for amyloid-like structure formation within FUS^{FL} condensates in presence of PEG8000 (150 mg/mL), we used a well-known amyloid reporter dye-Thioflavin T (ThT) [14]. 2–10 µM ThT probe was premixed with the experimental buffer (25 mM Tris. HCl, pH 7.5, 150 mM NaCl) used for FUS^{FL} (10 µM) droplet formation in presence of the crowder. Simultaneous fluorescence imaging of FUS droplets were performed by using Alex594 labeled FUS^{PrD}. Fluorescence imaging was performed using a Zeiss LSM 710 laser scanning confocal microscope. The excitation and emission wavelengths were 458 nm and 490 nm, respectively, with the exictation laser set at the same power as the Alexa594 channel.

Supplementary Materials: The following are available online at http://www.mdpi.com/2218-273X/9/2/71/s1. Table S1: Amino acid sequences of various constructs. Figure S1: Determination of biomolecular diffusion by fluorescence recovery after photobleaching (FRAP), Figure S2: Representative normalized force relaxation curve during trap-induced coalescence of suspended FUS^{FL} droplets, Figure S3: Aggregation of FUS^{FL} condensates in the optical trap in presence of 150 mg/mL PEG8000, Figure S4: FUS^{FL} condensates are ThT negative, Figure S5: FUS^{LCD} condensation is reversible and exhibit upper critical solution temperature (UCST), Figure S6: Clustering and morphological changes of FUS^{PrD} droplets with increasing concentration of PEG8000, Figure S7: FRAP analyses of FUS droplets in presence of various crowders, Figure S8: Representation of relative free-energy curves as a function of increasing crowder concentration showing transition of a stable homogeneous solution of FUS into a phase separated state, Note S1: A thermodynamic model describing the effect of a polymer crowder on the LLPS of FUS, Movie S1: Controlled fusion of suspended FUS^{FL} droplets by a dual-trap optical tweezer in the presence of 0 mg/mL of PEG8000, Movie S2: Controlled fusion of suspended FUS^{FL} droplets by a dual-trap optical tweezer in the presence of 25 mg/mL of PEG8000, Movie S3: Controlled fusion of suspended FUS^{FL} droplets by a dual-trap optical tweezer in the presence of 150 mg/mL of PEG8000.

Author Contributions: P.R.B. designed the study. T.K., I.A., and P.R.B. designed the experimental strategies with occasional input from M.M.M. W.W. expressed and purified recombinant proteins. T.K., W.W., and P.R.B. performed the phase diagram analysis. T.K. and I.A. collected confocal microscopy experiments, partitioning, FRAP measurements, and trap-induced droplet fusion with help from P.R.B. T.K., I.A., and J.N. analyzed all the data. P.R.B., T.K., and I.A. wrote the manuscript.

Funding: We gratefully acknowledge support for this work from University at Buffalo, SUNY, College of Arts and Sciences to P.R.B.

Acknowledgments: The authors gratefully acknowledge UB north campus confocal imaging facility (supported by National Science Foundation MRI Grant: DBI 0923133) and its director, Mr. Alan Siegel for helpful assistance. The authors are grateful to Dr. Gerald Koudelka for his generous help with protein expression and purification.

Conflicts of Interest: The authors declare no conflict of interest.

References

1. Banani, S.F.; Lee, H.O.; Hyman, A.A.; Rosen, M.K. Biomolecular condensates: Organizers of cellular biochemistry. *Nat. Rev. Mol. Cell Biol.* **2017**. [CrossRef] [PubMed]

2. Shin, Y.; Brangwynne, C.P. Liquid phase condensation in cell physiology and disease. *Science* **2017**, *357*, eaaf4382. [CrossRef] [PubMed]
3. Alberti, S. The wisdom of crowds: Regulating cell function through condensed states of living matter. *J. Cell Sci.* **2017**, *130*, 2789–2796. [CrossRef] [PubMed]
4. Meng, F.; Na, I.; Kurgan, L.; Uversky, V.N. Compartmentalization and Functionality of Nuclear Disorder: Intrinsic Disorder and Protein-Protein Interactions in Intra-Nuclear Compartments. *Int. J. Mol. Sci.* **2016**, *17*, 24. [CrossRef] [PubMed]
5. Uversky, V.N.; Kuznetsova, I.M.; Turoverov, K.K.; Zaslavsky, B. Intrinsically disordered proteins as crucial constituents of cellular aqueous two phase systems and coacervates. *FEBS Lett.* **2015**, *589*, 15–22. [CrossRef] [PubMed]
6. Uversky, V.N. Protein intrinsic disorder-based liquid-liquid phase transitions in biological systems: Complex coacervates and membrane-less organelles. *Adv. Colloid Interface Sci.* **2016**. [CrossRef] [PubMed]
7. Brangwynne, C.P.; Tompa, P.; Pappu, R.V. Polymer physics of intracellular phase transitions. *Nat. Phys.* **2015**, *11*, 899–904. [CrossRef]
8. Feric, M.; Vaidya, N.; Harmon, T.S.; Mitrea, D.M.; Zhu, L.; Richardson, T.M.; Kriwacki, R.W.; Pappu, R.V.; Brangwynne, C.P. Coexisting Liquid Phases Underlie Nucleolar Subcompartments. *Cell* **2016**, *165*, 1686–1697. [CrossRef] [PubMed]
9. Mittag, T.; Parker, R. Multiple Modes of Protein-Protein Interactions Promote RNP Granule Assembly. *J. Mol. Biol.* **2018**, *430*, 4636–4649. [CrossRef] [PubMed]
10. Protter, D.S.W.; Rao, B.S.; Van Treeck, B.; Lin, Y.; Mizoue, L.; Rosen, M.K.; Parker, R. Intrinsically Disordered Regions Can Contribute Promiscuous Interactions to RNP Granule Assembly. *Cell Rep.* **2018**, *22*, 1401–1412. [CrossRef] [PubMed]
11. Alberti, S.; Hyman, A.A. Are aberrant phase transitions a driver of cellular aging? *Bioessays* **2016**, *38*, 959–968. [CrossRef] [PubMed]
12. Patel, A.; Malinovska, L.; Saha, S.; Wang, J.; Alberti, S.; Krishnan, Y.; Hyman, A.A. ATP as a biological hydrotrope. *Science* **2017**, *356*, 753–756. [CrossRef] [PubMed]
13. Franzmann, T.M.; Jahnel, M.; Pozniakovsky, A.; Mahamid, J.; Holehouse, A.S.; Nuske, E.; Richter, D.; Baumeister, W.; Grill, S.W.; Pappu, R.V.; et al. Phase separation of a yeast prion protein promotes cellular fitness. *Science* **2018**, *359*, eaao5654. [CrossRef] [PubMed]
14. Choi, K.J.; Tsoi, P.S.; Moosa, M.M.; Paulucci-Holthauzen, A.; Liao, S.J.; Ferreon, J.C.; Ferreon, A.C.M. A Chemical Chaperone Decouples TDP-43 Disordered Domain Phase Separation from Fibrillation. *Biochemistry* **2018**, *57*, 6822–6826. [CrossRef] [PubMed]
15. Ellis, R.J. Macromolecular crowding: Obvious but underappreciated. *Trends Biochem. Sci.* **2001**, *26*, 597–604. [CrossRef]
16. Albertsson, P.A. Partition of cell particles and macromolecules in polymer two-phase systems. *Adv. Protein Chem.* **1970**, *24*, 309–341. [PubMed]
17. Abbott, N.L.; Blankschtein, D.; Hatton, T.A. On protein partitioning in two-phase aqueous polymer systems. *Bioseparation* **1990**, *1*, 191–225. [PubMed]
18. McPherson, A. Introduction to the Crystallization of Biological Macromolecules. *Membr. Protein Cryst.* **2009**, *63*, 5–23.
19. Roberts, M.J.; Bentley, M.D.; Harris, J.M. Chemistry for peptide and protein PEGylation. *Adv. Drug Deliv. Rev.* **2002**, *54*, 459–476. [CrossRef]
20. Minton, A.P.; Wilf, J. Effect of macromolecular crowding upon the structure and function of an enzyme: Glyceraldehyde-3-phosphate dehydrogenase. *Biochemistry* **1981**, *20*, 4821–4826. [CrossRef] [PubMed]
21. Sasahara, K.; McPhie, P.; Minton, A.P. Effect of dextran on protein stability and conformation attributed to macromolecular crowding. *J. Mol. Biol.* **2003**, *326*, 1227–1237. [CrossRef]
22. Tsao, D.; Minton, A.P.; Dokholyan, N.V. A didactic model of macromolecular crowding effects on protein folding. *PLoS ONE* **2010**, *5*, e11936. [CrossRef] [PubMed]
23. Banerjee, P.R.; Moosa, M.M.; Deniz, A.A. Two-Dimensional Crowding Uncovers a Hidden Conformation of alpha-Synuclein. *Angew. Chem. Int. Ed. Engl.* **2016**, *55*, 12789–12792. [CrossRef] [PubMed]
24. Paudel, B.P.; Fiorini, E.; Borner, R.; Sigel, R.K.O.; Rueda, D.S. Optimal molecular crowding accelerates group II intron folding and maximizes catalysis. *Proc. Natl. Acad. Sci. USA* **2018**, *115*, 11917–11922. [CrossRef] [PubMed]

25. Soranno, A.; Koenig, I.; Borgia, M.B.; Hofmann, H.; Zosel, F.; Nettels, D.; Schuler, B. Single-molecule spectroscopy reveals polymer effects of disordered proteins in crowded environments. *Proc. Natl. Acad. Sci. USA* **2014**, *111*, 4874–4879. [CrossRef] [PubMed]
26. Hatters, D.M.; Minton, A.P.; Howlett, G.J. Macromolecular crowding accelerates amyloid formation by human apolipoprotein C-II. *J. Biol. Chem.* **2002**, *277*, 7824–7830. [CrossRef] [PubMed]
27. Minton, A.P. Implications of macromolecular crowding for protein assembly. *Curr. Opin. Struct. Biol.* **2000**, *10*, 34–39. [CrossRef]
28. Rivas, G.; Fernandez, J.A.; Minton, A.P. Direct observation of the enhancement of noncooperative protein self-assembly by macromolecular crowding: Indefinite linear self-association of bacterial cell division protein FtsZ. *Proc. Natl. Acad. Sci. USA* **2001**, *98*, 3150–3155. [CrossRef] [PubMed]
29. Minton, A.P. Macromolecular crowding and molecular recognition. *J. Mol. Recognit.* **1993**, *6*, 211–214. [CrossRef] [PubMed]
30. Annunziata, O.; Asherie, N.; Lomakin, A.; Pande, J.; Ogun, O.; Benedek, G.B. Effect of polyethylene glycol on the liquid-liquid phase transition in aqueous protein solutions. *Proc. Natl. Acad. Sci. USA* **2002**, *99*, 14165–14170. [CrossRef] [PubMed]
31. Annunziata, O.; Ogun, O.; Benedek, G.B. Observation of liquid-liquid phase separation for eye lens gammaS-crystallin. *Proc. Natl. Acad. Sci. USA* **2003**, *100*, 970–974. [CrossRef] [PubMed]
32. Bloustine, J.; Virmani, T.; Thurston, G.M.; Fraden, S. Light scattering and phase behavior of lysozyme-poly(ethylene glycol) mixtures. *Phys. Rev. Lett.* **2006**, *96*. [CrossRef] [PubMed]
33. Wang, Y.; Annunziata, O. Comparison between protein-polyethylene glycol (PEG) interactions and the effect of PEG on protein-protein interactions using the liquid-liquid phase transition. *J. Phys. Chem. B* **2007**, *111*, 1222–1230. [CrossRef] [PubMed]
34. Asakura, S.; Oosawa, F. Interaction between particles suspended in solutions of macromolecules. *J. Polym. Sci.* **1958**, *33*, 183–192. [CrossRef]
35. Vivares, D.; Belloni, L.; Tardieu, A.; Bonnete, F. Catching the PEG-induced attractive interaction between proteins. *Eur. Phys. J. E Soft Matter* **2002**, *9*, 15–25. [CrossRef] [PubMed]
36. Uversky, V.N. Intrinsically disordered proteins and their environment: Effects of strong denaturants, temperature, pH, counter ions, membranes, binding partners, osmolytes, and macromolecular crowding. *Protein J.* **2009**, *28*, 305–325. [CrossRef] [PubMed]
37. Mitrea, D.M.; Cika, J.A.; Stanley, C.B.; Nourse, A.; Onuchic, P.L.; Banerjee, P.R.; Phillips, A.H.; Park, C.G.; Deniz, A.A.; Kriwacki, R.W. Self-interaction of NPM1 modulates multiple mechanisms of liquid-liquid phase separation. *Nat. Commun.* **2018**, *9*, 842. [CrossRef] [PubMed]
38. Ambadipudi, S.; Biernat, J.; Riedel, D.; Mandelkow, E.; Zweckstetter, M. Liquid-liquid phase separation of the microtubule-binding repeats of the Alzheimer-related protein Tau. *Nat. Commun.* **2017**, *8*, 275. [CrossRef] [PubMed]
39. Molliex, A.; Temirov, J.; Lee, J.; Coughlin, M.; Kanagaraj, A.P.; Kim, H.J.; Mittag, T.; Taylor, J.P. Phase separation by low complexity domains promotes stress granule assembly and drives pathological fibrillization. *Cell* **2015**, *163*, 123–133. [CrossRef] [PubMed]
40. Lin, Y.; Protter, D.S.; Rosen, M.K.; Parker, R. Formation and Maturation of Phase-Separated Liquid Droplets by RNA-Binding Proteins. *Mol. Cell* **2015**, *60*, 208–219. [CrossRef] [PubMed]
41. Hyman, A.A.; Weber, C.A.; Julicher, F. Liquid-liquid phase separation in biology. *Annu. Rev. Cell Dev. Biol.* **2014**, *30*, 39–58. [CrossRef] [PubMed]
42. Patel, A.; Lee, H.O.; Jawerth, L.; Maharana, S.; Jahnel, M.; Hein, M.Y.; Stoynov, S.; Mahamid, J.; Saha, S.; Franzmann, T.M.; et al. A Liquid-to-Solid Phase Transition of the ALS Protein FUS Accelerated by Disease Mutation. *Cell* **2015**, *162*, 1066–1077. [CrossRef] [PubMed]
43. Gitler, A.D.; Dhillon, P.; Shorter, J. Neurodegenerative disease: Models, mechanisms, and a new hope. *Dis. Models Mech.* **2017**, *10*, 499. [CrossRef] [PubMed]
44. Li, Y.R.; King, O.D.; Shorter, J.; Gitler, A.D. Stress granules as crucibles of ALS pathogenesis. *J. Cell Biol.* **2013**, *201*, 361–372. [CrossRef] [PubMed]
45. King, O.D.; Gitler, A.D.; Shorter, J. The tip of the iceberg: RNA-binding proteins with prion-like domains in neurodegenerative disease. *Brain Res.* **2012**, *1462*, 61–80. [CrossRef] [PubMed]
46. Gomes, E.; Shorter, J. The molecular language of membraneless organelles. *J. Biol. Chem.* **2018**. [CrossRef] [PubMed]

47. Wang, J.; Choi, J.M.; Holehouse, A.S.; Lee, H.O.; Zhang, X.; Jahnel, M.; Maharana, S.; Lemaitre, R.; Pozniakovsky, A.; Drechsel, D.; et al. A Molecular Grammar Governing the Driving Forces for Phase Separation of Prion-like RNA Binding Proteins. *Cell* **2018**, *174*, 688.e616–699.e616. [CrossRef] [PubMed]
48. Rivas, G.; Minton, A.P. Macromolecular Crowding In Vitro, In Vivo, and In Between. *Trends Biochem. Sci.* **2016**, *41*, 970–981. [CrossRef] [PubMed]
49. Burke, K.A.; Janke, A.M.; Rhine, C.L.; Fawzi, N.L. Residue-by-Residue View of In Vitro FUS Granules that Bind the C-Terminal Domain of RNA Polymerase II. *Mol. Cell* **2015**, *60*, 231–241. [CrossRef] [PubMed]
50. Harrison, A.F.; Shorter, J. RNA-binding proteins with prion-like domains in health and disease. *Biochem. J.* **2017**, *474*, 1417–1438. [CrossRef] [PubMed]
51. Maharana, S.; Wang, J.; Papadopoulos, D.K.; Richter, D.; Pozniakovsky, A.; Poser, I.; Bickle, M.; Rizk, S.; Guillen-Boixet, J.; Franzmann, T.M.; et al. RNA buffers the phase separation behavior of prion-like RNA binding proteins. *Science* **2018**, *360*, 918–921. [CrossRef] [PubMed]
52. Marenduzzo, D.; Finan, K.; Cook, P.R. The depletion attraction: An underappreciated force driving cellular organization. *J. Cell Biol.* **2006**, *175*, 681–686. [CrossRef] [PubMed]
53. Lu, P.J.; Zaccarelli, E.; Ciulla, F.; Schofield, A.B.; Sciortino, F.; Weitz, D.A. Gelation of particles with short-range attraction. *Nature* **2008**, *453*, 499–503. [CrossRef] [PubMed]
54. Mitrea, D.M.; Cika, J.A.; Guy, C.S.; Ban, D.; Banerjee, P.R.; Stanley, C.B.; Nourse, A.; Deniz, A.A.; Kriwacki, R.W. Nucleophosmin integrates within the nucleolus via multi-modal interactions with proteins displaying R-rich linear motifs and rRNA. *Elife* **2016**, *5*, e13571. [CrossRef] [PubMed]
55. Mitrea, D.M.; Kriwacki, R.W. Phase separation in biology; functional organization of a higher order. *Cell Commun. Signal.* **2016**, *14*, 1. [CrossRef] [PubMed]
56. Toretsky, J.A.; Wright, P.E. Assemblages: Functional units formed by cellular phase separation. *J. Cell Biol.* **2014**, *206*, 579–588. [CrossRef] [PubMed]
57. Castello, A.; Fischer, B.; Eichelbaum, K.; Horos, R.; Beckmann, B.M.; Strein, C.; Davey, N.E.; Humphreys, D.T.; Preiss, T.; Steinmetz, L.M.; et al. Insights into RNA biology from an atlas of mammalian mRNA-binding proteins. *Cell* **2012**, *149*, 1393–1406. [CrossRef] [PubMed]
58. Thandapani, P.; O'Connor, T.R.; Bailey, T.L.; Richard, S. Defining the RGG/RG motif. *Mol. Cell* **2013**, *50*, 613–623. [CrossRef] [PubMed]
59. Peng, K.; Radivojac, P.; Vucetic, S.; Dunker, A.K.; Obradovic, Z. Length-dependent prediction of protein intrinsic disorder. *BMC Bioinform.* **2006**, *7*, 208. [CrossRef] [PubMed]
60. Kato, M.; Han, T.W.; Xie, S.; Shi, K.; Du, X.; Wu, L.C.; Mirzaei, H.; Goldsmith, E.J.; Longgood, J.; Pei, J.; et al. Cell-free formation of RNA granules: Low complexity sequence domains form dynamic fibers within hydrogels. *Cell* **2012**, *149*, 753–767. [CrossRef] [PubMed]
61. Murray, D.T.; Kato, M.; Lin, Y.; Thurber, K.R.; Hung, I.; McKnight, S.L.; Tycko, R. Structure of FUS Protein Fibrils and Its Relevance to Self-Assembly and Phase Separation of Low-Complexity Domains. *Cell* **2017**, *171*, 615.e616–627.e616.
62. Franzmann, T.; Alberti, S. Prion-like low-complexity sequences: Key regulators of protein solubility and phase behavior. *J. Biol. Chem.* **2018**. [CrossRef] [PubMed]
63. Wei, M.T.; Elbaum-Garfinkle, S.; Holehouse, A.S.; Chen, C.C.; Feric, M.; Arnold, C.B.; Priestley, R.D.; Pappu, R.V.; Brangwynne, C.P. Phase behaviour of disordered proteins underlying low density and high permeability of liquid organelles. *Nat. Chem.* **2017**, *9*, 1118–1125. [CrossRef] [PubMed]
64. Sharp, K.A. Analysis of the size dependence of macromolecular crowding shows that smaller is better. *Proc. Natl. Acad. Sci. USA* **2015**, *112*, 7990–7995. [CrossRef] [PubMed]
65. Zhu, L.; Brangwynne, C.P. Nuclear bodies: The emerging biophysics of nucleoplasmic phases. *Curr. Opin. Cell Biol.* **2015**, *34*, 23–30. [CrossRef] [PubMed]
66. Schmidt, H.B.; Gorlich, D. Nup98 FG domains from diverse species spontaneously phase-separate into particles with nuclear pore-like permselectivity. *eLife* **2015**, *4*, e04251. [CrossRef] [PubMed]
67. Woodruff, J.B.; Ferreira Gomes, B.; Widlund, P.O.; Mahamid, J.; Honigmann, A.; Hyman, A.A. The Centrosome Is a Selective Condensate that Nucleates Microtubules by Concentrating Tubulin. *Cell* **2017**, *169*, 1066.e1010–1077.e1010. [CrossRef] [PubMed]
68. Wang, X.; Schwartz, J.C.; Cech, T.R. Nucleic acid-binding specificity of human FUS protein. *Nucleic Acids Res.* **2015**, *43*, 7535–7543. [CrossRef] [PubMed]

69. Schwartz, J.C.; Wang, X.; Podell, E.R.; Cech, T.R. RNA seeds higher-order assembly of FUS protein. *Cell Rep.* **2013**, *5*, 918–925. [CrossRef] [PubMed]
70. Schindelin, J.; Arganda-Carreras, I.; Frise, E.; Kaynig, V.; Longair, M.; Pietzsch, T.; Preibisch, S.; Rueden, C.; Saalfeld, S.; Schmid, B.; et al. Fiji: An open-source platform for biological-image analysis. *Nat. Methods* **2012**, *9*, 676–682. [CrossRef] [PubMed]
71. Phair, R.D.; Gorski, S.A.; Misteli, T. Measurement of dynamic protein binding to chromatin in vivo, using photobleaching microscopy. *Methods Enzymol.* **2003**, *375*, 393–414.
72. Kang, M.; Day, C.A.; Kenworthy, A.K.; DiBenedetto, E. Simplified equation to extract diffusion coefficients from confocal FRAP data. *Traffic* **2012**, *13*, 1589–1600. [CrossRef] [PubMed]
73. Day, C.A.; Kraft, L.J.; Kang, M.; Kenworthy, A.K. Analysis of protein and lipid dynamics using confocal fluorescence recovery after photobleaching (FRAP). *Curr. Prot. Cytom.* **2012**, *62*, 10–1002. [CrossRef] [PubMed]
74. Elbaum-Garfinkle, S.; Kim, Y.; Szczepaniak, K.; Chen, C.C.; Echmann, C.R.; Myong, S.; Brangwynne, C.P. The disordered P granule protein LAF-1 drives phase separation into droplets with tunable viscosity and dynamics. *Proc. Natl. Acad. Sci. USA* **2015**, *112*, 7189–7194. [CrossRef] [PubMed]

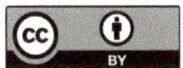

© 2019 by the authors. Licensee MDPI, Basel, Switzerland. This article is an open access article distributed under the terms and conditions of the Creative Commons Attribution (CC BY) license (http://creativecommons.org/licenses/by/4.0/).

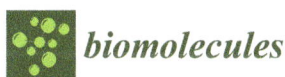

Article

Structural and Dynamical Order of a Disordered Protein: Molecular Insights into Conformational Switching of PAGE4 at the Systems Level

Xingcheng Lin [1,2,3], Prakash Kulkarni [4,*], Federico Bocci [1,5], Nicholas P. Schafer [1,5], Susmita Roy [1], Min-Yeh Tsai [1,5,6], Yanan He [7], Yihong Chen [7], Krithika Rajagopalan [8], Steven M. Mooney [9], Yu Zeng [10], Keith Weninger [11], Alex Grishaev [7,12], José N. Onuchic [1,2,5,13,*], Herbert Levine [1,20], Peter G. Wolynes [1,5], Ravi Salgia [4], Govindan Rangarajan [14,15], Vladimir Uversky [16,17], John Orban [7,18,*] and Mohit Kumar Jolly [1,19,*]

1. Center for Theoretical Biological Physics, Rice University, Houston, TX 77030, USA; xclin@mit.edu (X.L.); fb20@rice.edu (F.B.); npschafer@gmail.com (N.P.S.); susmitajanaroy@gmail.com (S.R.); mytsai886@gmail.com (M.-Y.T.); herbert.levine@rice.edu (H.L.); pwolynes@rice.edu (P.G.W.)
2. Department of Physics and Astronomy, Rice University, Houston, TX 77005, USA
3. Department of Chemistry, Massachusetts Institute of Technology, Cambridge, MA 02139, USA
4. Department of Medical Oncology and Therapeutics Research, City of Hope National Medical Center, Duarte, CA 91010, USA; rsalgia@coh.org
5. Department of Chemistry, Rice University, Houston, TX 77005, USA
6. Department of Chemistry, Tamkang University, New Taipei City 25137, Taiwan
7. Institute for Bioscience and Biotechnology Research, University of Maryland, Rockville, MD 20850, USA; hey@umd.edu (Y.H.); yihong@umd.edu (Y.C.); agrishaev@ibbr.umd.edu (A.G.)
8. Division of Biological Sciences, University of California, San Diego, La Jolla, CA 92093, USA; krrajagopalan@ucsd.edu
9. Department of Biology, University of Waterloo, Waterloo, ON N2L 3G1, Canada; steve.mooney@uwaterloo.ca
10. Department of Urology, The First Hospital of China Medical University Shenyang, Shenyang 110001, China; zengyud@hotmail.com
11. Department of Physics, North Carolina State University, Raleigh, NC 27695, USA; krwening@ncsu.edu
12. National Institute of Standards and Technology, Gaithersburg, MD 20899, USA
13. Department of BioSciences, Rice University, Houston, TX 77005, USA
14. Department of Mathematics, Indian Institute of Science, Bangalore 560012, India; rangaraj@iisc.ac.in
15. Center for Neuroscience, Indian Institute of Science, Bangalore 560012, India
16. Department of Molecular Medicine, Morsani College of Medicine, University of South Florida, Tampa, FL 33612, USA; vuversky@health.usf.edu
17. Laboratory of New methods in Biology, Institute for Biological Instrumentation, Russian Academy of Sciences, 142290 Pushchino, Moscow Region, Russia
18. Department of Chemistry and Biochemistry, University of Maryland, College Park, MD 20742, USA
19. Center for BioSystems Science and Engineering, Indian Institute of Science, Bangalore 560012, India
20. Department of Physics, Northeastern University, Boston, MA 02115, USA
* Correspondence: pkulkarni@coh.org (P.K.); jonuchic@rice.edu (J.N.O.); jorban@umd.edu (J.O.); mkjolly@iisc.ac.in (M.K.J.)

Received: 7 January 2019; Accepted: 10 February 2019; Published: 22 February 2019

Abstract: Folded proteins show a high degree of structural order and undergo (fairly constrained) collective motions related to their functions. On the other hand, intrinsically disordered proteins (IDPs), while lacking a well-defined three-dimensional structure, do exhibit some structural and dynamical ordering, but are less constrained in their motions than folded proteins. The larger structural plasticity of IDPs emphasizes the importance of entropically driven motions. Many IDPs undergo function-related disorder-to-order transitions driven by their interaction with specific binding partners. As experimental techniques become more sensitive and become better integrated with computational simulations, we are beginning to see how the modest structural ordering and large amplitude collective motions of IDPs endow them with an ability to mediate multiple interactions with different partners in the cell. To illustrate these points, here, we use Prostate-associated gene 4 (PAGE4), an IDP implicated in prostate cancer (PCa) as an example. We first review our previous efforts using molecular dynamics simulations based on atomistic AWSEM to study the conformational dynamics of PAGE4 and how its motions change in its different physiologically relevant phosphorylated forms. Our simulations quantitatively reproduced experimental observations and revealed how structural and dynamical ordering are encoded in the sequence of PAGE4 and can be modulated by different extents of phosphorylation by the kinases HIPK1 and CLK2. This ordering is reflected in changing populations of certain secondary structural elements as well as in the regularity of its collective motions. These ordered features are directly correlated with the functional interactions of WT-PAGE4, HIPK1-PAGE4 and CLK2-PAGE4 with the AP-1 signaling axis. These interactions give rise to repeated transitions between (high HIPK1-PAGE4, low CLK2-PAGE4) and (low HIPK1-PAGE4, high CLK2-PAGE4) cell phenotypes, which possess differing sensitivities to the standard PCa therapies, such as androgen deprivation therapy (ADT). We argue that, although the structural plasticity of an IDP is important in promoting promiscuous interactions, the modulation of the structural ordering is important for sculpting its interactions so as to rewire with agility biomolecular interaction networks with significant functional consequences.

Keywords: PAGE4; intrinsically disordered proteins; conformational plasticity; order–disorder transition; phosphorylation

1. Introduction

Strictly speaking, both canonically folded proteins and intrinsically disordered proteins (IDPs) lack unique three-dimensional (3D) structures [1]. Folded proteins undergo structural fluctuations on timescales ranging from femtoseconds to seconds, while IDPs exhibit dynamics on times ranging up to milliseconds. Thermal motions explore low-lying states on the energy landscapes of proteins. These low-lying states are simply more numerous and more structurally diverse in the case of IDPs. Despite their lack of stable structures, IDPs are indispensable in regulating various cellular functions. The greater structural plasticity of IDPs facilitates their interactions with multiple binding partners, leading to "one-to-many" and "many-to-one" binding strategies [2]. This functional plasticity coming from their structural diversity allows IDPs to function as hubs in protein–protein interaction networks, thereby regulating in a more complex fashion cellular decision making [3,4].

Although some studies have shown that IDPs can remain structurally disordered even when they interact with a cognate partner [5], this disorder is far from the complete randomness envisioned in elementary polymer physics models as self-avoiding random walks in 3D space, without any structural preferences [6]. In contrast to that elementary picture, many IDPs exhibit both local structural and dynamical ordering. IDPs undergo transitions among a diversity of metastable states that may be differentially stabilized by binding to interaction partners [7]. By being shrouded by a relatively high degree of structural plasticity, this ordering is difficult to discern using standard biophysical techniques. Furthermore, due to their intrinsically diverse conformational ensembles, IDPs are more susceptible to perturbation when compared to folded proteins. They therefore undergo larger structural modulation by the binding of ligands or by post-translational modifications (PTMs) [8,9], which can thereby perturb the balance between different functional states. The plasticity of IDPs is reflected by a set of activities of proteins that are driven by entropy [10–12]. Furthermore, it has recently been recognized that some IDPs can engage in polyvalent and highly dynamic interactions that drive large-scale liquid–liquid phase transitions that may be crucial in the generation of membrane-less organelles [13–16].

The existence of plasticity in structural conformations of proteins has long been recognized. It is now well-established that many proteins are polymorphic, changing from one folded state to another as a part of their functional repertoire [17]. Conformational switching, as well as the associated allosteric transitions, enables different functional behaviors that depend on environmental conditions. This conformational plasticity is especially prominent in metamorphic proteins [18], where multiple conformations with widely different structures exist for a single encoded sequence [19–21]. Therefore, IDPs do not stand entirely apart from their folded brethren. However, clearly we must recognize that IDPs have a qualitatively lower degree of structural order than folded proteins and they are more competent to perform their functions through frequent disorder-to-order transitions [22–28].

Prostate-associated gene 4 (PAGE4) is an archetypal IDP implicated in human prostate cancer (PCa) [29,30] (Figure 1). PAGE4 binds to and potentiates the oncoprotein c-Jun, which heterodimerizes with members of the Fos family to form the Activator Protein-1 (AP-1) transcription factor complex [31,32]. AP-1 is a negative regulator of the androgen receptor (AR) [33]. In PCa cells, the interactions among PAGE4, AP-1, Fos, and AR comprise a regulatory circuit module. Theoretical studies suggest that the nonlinear dynamics of this circuit underlie phenotypic switching in PCa cells [34,35]. Bioinformatic algorithms predict that the PAGE4 protein is expected to be highly disordered [36]. Figure 1 represents results of the multiparametric analysis of human PAGE4 intrinsic disorder predisposition by four algorithms from the PONDR family, PONDR® FIT, PONDR® VLXT, PONDR® VSL2, and PONDR® VL3 [37–41], as well as the IUPred web server for prediction of short and long disordered regions [42]. Furthermore, the outputs of all these predictors were averaged to generate the mean disorder profile, since averaging usually increases the predictive performance compared to using any single predictor [43,44]. According to these analyses, PAGE4, although highly disordered, is expected to possess several regions with somewhat increased propensity to order (most notably residues 13–19 and 86–92, and to a lesser degree 49–61). Nuclear magnetic resonance (NMR) experiments also indicate that PAGE4 has metastable secondary structures (Figure 9 of [45]). Two kinases are found to modulate the structure of the PAGE4 ensemble by phosphorylation, specifically, the Homeodomain-interacting Protein Kinase 1 (HIPK1) and the CDC-Like Kinase 2 (CLK2) [34]. The phosphorylated PAGE4 ensembles have different conformational preferences; the structures are relatively more compact for the wildtype form (WT-PAGE4) and for the HIPK1-phosphorylated form (HIPK1-PAGE4) but are more expanded in the CLK2-phosphorylated form (CLK2-PAGE4). PAGE4, although plastic compared to folded proteins, is clearly thus not structurally random. In order for the phosphorylation-induced conformational shift of the PAGE4 ensemble to modulate the binding affinity towards its transcriptional partner, the AP-1 complex, there must be some significant degree of order in the structures and motions of PAGE4 to begin with.

The flexibility of IDPs complicates the detailed characterization of their residual structure and their dynamics with currently available experimental methods. On the other hand, several biophysical techniques such as small angle X-ray scattering (SAXS), single-molecule fluorescence resonance energy transfer (smFRET), and nuclear magnetic resonance (NMR) are able to capture aspects of both the instantaneous and the ensemble-averaged properties of IDPs [46–49]. Specifically, solution X-ray scattering (SAXS) data enable us to determine the ensemble averaged radii of gyration (Rgs) of IDPs. The chemical shifts from NMR experiments give more local information indicating the preferences of parts of IDPs for different secondary structure elements. NMR paramagnetic relaxation enhancement (PRE) experiments can provide important information about long-range contacts. Changes in the energy transfer efficiency in the smFRET measurements encode the changes of distance between the donor and acceptor probes attached at different locations of the proteins, and can thus be utilized to measure the time-resolved dynamics of different domains within IDPs. The information attained from these experiments about the ensembles of structures of IDPs, and their changes upon post-translational modification, is however somewhat limited and insufficient for correlating the ensemble characteristics with changes in function. One can observe the effects on the ensemble arising from a structural change, but one cannot follow the conformational transition itself in most cases. Therefore, to understand these functionally important structural changes, it is useful to combine experimental measurements with structurally detailed computational simulations.

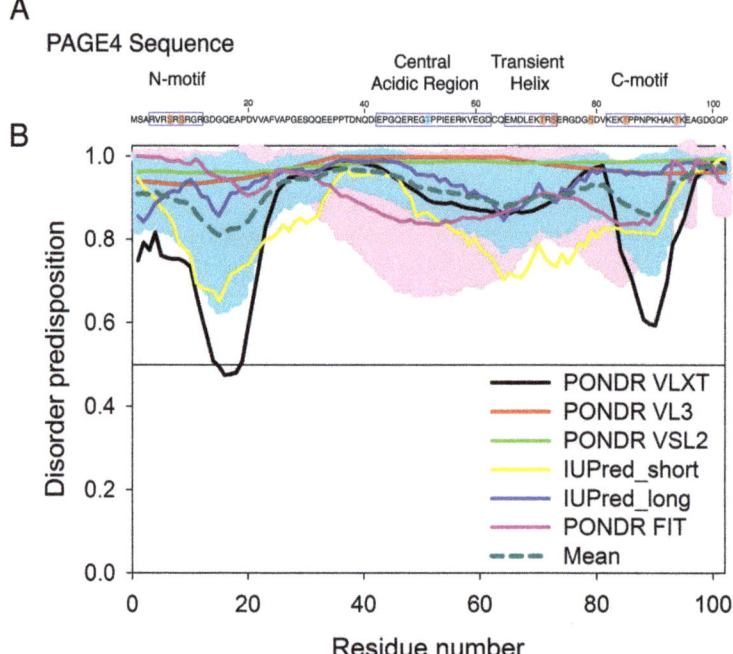

Figure 1. The sequence of prostate-associated gene 4 (PAGE4) and the evaluation of its intrinsic disorder propensity. (**A**) The sequence of PAGE4. The sites phosphorylated by HIPK1 are highlighted in blue, and those phosphorylated sites by CLK2 are highlighted in red. All phosphorylated sites were modeled in the AAWSEM simulation [35]. The N-motif (residues 4–12), Central acidic region (residues 43–62), transiently helical region (residues 65–73) and C-motif (residues 82–95) are also indicated by square box. (**B**) The disorder propensity of PAGE4 was calculated by several per-residue disorder predictors, such as PONDR® VLXT (black line), PONDR® VL3 (red line), PONDR® VSL2 (green line), IUPred_short (yellow line), IUPred_long (blue line) and PONDR® FIT (pink line). The dark cyan dashed line shows the mean disorder propensity calculated by averaging disorder profiles of individual predictors. Light pink and cyan shadows around the PONDR® FIT and mean curve show the error distribution. In these analyses, the predicted intrinsic disorder scores above 0.5 were considered to correspond to the disordered regions.

Molecular dynamics (MD) simulations complement experimental studies and can capture detailed structural dynamics of IDPs. Conventional all-atom simulations, in principle, enable the simulation of IDPs in different environmental conditions [50], but the structural plasticity of IDPs requires that a more substantial part of conformational space be covered by simulations than is needed for well-folded proteins. Sampling IDP ensembles presents a demanding challenge for all-atom simulations. Coarse-grained techniques overcome this problem by integrating out some non-backbone degrees of freedom, leading to much higher computational efficiency [51–53]. Furthermore, coarse-grained models allow for flexibility in incorporating the effects of post-translational modifications, such as phosphorylation [54,55].

When examining the structural ensembles for IDPs in simulation, one would like to be able to reproduce experimental observables, sparse as they are. Even though these observables are by themselves insufficient for full specification of the structural ensembles of IDPs, they are important benchmarks for reconciling the results of computational modeling with observations. We must bear in mind, however, that the existence of large conformational fluctuations makes it intrinsically difficult to predict certain properties of IDPs [53]. Small changes in modeling parameters are amplified due to their high effective susceptibility to perturbation, an effect that is less pronounced in the case of the less fluctuating class of folded proteins. Moreover, the majority of the force fields used in protein MD simulations have been tuned to minimize deviations from the folded crystal structure targets. Therefore, we might expect them to over-stabilize intra-chain hydrophobic and hydrogen bonding interactions relative to the interactions with the solvent to keep the molecule folded. These issues are reflected in the over-collapsed nature of the ensemble for IDPs that have been obtained in all-atom MD simulations when compared to measurements from SAXS experiments [56]. To correct this problem and to further control these fluctuations, we can tune the modeling parameters [35,56] or add an external compensatory biasing potential based on the experimental measurements to better represent the ensemble in the laboratory [53,57].

2. AAWSEM: A Coarse-Grained Modeling Framework to Simulate Intrinsically Disordered Proteins

The associative memory, water-mediated, structure and energy model (AWSEM) is a coarse-grained model whose parameters have been optimized using the principle of minimal frustration as a machine learning algorithm [58,59]. AWSEM has been successfully applied to the prediction of protein folding and protein structures [60–66], mechanisms of protein aggregation [67,68], as well as protein–protein and protein–DNA interactions [69–71]. AWSEM's Hamiltonian contains energy terms describing bonded and non-bonded interactions, and an associative memory term [60]:

$$V_{total} = V_{backbone} + V_{non-backbone} + V_{FM} + V_{elec} \qquad (1)$$

The non-bonded interactions of AWSEM, $V_{non-backbone}$, were learned using the principle of minimal frustration, which provides a quantitative framework for ensuring that the interactions between residue pairs that are close in the native state are dominant in the process of protein folding [72,73]. The associative memory term, V_{FM}, motivated by neural network theory [74], modulates the local structures of protein by using as biases input memories that are structures from the protein database or that have been found using the clustered structures from explicitly simulated protein trajectories through atomistic AWSEM (AAWSEM) [63,64]. Since the structures from the protein database are dominated by globular folded proteins, we use atomistic simulations to generate associative memories for the simulations of IDPs using the AAWSEM model.

The use of the coarse-grained AAWSEM, including the explicit treatment of electrostatic interactions, allows us to investigate the dynamics of IDPs where the effect of charges is predominant. Thus, we used AAWSEM to simulate the WT- and two phospho-forms of PAGE4. The phosphorylated residues are explicitly patched with phosphoryl groups in all-atom simulations for the generation of associative memories, and as far as their long-range interactions are concerned are simulated as hyper-charged (−2.0e) glutamic acid (Glu) residues in the subsequent coarse-grained simulations [54,55]. The electrostatic interactions were simulated by using the Debye-Hückel potential [75] in V_{elec}. Details of the simulation setup can be found in [35].

Similar to the case of explicit-solvent force fields, AWSEM simulation with standard parameters produce an over-collapsed structural ensemble of IDPs [53]. The AAWSEM can partially remedy this issue by simulating segments of PAGE4 in an atomistic force field CHARMM36m, which is known to work well for IDPs [56]. The clustered structures from the all-atom simulations were used as associative memories to guide the local structure formation of PAGE4 in the coarse-grained AWSEM simulation. Nevertheless, such a modified all-atom force field can still fail for larger proteins [76], probably due to the failure of the current functional form of the force field to capture the short-range London dispersion interactions of water molecules [77]. Therefore, to control the degree of collapse of the PAGE4 system, we shifted the γ parameters, which define the residue type based non-bonded interactions, in the non-bonded $V_{non-backbone}$ term of the AWSEM potential [35]. The modified parameters ensure that the average radius of gyration R_g values for WT-PAGE4 from our simulations match those from the SAXS measurements [34]. The AAWSEM model with these modified parameters then quantitatively predicts the average radii of gyration values for the two phosphoforms of PAGE4. This parameter tuning approach shares some similarity with the one in [77] where the dispersion forces of water molecules were tuned by effectively increasing the C6 term of LJ potential. An alternative approach would be to directly add an explicit biasing potential controlling the size of the simulated systems [53]. We stress that, even without explicitly controlling collapse in this way, the model still reproduces qualitatively the major experimental findings, such as the observed expansion of the size of the CLK2-PAGE4 ensemble upon hyper-phosphorylation [35].

3. AAWSEM-Based Simulations of PAGE4 Reveal Two Different Kinds of Order Underneath Its Disordered Cloak

3.1. Simulation Reproduces the Expansion of PAGE4 Upon Hyper-Phosphorylation

The free energy profiles generated from the AAWSEM simulations show a shift in the degree of collapse of PAGE4 upon phosphorylation (Figure 2A). HIPK1-PAGE4 (with an average R_g = 32.1 Å) has a similar size compared to WT-PAGE4 (with an average R_g = 32.9 Å), while CLK2-PAGE4 (with an average R_g = 41.8 Å) is greatly expanded in size after hyper-phosphorylation. These combined observations are in line with the experimental SAXS data (WT-PAGE4: 36.2 Å, HIPK1-PAGE4: 34.7 Å and CLK2-PAGE4: 49.8 Å) [34]. In addition, the simulation quantitatively reproduces the smFRET results that the size expansion of CLK2-PAGE4 arises from its expanded N-terminal portion [34] (Figure 2B). The ability to recapitulate experimental results allows one to reliably query the structural details of the WT- and two phospho-forms of PAGE4.

3.2. Simulations Reveal Structural Order in PAGE4

The simulations uncovered a hidden layer of order underlying the apparent disordered features of PAGE4. Our simulations indicated a change in the preference for forming turn-like structures (as determined using the Stride algorithm [78]) in the central acidic region of PAGE4 upon different levels of phosphorylation (Figure 3A). This structural change is in line with the observations from the NMR experiments (Figure 5 of [45]). Although the AAWSEM simulations agree with the bioinformatic predictions that the overall structure of PAGE4 is disordered, they suggest that some regions of PAGE4 exhibit more structural ordering than do others. Such ordering features are reflected by the population of secondary turn-like structures during simulations. The preference for forming the turn-like structure changes with differing levels of phosphorylation, and the change of the preference of secondary-structure formation suggests an order-to-disorder transition prevalent in the conformational transition of both globular proteins and IDPs [2,17]. Specifically, the increased presence of turn-like structures in the central acidic region of PAGE4 (residues 43 to 62) is consistent with the NMR experiments, which showed a decreased flexibility in the same region upon the phosphorylation of Thr-51 (Figure 9 of [45]). The change in the element of stable turn-like structure also correlates with the change of stability of the binding interface between PAGE4 and its transcriptional partner AP-1 complex. It has been hypothesized that the "transiently helical region" (residues 65–73), a nine-residue region of PAGE4, comprises the binding site towards the AP-1 complex. The simulations of CLK2-PAGE4 suggest a lesser extent of ordering in this region, reflected by a reduced propensity for forming turns after being hyper-phosphorylated (Figure 3A). Therefore, our simulations suggest that there is a hyper-phosphorylation-induced disorder that is associated with the loss of binding affinity of PAGE4 towards its binding partner AP-1 complex. Admittedly, the simulations suggest some changes of the turn-like preference in the N and C termini of PAGE4 upon phosphorylation that were not observed in the NMR experiments. The difference between the simulations and experiment may be attributed to statistical noise coming from poor sampling during the all-atom simulations that are used as input to the AAWSEM simulations.

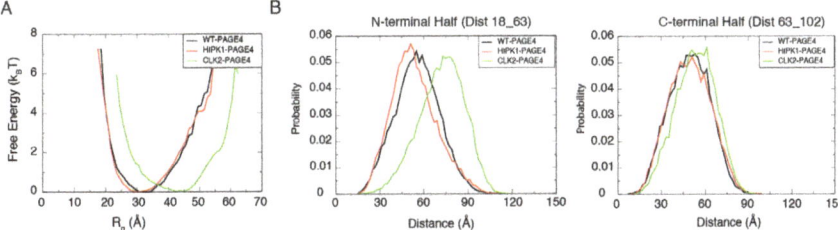

Figure 2. The simulations reproduce the size preference of PAGE4 ensembles at different phosphorylation states. (**A**) The free energy profiles as a function of the radius of gyration (R_g) of the simulated ensemble of PAGE4. The free energy F was calculated as $F = -k_B T log(P)$ where P is the probability for the protein to have a specific value of the R_g. The CLK2-PAGE4 exhibits a significant size expansion compared with the HIPK1-PAGE4 and WT-PAGE4. (**B**) The probability distributions for the distances within the two residue pairs that were previously measured in the smFRET experiments [34]. Residues 18 and 63 are located in the N-terminal half while Residues 63 and 102 are in the C-terminal half of PAGE4. The data indicate a more dramatic size expansion in the N-terminal half of CLK2-PAGE4 compared with that in the C-terminal half. Reproduced from [35] with permission.

We also observed the formation of a stable N-terminal loop in WT-PAGE4 and HIPK1-PAGE4, while it disappears in CLK2-PAGE4. The 3D structural ensemble, as well as the constructed average contact map from our simulations (Figure 3B), both show a preference for the N-terminal motif (N-motif, residues 4–12) to form a contact with the central acidic region (residues 43–62) of the WT-PAGE4 and HIPK1-PAGE4 molecules, consistent with the NMR and smFRET experiments (Figure 7 of [45] and Figure 6 of [34]). This stable N-terminal loop formation explains the reduced overall size of PAGE4 in WT-PAGE4 and HIPK1-PAGE4. This loop formation accounts for another level of structural order underlying the disordered dynamics of this IDP molecule.

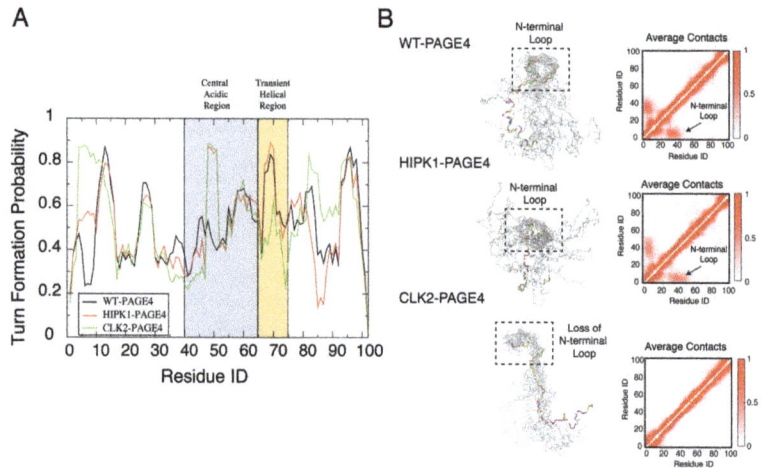

Figure 3. Orderly features behind the disordered PAGE4 ensembles. (**A**) The probability for each residue of PAGE4 to adopt a turn-like structure upon different levels of phosphorylation. The central acidic region and transient helical region are shaded in blue and orange, respectively. The secondary structure was calculated using the Stride algorithm based on the simulated trajectories [78]. Phosphorylations stabilize the turn-like structure in the central acidic region of PAGE4, while hyper-phosphorylation decreases the degree of order in the transiently helical region. (**B**) (**Left**) Representative structural snapshots collected from our simulations generated by AAWSEM. Randomly picked structures are aligned to minimize the root-mean-square deviations (RMSDs) among their N-motifs [79]. (**B**) (**Right**) The average contact maps generated from the simulated ensembles. Contacts are defined as two residues in close spatial proximity to each other. The color bar shows the probability of contact formation. There are non-zero probabilities of contacts formed between the N-motif and the central acidic region in WT-PAGE4 and HIPK1-PAGE4 (indicated by arrows in plots), indicating a metastable structural loop formation in this region. Hyper-phosphorylation eradicates this loop formation in the CLK2 form. Reproduced from [35] with permission.

3.3. Collective Motions of PAGE4 Are Associated with Its Functions

In addition to the residual structural order described above, organized dynamics of PAGE4 is revealed by principal component analysis (PCA) of the AAWSEM simulations. We performed PCA based on the contact maps of the simulated ensembles [54,55]. This analysis allows one to classify the collective motions and to understand how correlated movements of different domains of PAGE4 allow long-range interactions to form. The analysis (Figure 4) shows that there are correlated motions at the N-terminal half of WT-PAGE4, where the positively charged N-motif forms a loop with the central acidic region of the protein (shown as blue blobs of the first two principal modes in the top panel of Figure 4B). Interestingly, when WT-PAGE4 becomes phosphorylated by HIPK1, the molecule acquires a second type of motion involving loop formation in the C-terminus (C-motif, residues 82 to 95). The C-terminal motion is anti-correlated with the movement of the N-terminus (shown as additional red blobs of the first two principal modes in the middle panel of Figure 4B). This anti-correlation suggests that the two termini take turns forming a loop with the central acidic region of HIPK1-PAGE4. After PAGE4 is hyper-phosphorylated into CLK2-PAGE4, however, the overall magnitude of disorder increases accompanied by a loss of both types of correlated motions, except for the correlated local motions among these residues that are close in sequence, reflected by randomization of the long-range PC pattern (bottom panel of Figure 4B). The motions associated with the formation of loops by the N- and C-termini of the WT- and HIPK1-PAGE4 may facilitate the binding of PAGE4 to its cognate DNAs or the AP-1 protein complex. The structural plasticity of N- and C-termini enlarges the scope of interactions for PAGE4 to find its binding partners, while looping motion assists in the following binding processes. Such a mechanism is reminiscent of the "fly-casting" motion frequently observed in the studies of IDPs, where the plasticity of the proteins allows them to enlarge their scope of interactions and lowers the free energy barriers for IDPs for finding their binding partners [80,81]. After hyper-phosphorylation of PAGE4, however, a more randomized CLK2-PAGE4 loses its ability to approach and bind to its transactivation partners, resulting in a the loss of function and the degradation of PAGE4 in the end.

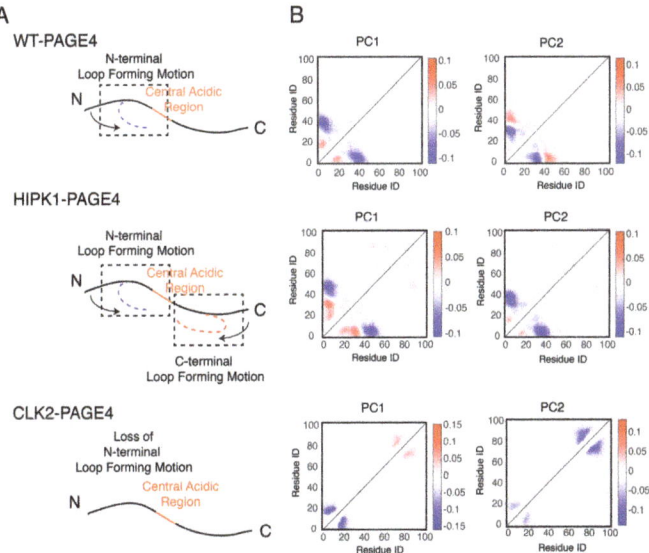

Figure 4. The collective motions revealed from the principal component analysis of PAGE4 simulations are shown. (**A**) Representative cartoon summarizes the collective motions of different phospho-forms of PAGE4. (**Top**) WT-PAGE4 has a collective motion of contacts formed between the N-terminal end and the central acidic region, resulting in a regulated loop formation. (**Middle**) In addition to that, HIPK1-PAGE4 has another loop motion in the C-terminal end that is anti-correlated with that in the N-terminus. (**Bottom**) Hyper-phosphorylation causes the loss of N-terminal loop motion in CLK2-PAGE4. (**B**) The top two principal component modes generated by the contact-based principal component analysis. We plot the coefficients of the first two principal components PC1 and PC2. Larger coefficients indicate a more significant variation of contact formation in that specific principal mode. The relative sign (shown in colors) of two coefficients corresponds to either correlated (same sign) or anti-correlated (opposite signs) formation of contacts. Here, in HIPK1-PAGE4, the C-terminal loop formation has an anti-correlated behavior compared with the N-terminal loop formation. When PAGE4 becomes hyper-phosphorylated, CLK2-PAGE4 loses both N- and C-terminal motion in the first two principal modes. Reproduced from [35] with permission.

4. From Structure to Function: PAGE4 Conformational Switching May Underlie Therapy Resistance in Prostate Cancer (PCa)

4.1. PAGE4 Conformational Switching Can Give Rise to Oscillations between an Androgen-Dependent Cell Phenotype and An Androgen-Independent Cell Phenotype

The conformational switching of PAGE4 can have important consequences in regulating cellular plasticity in the context of PCa. Double-phosphorylated PAGE4 (HIPK1-PAGE4) can potentiate c-Jun, hence leading to suppression of the androgen receptor (AR) activity. Cells resistant to androgen-deprivation therapy (ADT) typically have high levels of androgen receptor activity [34]. Therefore, high levels of HIPK1-PAGE4 typically correspond to an androgen-dependent (AD) cell phenotype that is sensitive to standard treatment for PCa such as ADT. Conversely, hyper-phosphorylated PAGE4 (CLK2-PAGE4) does not modulate AR activity, and high CLK2-PAGE4 levels can lead to an androgen-independent (AI) cell phenotype that is resistant to androgen deprivation [34].

A mechanism-based mathematical model helps to unravel the role of PAGE4 dynamics in regulating cellular plasticity. The model considers: (1) the different structural conformations of PAGE4: wild-type PAGE4 (WT-PAGE4), HIPK1-PAGE4, and CLK2-PAGE4; and (2) their modulation of AR activity. In the model, the HIPK1 kinase catalyses the switch from WT-PAGE4 to HIPK1-PAGE4, while the CLK2 kinase catalyses the conversion of HIPK1-PAGE4 into CLK2-PAGE4 (Figure 5A). Furthermore, HIPK1-PAGE4 indirectly inhibits AR activity via c-Jun as already discussed. AR activity, however, suppresses the expression of the CLK2 kinase, hence giving rise to a negative feedback between HIPK1-PAGE4 and CLK2 (Figure 5A). This negative feedback can result in oscillations between an AD cell phenotype with (high HIPK1-PAGE4, low CLK2-PAGE4) and an AI cell phenotype with (low HIPK1-PAGE4, high CLK2-PAGE4) (Figure 5B, non-shaded region). These oscillations are largely robust to parameter variation; details of the model setup can be found in [35]. The half-life of WT-PAGE4 is approximately 150 hours, which represents the longer reaction timescale in the system [32]. This timescale is reflected in an oscillation period of approximately one week (Figure 5B). Most androgen-deprivation therapies are applied on a similar timescale of one to several weeks [82,83], therefore indicating the potential role of interactions between treatments and the PAGE4 signaling axis. It should be noted that this prediction about repeated transitions between different cell states needs to be experimentally validated. Further, some modifications in the model topology introduced by additional players can alter the system dynamics so as to be multistable [84], which can also enable cell-state transitions in the presence of biological noise [85].

4.2. Androgen Deprivation Restricts the Phenotypic Heterogeneity by Damping PAGE4 Oscillations

The framework has been extended to include a constant inhibitory signal on AR activity (Figure 5A) in order to model the application of Androgen Deprivation Therapy (ADT), the standard care of treatment for locally advanced and metastatic PCa [82]. One finds that ADT quenches the oscillatory dynamics and can stabilize the AI, therapy-resistant cell phenotype (Figure 5B, orange-shaded part). To understand the implications of ADT at a cell population level, PAGE4 oscillations in a cohort of 10,000 PCa cells were simulated. In the cell population, oscillations are not synchronized: at any given time, some cells will be in the AI phase of the PAGE4 oscillation cycle, while others will be in the AD phase of the PAGE4 oscillation cycle. Therefore, the distribution of intracellular CLK2 (or any other variable in the model) in the population is quite broad (Figure 5C, Day 0 case). Introducing ADT, however, restricts cell heterogeneity by forcing the cells generally to have a very similar intracellular CLK2 level in approximately two weeks (Figure 5C, Day 7 and Day 14 cases). Thus, the model predicts that ADT can reduce the extent of non-genetic heterogeneity of a PCa cell population. Importantly, this model does not explicitly consider cell death. It is reasonable to hypothesize that, in the presence of ADT, some PCa cells would undergo therapy-induced apoptosis, but that any surviving cells can exhibit resistance. Therefore, the model predicts that the surviving PCa cell population is likely to consist of a much more homogeneous cohort of androgen-independent (or ADT-resistant) cells, due to synchronization of oscillations across the population.

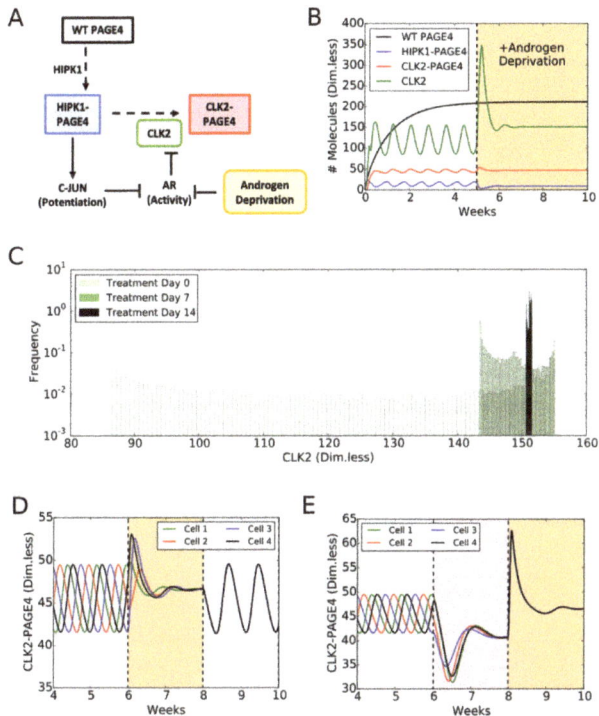

Figure 5. PAGE4 conformational switching gives rise to cell phenotypic oscillations which are suppressed by Androgen Deprivation treatments. (**A**) The PAGE4 phosphorylation circuit and its connection with androgen receptor (AR) activity. Wild-type PAGE4 is double-phosphorylated at two residues by HIPK1 kinase, and HIPK1-PAGE4 is hyper-phosphorylated by the CLK2 kinase. CLK2 is downregulated by AR, which in turn is inhibited by HIPK1-PAGE4 via the intermediates c-Jun. Androgen Deprivation treatment is introduced as an inhibitory signal on AR activity. (**B**) Temporal dynamics of the cellular level of WT PAGE4, HIPK1-PAGE4, CLK2-PAGE4 and CLK2. Without androgen-deprivation therapy (ADT), the oscillatory behavior exhibits a period of approximately one week (left area without shading). ADT (orange-shaded area) quenches oscillations within approximately two weeks. WT PAGE4, HIPK1-PAGE4, CLK2-PAGE4 and CLK2 are represented in dimensionless units. (**C**) Distribution of CLK2 intracellular levels in a simulated cohort of 10,000 prostate cancer (PCa) cells. In the absence of treatment, the distribution of CLK2 levels is broad ("Day 0" case). One week of treatment considerably shrinks the distribution ("Day 7" case). After two weeks of treatment, all cells have a similar level of CLK2 ("Day 14" case). (**D**) Temporal dynamics of CLK2-PAGE4 in four initially unsynchronized cells under intermittent ADT. The orange shading represents the periods of ADT. (**E**) Temporal dynamics of CLK2-PAGE4 in four initially unsynchronized cells under the BAT. The pink and orange shadings represent the periods of AR overexpression and ADT, respectively. Reproduced from [35] with permission.

A number of promising treatments for PCa besides ADT have been proposed in recent years, including intermittent ADT [82]. Intermittent ADT considers periodic ADT separated by "drug holiday" periods when no treatment is applied. As already discussed, a timescale of a week of ADT is sufficient to suppress oscillations in a cell population. These oscillations, however, emerge again during the holiday periods when AR activity is not inhibited (Figure 5D). Intriguingly, the on-off treatment cycle synchronizes the oscillations in cells that were initially unsynchronized (Figure 5D). This prediction, which still needs detailed experimental validation, lends further support to the idea that treatments such as ADT can restrict the phenotypic heterogeneity of a PCa cell population. Several independent investigations have considered various durations of ADT and holiday periods in both xenograft models and the clinic [86]. Based on our simulation results, a period of at least one week appears necessary since the switch of cell states is on a similar timescale.

As another example of alternative therapy, Bipolar Androgen Treatment (BAT), alternates two weeks of AR overexpression and two weeks of regular ADT [82]. Similar to the intermittent ADT, BAT is predicted to synchronize PCa cells that are otherwise out of phase prior to treatment (Figure 5E). Interestingly, the period of AR overexpression enforces an androgen-dependent phenotype (pink-shaded area in Figure 5E), while the two weeks of ADT lead to the already observed AI phenotype (orange-shaded area in Figure 5E). Therefore, the effectiveness of this treatment might lie in its ability to establish a treatment-sensitive phenotype first, which afterwards makes PCa cells more vulnerable to ADT.

5. Discussion and Conclusions

Intrinsically disordered proteins (IDPs) play a number of key roles in mediating interactions among the molecular components of the cell [2]. Their malleable structural properties enlarge their scope of interactions and lower the thermodynamic barriers for finding and associating with their interacting partners [80], which ranges from proteins to DNA. Intrinsically disordered proteins stand on the brink of stability and thus have more flexibility in sampling relevant conformational space [18]. On the other hand, an IDP is certainly not a completely disordered Gaussian polymer chain. Its underlying sequences encodes a certain level of order manifested in its specificity for the purpose of its function and stabilization upon binding to its interaction partners [7]. Even for a protein such as PAGE4, which has been identified as a near-complete random coil by bioinformatic tools [36], there are underlying structural features that confer on it the ability to respond differently to different levels of post-translational phosphorylation [35]. Therefore, under the cloak of its generally disordered nature, it is the residual order that bestows each IDP with its characteristic functions in the cell.

The presence of order-to-disorder conformational transitions with functional implications is not a unique trait of IDPs. Instead, we can gain insights from multiple examples well-studied in the realm of globular proteins as well [87–91]. On a local scale, a "cracking" motion features an order–disorder–order transition that is utilized by some proteins as a way to lower the barrier of conformational transition, or to facilitate the allosteric transitions [87,88,92]. On a global scale, a complete structural rearrangement of the system is sometimes needed to deliver the functional parts of a protein into its target location [91]. The plasticity of protein structures typically facilitates such transitions, but it is the ordering of the structure that eventually enables the functions. By the same token, although the sensitivity of IDP structure to perturbations indicates that modeling errors are amplified, the currently available force fields developed for folded proteins may already be accurate enough to capture the essential properties of IDPs, especially their thermodynamics, which is less sensitive. The fact that we can use a slightly modified version of the AWSEM model, which was initially optimized for folding globular proteins [60], to accurately capture the existing experimental data on PAGE4 [35], demonstrates that the key components built into this globular protein-derived force field do not differ too much from the actual forces at work in IDPs. Future work, however, is required to unify the modeling of IDPs and globular proteins for the simulations of an extensive network of protein complexes involving different types of proteins and other critical cellular components.

Another research area that needs further investigation is integrating structural insights into mechanism-based systems biology models. Here, the findings from our systems biology based model for PAGE4 and its interacting partners emphasize the role that conformational dynamics of proteins can play in rewiring regulatory networks, which in turn has important consequences for phenotypic plasticity. Such plasticity is thought to be related to transcriptional noise (i.e., stochastic gene expression [93–95]), but our analysis suggests that "conformational noise" may also modulate cell-fate [96]. Particularly, in the context of cancer progression, many oncogenes, tumor-suppressor genes, and regulators of metastatic spread have been identified as IDPs [97–99]. Comparing the conformational ensembles of cancer-specific mutant forms with those of their wild-type counterparts can yield important insights for therapeutic strategies.

Author Contributions: writing, review and editing, X.L., F.B., N.P.S.; review and editing, S.R., M.T., Y.H., Y.C., K.R., S.M.M., Y.Z., K.W., A.G., R.S., G.R., V.U.; supervision, review and editing, P.K., J.N.O., H.L., P.G.W., J.O., M.K.J.

Funding: This work was supported by National Science Foundation (NSF) through the Center for Theoretical Biological Physics (NSF-PHY-1427654, NSF MCB-1241332, and NSF-CHE-1614101). We also wish to acknowledge support from National Institutes of Health (NIH) grants GM062154 (J.O.) and CA181730 (J.O. and P.K.). P.G.W. was supported by Grant R01 GM44557 from the National Institute of General Medical Sciences. Additional support was also provided by the D.R. Bullard-Welch Chair at Rice University, Grant C-0016. G.R. was supported by JC Bose Fellowship and SERB Centre for Mathematical Biology Phase II grant. F.B. was supported by the Marjory Meyer Hasselmann Fellowship. M.K.J. was supported by Ramanujan Fellowship, SERB, DST, Government of India (SB/S2/RJN-049/2018).

Acknowledgments: Certain commercial equipment, instruments, and materials are identified in this paper in order to specify the experimental procedure. Such identification does not imply recommendation or endorsement by the National Institute of Standards and Technology, nor does it imply that the material or equipment identified is necessarily the best available for the purpose.

Conflicts of Interest: The authors declare no conflict of interest. The funders had no role in the design of the study; in the collection, analyses, or interpretation of data; in the writing of the manuscript, or in the decision to publish the results.

References

1. Frauenfelder, H.; Sligar, S.G.; Wolynes, P.G. The energy landscapes and motions of proteins. *Science* **1991**, *254*, 1598–1603. [CrossRef] [PubMed]
2. Oldfield, C.J.; Dunker, A.K. Intrinsically Disordered Proteins and Intrinsically Disordered Protein Regions. *Ann. Rev. Biochem.* **2014**, *83*, 553–584. [CrossRef] [PubMed]
3. Patil, A.; Kinoshita, K.; Nakamura, H. Hub Promiscuity in Protein-Protein Interaction Networks. *Int. J. Mol. Sci.* **2010**, *11*, 1930–1943. [CrossRef] [PubMed]
4. Haynes, C.; Oldfield, C.J.; Ji, F.; Klitgord, N.; Cusick, M.E.; Radivojac, P.; Uversky, V.N.; Vidal, M.; Iakoucheva, L.M. Intrinsic disorder is a common feature of hub proteins from four eukaryotic interactomes. *PLoS Comput. Biol.* **2006**, *2*, e100. [CrossRef] [PubMed]
5. Borgia, A.; Borgia, M.B.; Bugge, K.; Kissling, V.M.; Heidarsson, P.O.; Fernandes, C.B.; Sottini, A.; Soranno, A.; Buholzer, K.J.; Nettels, D.; et al. Extreme disorder in an ultrahigh-affinity protein complex. *Nature* **2018**, *555*, 61–66. [CrossRef] [PubMed]
6. Phillips, R. *Physical Biology of the Cell*, 2nd ed.; Garland Science: London, UK; New York, NY, USA, 2013.
7. Dyson, H.J.; Wright, P.E. Intrinsically unstructured proteins and their functions. *Nat. Rev. Mol. Cell Biol.* **2005**, *6*, 197–208. [CrossRef] [PubMed]
8. Wright, P.E.; Dyson, H.J. Intrinsically disordered proteins in cellular signalling and regulation. *Nat. Rev. Mol. Cell Biol.* **2015**, *16*, 18–29. [CrossRef]

9. Berlow, R.B.; Dyson, H.J.; Wright, P.E. Expanding the Paradigm: Intrinsically Disordered Proteins and Allosteric Regulation. *J. Mol. Biol.* **2018**, *430*, 2309–2320. [CrossRef]
10. Dunker, A.K.; Brown, C.J.; Lawson, J.D.; Iakoucheva, L.M.; Obradović, Z. Intrinsic disorder and protein function. *Biochemistry* **2002**, *41*, 6573–6582. [CrossRef]
11. Tompa, P. Intrinsically unstructured proteins. *Trends Biochem. Sci.* **2002**, *27*, 527–533. [CrossRef]
12. Tompa, P. The interplay between structure and function in intrinsically unstructured proteins. *FEBS Lett.* **2005**, *579*, 3346–3354. [CrossRef] [PubMed]
13. Darling, A.L.; Liu, Y.; Oldfield, C.J.; Uversky, V.N. Intrinsically Disordered Proteome of Human Membrane-Less Organelles. *Proteomics* **2018**, *18*, 1700193. [CrossRef] [PubMed]
14. Uversky, V.N. Intrinsically disordered proteins in overcrowded milieu: Membrane-less organelles, phase separation, and intrinsic disorder. *Curr. Opin. Struct. Biol.* **2017**, *44*, 18–30. [CrossRef] [PubMed]
15. Uversky, V.N. Protein intrinsic disorder-based liquid–liquid phase transitions in biological systems: Complex coacervates and membrane-less organelles. *Adv. Colloid Interface Sci.* **2017**, *239*, 97–114. [CrossRef] [PubMed]
16. Uversky, V.N.; Kuznetsova, I.M.; Turoverov, K.K.; Zaslavsky, B. Intrinsically disordered proteins as crucial constituents of cellular aqueous two phase systems and coacervates. *FEBS Lett.* **2015**, *589*, 15–22. [CrossRef] [PubMed]
17. Whitford, P.C.; Sanbonmatsu, K.Y.; Onuchic, J.N. Biomolecular dynamics: order-disorder transitions and energy landscapes. *Rep. Progr. Phys. Phys. Soc.* **2012**, *75*, 076601. [CrossRef] [PubMed]
18. Kulkarni, P.; Solomon, T.L.; He, Y.; Chen, Y.; Bryan, P.N.; Orban, J. Structural metamorphism and polymorphism in proteins on the brink of thermodynamic stability: Continuum of Order/Disorder Transitions. *Protein Sci.* **2018**, *27*, 1557–1567. [CrossRef] [PubMed]
19. Bryan, P.N.; Orban, J. Proteins that switch folds. *Curr. Opin. Struct. Biol.* **2010**, *20*, 482–488. [CrossRef]
20. Bryan, P.N.; Orban, J. Implications of protein fold switching. *Curr. Opin. Struct. Biol.* **2013**, *23*, 314–316. [CrossRef]
21. Goodchild, S.C.; Curmi, P.M.G.; Brown, L.J. Structural gymnastics of multifunctional metamorphic proteins. *Biophys. Rev.* **2011**, *3*, 143. [CrossRef]
22. Oldfield, C.J.; Cheng, Y.; Cortese, M.S.; Romero, P.; Uversky, V.N.; Dunker, A.K. Coupled folding and binding with alpha-helix-forming molecular recognition elements. *Biochemistry* **2005**, *44*, 12454–12470. [CrossRef] [PubMed]
23. Mohan, A.; Oldfield, C.J.; Radivojac, P.; Vacic, V.; Cortese, M.S.; Dunker, A.K.; Uversky, V.N. Analysis of molecular recognition features (MoRFs). *J. Mol. Biol.* **2006**, *362*, 1043–1059. [CrossRef] [PubMed]
24. Cheng, Y.; Oldfield, C.J.; Meng, J.; Romero, P.; Uversky, V.N.; Dunker, A.K. Mining alpha-helix-forming molecular recognition features with cross species sequence alignments. *Biochemistry* **2007**, *46*, 13468–13477. [CrossRef] [PubMed]
25. Vacic, V.; Oldfield, C.J.; Mohan, A.; Radivojac, P.; Cortese, M.S.; Uversky, V.N.; Dunker, A.K. Characterization of molecular recognition features, MoRFs, and their binding partners. *J. Proteome Res.* **2007**, *6*, 2351–2366. [CrossRef] [PubMed]
26. Miskei, M.; Gregus, A.; Sharma, R.; Duro, N.; Zsolyomi, F.; Fuxreiter, M. Fuzziness enables context dependence of protein interactions. *FEBS Lett.* **2017**, *591*, 2682–2695. [CrossRef] [PubMed]
27. Pauwels, K.; Lebrun, P.; Tompa, P. To be disordered or not to be disordered: is that still a question for proteins in the cell? *Cell. Mol. Life Sci.* **2017**, *74*, 3185–3204. [CrossRef] [PubMed]
28. Ahrens, J.B.; Nunez-Castilla, J.; Siltberg-Liberles, J. Evolution of intrinsic disorder in eukaryotic proteins. *Cell. Mol. Life Sci.* **2017**, *74*, 3163–3174. [CrossRef] [PubMed]
29. Kulkarni, P.; Dunker, A.; Weninger, K.; Orban, J. Prostate-associated gene 4 (PAGE4), an intrinsically disordered cancer/testis antigen, is a novel therapeutic target for prostate cancer. *Asian J. Androl.* **2016**, *18*, 695. [CrossRef] [PubMed]
30. Salgia, R.; Jolly, M.K.; Dorff, T.; Lau, C.; Weninger, K.; Orban, J.; Kulkarni, P. Prostate-Associated Gene 4 (PAGE4): Leveraging the Conformational Dynamics of a Dancing Protein Cloud as a Therapeutic Target. *J. Clin. Med.* **2018**, *7*. [CrossRef] [PubMed]

31. Rajagopalan, K.; Qiu, R.; Mooney, S.M.; Rao, S.; Shiraishi, T.; Sacho, E.; Huang, H.; Shapiro, E.; Weninger, K.R.; Kulkarni, P. The Stress-response protein prostate-associated gene 4, interacts with c-Jun and potentiates its transactivation. *Biochim. Biophys. Acta (BBA) Mol. Basis Dis.* **2014**, *1842*, 154–163. [CrossRef] [PubMed]
32. Mooney, S.M.; Qiu, R.; Kim, J.J.; Sacho, E.J.; Rajagopalan, K.; Johng, D.; Shiraishi, T.; Kulkarni, P.; Weninger, K.R. Cancer/Testis Antigen PAGE4, a Regulator of c-Jun Transactivation, Is Phosphorylated by Homeodomain-Interacting Protein Kinase 1, a Component of the Stress-Response Pathway. *Biochemistry* **2014**, *53*, 1670–1679. [CrossRef] [PubMed]
33. Sato, N.; Sadar, M.D.; Bruchovsky, N.; Saatcioglu, F.; Rennie, P.S.; Sato, S.; Lange, P.H.; Gleave, M.E. Androgenic induction of prostate-specific antigen gene is repressed by protein-protein interaction between the androgen receptor and AP-1/c-Jun in the human prostate cancer cell line LNCaP. *J. Biol. Chem.* **1997**, *272*, 17485–17494. [CrossRef] [PubMed]
34. Kulkarni, P.; Jolly, M.K.; Jia, D.; Mooney, S.M.; Bhargava, A.; Kagohara, L.T.; Chen, Y.; Hao, P.; He, Y.; Veltri, R.W.; et al. Phosphorylation-induced conformational dynamics in an intrinsically disordered protein and potential role in phenotypic heterogeneity. *Proc. Nat. Acad. Sci. USA* **2017**, *114*, E2644–E2653. [CrossRef]
35. Lin, X.; Roy, S.; Jolly, M.K.; Bocci, F.; Schafer, N.P.; Tsai, M.Y.; Chen, Y.; He, Y.; Grishaev, A.; Weninger, K.; et al. PAGE4 and Conformational Switching: Insights from Molecular Dynamics Simulations and Implications for Prostate Cancer. *J. Mol. Biol.* **2018**, *430*, 2422–2438. [CrossRef] [PubMed]
36. Yan, R.; Xu, D.; Yang, J.; Walker, S.; Zhang, Y. A comparative assessment and analysis of 20 representative sequence alignment methods for protein structure prediction. *Sci. Rep.* **2013**, *3*. [CrossRef]
37. Romero, P.; Obradovic, Z.; Li, X.; Garner, E.C.; Brown, C.J.; Dunker, A.K. Sequence complexity of disordered protein. *Proteins* **2001**, *42*, 38–48. [CrossRef]
38. Li, X.; Romero, P.; Rani, M.; Dunker, A.K.; Obradovic, Z. Predicting Protein Disorder for N-, C-, and Internal Regions. *Genome Informat. Workshop Genome Informat.* **1999**, *10*, 30–40.
39. Xue, B.; Dunbrack, R.L.; Williams, R.W.; Dunker, A.K.; Uversky, V.N. PONDR-FIT: A meta-predictor of intrinsically disordered amino acids. *Biochim. Biophys. Acta (BBA) Proteins Proteom.* **2010**, *1804*, 996–1010. [CrossRef] [PubMed]
40. Obradovic, Z.; Peng, K.; Vucetic, S.; Radivojac, P.; Dunker, A.K. Exploiting heterogeneous sequence properties improves prediction of protein disorder. *Proteins* **2005**, *61*, 176–182. [CrossRef] [PubMed]
41. Peng, K.; Radivojac, P.; Vucetic, S.; Dunker, A.K.; Obradovic, Z. Length-dependent prediction of protein intrinsic disorder. *BMC Bioinformat.* **2006**, *7*, 208. [CrossRef]
42. Dosztányi, Z.; Csizmok, V.; Tompa, P.; Simon, I. IUPred: web server for the prediction of intrinsically unstructured regions of proteins based on estimated energy content. *Bioinformatics* **2005**, *21*, 3433–3434. [CrossRef]
43. Walsh, I.; Giollo, M.; Di Domenico, T.; Ferrari, C.; Zimmermann, O.; Tosatto, S.C.E. Comprehensive large-scale assessment of intrinsic protein disorder. *Bioinformatics* **2015**, *31*, 201–208. [CrossRef] [PubMed]
44. Fan, X.; Kurgan, L. Accurate prediction of disorder in protein chains with a comprehensive and empirically designed consensus. *J. Biomol. Struct. Dyn.* **2014**, *32*, 448–464. [CrossRef] [PubMed]
45. He, Y.; Chen, Y.; Mooney, S.M.; Rajagopalan, K.; Bhargava, A.; Sacho, E.; Weninger, K.; Bryan, P.N.; Kulkarni, P.; Orban, J. Phosphorylation-induced Conformational Ensemble Switching in an Intrinsically Disordered Cancer/Testis Antigen. *J. Biol. Chem.* **2015**, *290*, 25090–25102. [CrossRef] [PubMed]
46. Bernadó, P.; Svergun, D.I. Structural analysis of intrinsically disordered proteins by small-angle X-ray scattering. *Mol. BioSyst.* **2012**, *8*, 151–167. [CrossRef]
47. Schneider, R.; Huang, J.R.; Yao, M.; Communie, G.; Ozenne, V.; Mollica, L.; Salmon, L.; Ringkjøbing Jensen, M.; Blackledge, M. Towards a robust description of intrinsic protein disorder using nuclear magnetic resonance spectroscopy. *Mol. BioSyst.* **2012**, *8*, 58–68. [CrossRef]
48. Schuler, B.; Soranno, A.; Hofmann, H.; Nettels, D. Single-Molecule FRET Spectroscopy and the Polymer Physics of Unfolded and Intrinsically Disordered Proteins. *Annu. Rev. Biophys.* **2016**, *45*, 207–231. [CrossRef]
49. Jemth, P.; Karlsson, E.; Vögeli, B.; Guzovsky, B.; Andersson, E.; Hultqvist, G.; Dogan, J.; Güntert, P.; Riek, R.; Chi, C.N. Structure and dynamics conspire in the evolution of affinity between intrinsically disordered proteins. *Sci. Adv.* **2018**, *4*, eaau4130. [CrossRef]

50. Zheng, W.; Borgia, A.; Buholzer, K.; Grishaev, A.; Schuler, B.; Best, R.B. Probing the Action of Chemical Denaturant on an Intrinsically Disordered Protein by Simulation and Experiment. *J. Am. Chem. Soc.* **2016**, *138*, 11702–11713. [CrossRef]
51. Dignon, G.L.; Zheng, W.; Kim, Y.C.; Best, R.B.; Mittal, J. Sequence determinants of protein phase behavior from a coarse-grained model. *PLoS Comput. Biol.* **2018**, *14*, e1005941. [CrossRef]
52. Dignon, G.L.; Zheng, W.; Best, R.B.; Kim, Y.C.; Mittal, J. Relation between single-molecule properties and phase behavior of intrinsically disordered proteins. *Proc. Natl. Acad. Sci. USA* **2018**, *115*, 9929–9934. [CrossRef] [PubMed]
53. Wu, H.; Wolynes, P.G.; Papoian, G.A. AWSEM-IDP: A Coarse-Grained Force Field for Intrinsically Disordered Proteins. *J. Phys. Chem. B* **2018**, *122*, 11115–11125. [CrossRef] [PubMed]
54. Shen, T.; Zong, C.; Hamelberg, D.; McCammon, J.A.; Wolynes, P.G. The folding energy landscape and phosphorylation: modeling the conformational switch of the NFAT regulatory domain. *FASEB J.* **2005**, *19*, 1389–1395. [CrossRef] [PubMed]
55. Lätzer, J.; Shen, T.; Wolynes, P.G. Conformational Switching upon Phosphorylation: A Predictive Framework Based on Energy Landscape Principles. *Biochemistry* **2008**, *47*, 2110–2122. [CrossRef] [PubMed]
56. Huang, J.; Rauscher, S.; Nawrocki, G.; Ran, T.; Feig, M.; de Groot, B.L.; Grubmüller, H.; MacKerell, A.D., Jr. CHARMM36m: an improved force field for folded and intrinsically disordered proteins. *Nat. Methods* **2016**, *14*, 71. [CrossRef] [PubMed]
57. Latham, A.P.; Zhang, B. Improving Coarse-Grained Protein Force Fields with Small-Angle X-ray Scattering Data. *J. Phys. Chem. B* **2019**, *123(5)*, 1026–1034. [CrossRef] [PubMed]
58. Bryngelson, J.D.; Wolynes, P.G. Spin glasses and the statistical mechanics of protein folding. *Proc. Natl. Acad. Sci. USA* **1987**, *84*, 7524–7528. [CrossRef] [PubMed]
59. Goldstein, R.A.; Luthey-Schulten, Z.A.; Wolynes, P.G. Optimal protein-folding codes from spin-glass theory. *Proc. Natl. Acad. Sci. USA* **1992**, *89*, 4918–4922. [CrossRef]
60. Davtyan, A.; Schafer, N.P.; Zheng, W.; Clementi, C.; Wolynes, P.G.; Papoian, G.A. AWSEM-MD: Protein Structure Prediction Using Coarse-Grained Physical Potentials and Bioinformatically Based Local Structure Biasing. *J. Phys. Chem. B* **2012**, *116*, 8494–8503. [CrossRef]
61. Zheng, W.; Schafer, N.P.; Davtyan, A.; Papoian, G.A.; Wolynes, P.G. Predictive energy landscapes for protein-protein association. *Proc. Natl. Acad. Sci. USA* **2012**, *109*, 19244–19249. [CrossRef]
62. Kim, B.L.; Schafer, N.P.; Wolynes, P.G. Predictive energy landscapes for folding -helical transmembrane proteins. *Proc. Natl. Acad. Sci. USA* **2014**, *111*, 11031–11036. [CrossRef] [PubMed]
63. Chen, M.; Lin, X.; Zheng, W.; Onuchic, J.N.; Wolynes, P.G. Protein Folding and Structure Prediction from the Ground Up: The Atomistic Associative Memory, Water Mediated, Structure and Energy Model. *J. Phys. Chem. B* **2016**, *120*, 8557–8565. [CrossRef] [PubMed]
64. Chen, M.; Lin, X.; Lu, W.; Onuchic, J.N.; Wolynes, P.G. Protein Folding and Structure Prediction from the Ground Up II: AAWSEM for α/β Proteins. *J. Phys. Chem. B* **2017**, *121*, 3473–3482. [CrossRef] [PubMed]
65. Sirovetz, B.J.; Schafer, N.P.; Wolynes, P.G. Protein structure prediction: making AWSEM AWSEM-ER by adding evolutionary restraints. *Proteins Struct. Funct. Bioinformat.* **2017**, *85*, 2127–2142. [CrossRef] [PubMed]
66. Chen, M.; Lin, X.; Lu, W.; Schafer, N.P.; Onuchic, J.N.; Wolynes, P.G. Template-Guided Protein Structure Prediction and Refinement Using Optimized Folding Landscape Force Fields. *J. Chem. Theory Comput.* **2018**, *14*, 6102–6116. [CrossRef] [PubMed]
67. Zheng, W.; Tsai, M.Y.; Chen, M.; Wolynes, P.G. Exploring the aggregation free energy landscape of the amyloid-β protein (1–40). *Proc. Natl. Acad. Sci. USA* **2016**, *113*, 11835–11840. [CrossRef] [PubMed]
68. Chen, M.; Tsai, M.; Zheng, W.; Wolynes, P.G. The Aggregation Free Energy Landscapes of Polyglutamine Repeats. *J. Am. Chem. Soc.* **2016**, *138*, 15197–15203. [CrossRef]
69. Potoyan, D.A.; Zheng, W.; Komives, E.A.; Wolynes, P.G. Molecular stripping in the *NF-κB/IκB/DNA* genetic regulatory network. *Proc. Natl. Acad. Sci. USA* **2016**, *113*, 110–115. [CrossRef]

70. Potoyan, D.A.; Bueno, C.; Zheng, W.; Komives, E.A.; Wolynes, P.G. Resolving the NFκB Heterodimer Binding Paradox: Strain and Frustration Guide the Binding of Dimeric Transcription Factors. *J. Am. Chem. Soc.* **2017**, *139*, 18558–18566. [CrossRef]
71. Tsai, M.Y.; Zhang, B.; Zheng, W.; Wolynes, P.G. Molecular Mechanism of Facilitated Dissociation of Fis Protein from DNA. *J. Am. Chem. Soc.* **2016**, *138*, 13497–13500. [CrossRef]
72. Koretke, K.K.; Luthey-Schulten, Z.; Wolynes, P.G. Self-consistently optimized energy functions for protein structure prediction by molecular dynamics. *Proc. Natl. Acad. Sci. USA* **1998**, *95*, 2932–2937. [CrossRef] [PubMed]
73. Schafer, N.P.; Kim, B.L.; Zheng, W.; Wolynes, P.G. Learning To Fold Proteins Using Energy Landscape Theory. *Israel J. Chem.* **2014**, *54*, 1311–1337. [CrossRef] [PubMed]
74. Friedrichs, M.S.; Wolynes, P.G. Toward protein tertiary structure recognition by means of associative memory hamiltonians. *Science* **1989**, *246*, 371–373. [CrossRef] [PubMed]
75. Tsai, M.Y.; Zheng, W.; Balamurugan, D.; Schafer, N.P.; Kim, B.L.; Cheung, M.S.; Wolynes, P.G. Electrostatics, structure prediction, and the energy landscapes for protein folding and binding: Electrostatic Energy Landscapes for Folding and Binding. *Protein Sci.* **2016**, *25*, 255–269. [CrossRef] [PubMed]
76. Robustelli, P.; Piana, S.; Shaw, D.E. Developing a molecular dynamics force field for both folded and disordered protein states. *Proc. Natl. Acad. Sci. USA* **2018**, *115*, E4758–E4766. [CrossRef] [PubMed]
77. Piana, S.; Donchev, A.G.; Robustelli, P.; Shaw, D.E. Water Dispersion Interactions Strongly Influence Simulated Structural Properties of Disordered Protein States. *J. Phys. Chem. B* **2015**, *119*, 5113–5123. [CrossRef]
78. Frishman, D.; Argos, P. Knowledge-based protein secondary structure assignment. *Proteins Struct. Funct. Genet.* **1995**, *23*, 566–579. [CrossRef]
79. Humphrey, W.; Dalke, A.; Schulten, K. VMD: Visual molecular dynamics. *J. Mol. Graph.* **1996**, *14*, 33–38. [CrossRef]
80. Levy, Y.; Onuchic, J.N.; Wolynes, P.G. Fly-Casting in Protein—DNA Binding: Frustration between Protein Folding and Electrostatics Facilitates Target Recognition. *J. Am. Chem. Soc.* **2007**, *129*, 738–739. [CrossRef]
81. Trizac, E.; Levy, Y.; Wolynes, P.G. Capillarity theory for the fly-casting mechanism. *Proc. Natl. Acad. Sci. USA* **2010**, *107*, 2746–2750. [CrossRef]
82. Kratiras, Z.; Konstantinidis, C.; Skriapas, K. A review of continuous vs intermittent androgen deprivation therapy: Redefining the gold standard in the treatment of advanced prostate cancer. Myths, facts and new data on a perpetual dispute. *Int. Braz J. Urol.* **2014**, *40*, 3–15. [CrossRef]
83. Schweizer, M.T.; Antonarakis, E.S.; Wang, H.; Ajiboye, A.S.; Spitz, A.; Cao, H.; Luo, J.; Haffner, M.C.; Yegnasubramanian, S.; Carducci, M.A.; et al. Effect of bipolar androgen therapy for asymptomatic men with castration-resistant prostate cancer: Results from a pilot clinical study. *Sci. Transl. Med.* **2015**, *7*, 269ra2. [CrossRef] [PubMed]
84. Goldbeter, A. Dissipative structures in biological systems: bistability, oscillations, spatial patterns and waves. *Philos. Trans. R. Soc. A* **2018**, *376*, 20170376. [CrossRef] [PubMed]
85. Jia, D.; Jolly, M.K.; Kulkarni, P.; Levine, H. Phenotypic Plasticity and Cell Fate Decisions in Cancer: Insights from Dynamical Systems Theory. *Cancers* **2017**, *9*, 70. [CrossRef] [PubMed]
86. Buchan, N.C.; Goldenberg, S.L. Intermittent androgen suppression for prostate cancer. *Nat. Rev. Urol.* **2010**, *7*, 552–560. [CrossRef] [PubMed]
87. Whitford, P.C.; Miyashita, O.; Levy, Y.; Onuchic, J.N. Conformational transitions of adenylate kinase: Switching by cracking. *J. Mol. Biol.* **2007**, *366*, 1661–1671. [CrossRef] [PubMed]
88. Whitford, P.C.; Gosavi, S.; Onuchic, J.N. Conformational Transitions in Adenylate Kinase: ALLOSTERIC COMMUNICATION REDUCES MISLIGATION. *J. Biol. Chem.* **2008**, *283*, 2042–2048. [CrossRef] [PubMed]
89. Noel, J.K.; Schug, A.; Verma, A.; Wenzel, W.; Garcia, A.E.; Onuchic, J.N. Mirror Images as Naturally Competing Conformations in Protein Folding. *J. Phys. Chem. B* **2012**, *116*, 6880–6888. [CrossRef]
90. Schug, A.; Whitford, P.C.; Levy, Y.; Onuchic, J.N. Mutations as trapdoors to two competing native conformations of the Rop-dimer. *Proc. Natl. Acad. Sci. USA* **2007**, *104*, 17674–17679. [CrossRef]

91. Lin, X.; Eddy, N.R.; Noel, J.K.; Whitford, P.C.; Wang, Q.; Ma, J.; Onuchic, J.N. Order and disorder control the functional rearrangement of influenza hemagglutinin. *Proc. Natl. Acad. Sci. USA* **2014**, *111*, 12049–12054. [CrossRef]
92. Miyashita, O.; Onuchic, J.N.; Wolynes, P.G. Nonlinear elasticity, proteinquakes, and the energy landscapes of functional transitions in proteins. *Proc. Natl. Acad. Sci. USA* **2003**, *100*, 12570–12575. [CrossRef] [PubMed]
93. Sasai, M.; Wolynes, P.G. Stochastic gene expression as a many-body problem. *Proc. Natl. Acad. Sci. USA* **2003**, *100*, 2374–2379. [CrossRef]
94. Raj, A.; van Oudenaarden, A. Nature, Nurture, or Chance: Stochastic Gene Expression and Its Consequences. *Cell* **2008**, *135*, 216–226. [CrossRef]
95. Jia, D.; Jolly, M.K.; Tripathi, S.C.; Den Hollander, P.; Huang, B.; Lu, M.; Celiktas, M.; Ramirez-Peña, E.; Ben-Jacob, E.; Onuchic, J.N.; et al. Distinguishing mechanisms underlying EMT tristability. *Cancer Converg.* **2017**, *1*. [CrossRef]
96. Mahmoudabadi, G.; Rajagopalan, K.; Getzenberg, R.H.; Hannenhalli, S.; Rangarajan, G.; Kulkarni, P. Intrinsically disordered proteins and conformational noise: Implications in cancer. *Cell Cycle* **2013**, *12*, 26–31. [CrossRef] [PubMed]
97. Jolly, M.K.; Kulkarni, P.; Weninger, K.; Orban, J.; Levine, H. Phenotypic Plasticity, Bet-Hedging, and Androgen Independence in Prostate Cancer: Role of Non-Genetic Heterogeneity. *Front. Oncol.* **2018**, *8*. [CrossRef] [PubMed]
98. Kumar, D.; Sharma, N.; Giri, R. Therapeutic Interventions of Cancers Using Intrinsically Disordered Proteins as Drug Targets: c-Myc as Model System. *Cancer Informat.* **2017**, *16*, 1176935117699408. [CrossRef]
99. Mooney, S.M.; Jolly, M.K.; Levine, H.; Kulkarni, P. Phenotypic plasticity in prostate cancer: role of intrinsically disordered proteins. *Asian J. Androl.* **2016**, *18*, 704–710. [CrossRef] [PubMed]

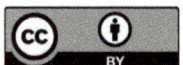

© 2019 by the authors. Licensee MDPI, Basel, Switzerland. This article is an open access article distributed under the terms and conditions of the Creative Commons Attribution (CC BY) license (http://creativecommons.org/licenses/by/4.0/).

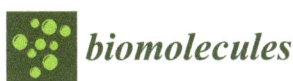

Review

Extreme Fuzziness: Direct Interactions between Two IDPs

Wenning Wang * and Dongdong Wang

Department of Chemistry, Institute of Biomedical Sciences and Multiscale Research Institute of Complex Systems, Fudan University, Shanghai 200438, China; 14110220035@fudan.edu.cn
* Correspondence: wnwang@fudan.edu.cn; Tel.: +86-21-31243985

Received: 15 December 2018; Accepted: 18 February 2019; Published: 26 February 2019

Abstract: Protein interactions involving intrinsically disordered proteins (IDPs) greatly extend the range of binding mechanisms available to proteins. In interactions employing coupled folding and binding, IDPs undergo disorder-to-order transitions to form a complex with a well-defined structure. In many other cases, IDPs retain structural plasticity in the final complexes, which have been defined as the fuzzy complexes. While a large number of fuzzy complexes have been characterized with variety of fuzzy patterns, many of the interactions are between an IDP and a structured protein. Thus, whether two IDPs can interact directly to form a fuzzy complex without disorder-to-order transition remains an open question. Recently, two studies of interactions between IDPs (4.1G-CTD/NuMA and H1/ProTα) have found a definite answer to this question. Detailed characterizations combined with nuclear magnetic resonance (NMR), single-molecule Förster resonance energy transfer (smFRET) and molecular dynamics (MD) simulation demonstrate that direct interactions between these two pairs of IDPs do form fuzzy complexes while retaining the conformational dynamics of the isolated proteins, which we name as the extremely fuzzy complexes. Extreme fuzziness completes the full spectrum of protein-protein interaction modes, suggesting that a more generalized model beyond existing binding mechanisms is required. Previous models of protein interaction could be applicable to some aspects of the extremely fuzzy interactions, but in more general sense, the distinction between native and nonnative contacts, which was used to understand protein folding and binding, becomes obscure. Exploring the phenomenon of extreme fuzziness may shed new light on molecular recognition and drug design.

Keywords: intrinsic disordered protein; extremely fuzzy complex; protein interaction; binding mechanism

---

1. Introduction

A stable three-dimensional structure of a protein is the key to understanding protein function in the conventional structure-function paradigm [1]. On the other hand, it has long been recognized that proteins are 'soft matter' whose conformational fluctuation has functional significance [2]. Generally speaking, proteins are dynamic across a wide range of time scales and amplitudes, from pico-second bond vibrations to second-minute folding process. For a well-structured protein, the conformational dynamics extensively studied include fast motion of side chains, flexibility of local segments (such as loops) or collective motions sampling the conformational space around the stable (native) structure [3]. By incorporating conformational dynamics, the 'structure-function' paradigm expands to a 'structure-dynamics-function' one [3–5]. Since two decades ago, this framework has been challenged by the recognition of the considerable amount and intriguing characteristics of proteins without well-folded structures, i.e., intrinsically disordered proteins (IDPs) [6–11].

Intrinsically disordered proteins do not have a unique stable structure, or a unique folding funnel on the free energy landscape [12]. Intrinsically disordered proteins or intrinsically disordered domains/regions (IDRs) are abundant in all organisms, especially in eukaryotic proteomes.

In the human genome, around 40% of protein-coding genes contain disordered regions of >30 amino acids in length [13–15]. Nevertheless, IDPs have been 'dark matter' in structural biology for a long time because they are difficult to characterize with traditional tools of biophysics. Today, increasing evidence has revealed that IDPs are implicated in various important biological functions, including signal transduction, regulation, gene transcription and replication. Probably due to the structural disorder, the predominant function of IDPs is protein-protein interaction although enzyme activity of IDP was discovered recently [16].

Understanding protein-protein interaction involving IDPs is a central theme for experimental and theoretical studies of IDPs [17]. Our knowledge about it has gone through several stages [18]. The early established prototype of IDP-mediated interaction is the so-called folding upon binding, or coupled folding and binding, in which the IDP folds into well-defined structure upon complex formation [19]. On the other hand, structural heterogeneity and flexibility have been found in many protein complexes involving IDPs. In one scenario referred to as polymorphism, the disordered protein/peptide folds into stable structure but forms alternative conformations in the final complex [20]. In other cases, however, part of the IDP retains structural flexibility, experiencing rapid conformational exchange [21–23]. In yet another situation, several binding sites on the IDP compete to bind a single site on the receptor, and the binding could be described as rapid switching among the interactions of the receptor with alternative sites on the IDP [24]. To describe all these binding modes other than the traditional interactions between structured proteins, Tompa and Fuxreiter proposed the notion of fuzziness and fuzzy complex [25]. Initially, the term 'fuzzy complex' was used to refer to all kinds of protein complexes involving structural heterogeneity and flexibility, which encompasses a broad spectrum of protein interactions mediated by IDPs [25]. Fuzziness also occurs in intramolecular interactions, functioning as a signal sensor [26]. Recently, Olsen et al., proposed that fuzziness should have a more strict definition, and they define it as 'two or more ligand binding sites on the receptor being able to bind to two or more receptor binding sites on the ligand' [27]. In other words, multivalency plays a central role in fuzzy interactions [28]. According to this definition, the binding interface remains highly dynamic in the complex, and the examples mentioned above do not belong to fuzzy complexes. For example, two complexes can be categorized to such strictly defined fuzzy complexes, which are complex between nucleoporins and nuclear transporter receptors [29,30], and complex between clathrin heavy chain and assembly protein 180 kDa (AP180) [31–33]. It is noticeable that almost all these IDP mediated protein interactions involve one well-structured protein. Early studies of the dimerization of the intracellular region of the T cell receptor subunit ζ had provided indications of fuzzy complex formation between IDPs [34,35], but it was questioned by later experimental evidence [36]. Therefore, whether two IDPs can interact directly to form a fuzzy complex while retaining structural plasticity remains an open question [37]. Recently, this question has been answered by two studies [38,39] with detailed characterizations of the interactions between two pairs of IDPs that form dynamic fuzzy complexes. In both cases, the structural disorder and conformational dynamics of the two interacting IDPs are preserved in the complexes. To distinguish this type of fuzzy complexes from those discovered before, we call them the extremely fuzzy complexes.

2. Interaction between 4.1G-CTD and NuMA

The first clearly characterized extremely fuzzy complex is 4.1G-CTD/NuMA [38]. Protein 4.1 is a ubiquitously expressed adaptor protein, which serves as a hub organizing signaling complexes involving many membrane proteins [40]. All members in protein 4.1 family (4.1R, 4.1G, 4.1N, and 4.1B) have two common functional domains: a four.one–ezrin–radixin–moesin (FERM) domain and a C-terminal domain (CTD) (Figure 1a) [40]. It was recently discovered that the interaction of 4.1G/4.1R-CTD with the nuclear mitotic apparatus (NuMA) protein plays a key role in NuMA localization during symmetric [41] and asymmetric [42] cell divisions. The C-terminal region of NuMA that interacts with 4.1G is a 26-amino acid disordered fragment (Figure 1a), while NMR shows that 4.1G-CTD is also intrinsically disordered (Figure 2a in [38]). Interestingly, the specific interaction between the two proteins does not induce structure formation in the complex. Titration of NuMA induces resonance line broadening on the heteronuclear single quantum coherence (HSQC) spectrum of 4.1G-CTD, but the chemical shift dispersion remained limited without obvious chemical shift changes (Figure S5 in [38]). Single-molecule Förster resonance energy transfer (smFRET) measurements also show that 4.1G-CTD exhibits similar stochastic conformational fluctuations in the free form and in the complex (Figure 5 in [38]). Atomic molecular dynamics (MD) simulations provide great details of the interaction between the two proteins. In contrast to the fuzzy binding between an IDP and a structured protein, the interaction between 4.1G-CTD and NuMA encompasses many contact spots on both 4.1G and NuMA without a fixed binding interface. Nevertheless, the binding sites could be clearly identified according to the statistics of the contact frequency from the MD simulation trajectories (Figure 3b in [38]). Several contact 'hot spots' on 4.1G-CTD and NuMA have been verified by point mutagenesis experiments (Figure 3c in [38]). Therefore, the binding could be described as dynamic and stochastic interactions between multiple sites on both proteins, conforming to the strict definition of fuzziness [27]. Moreover, the binding modulates the structures of both 4.1G-CTD and NuMA. Both smFRET measurement and MD simulation show that the conformational ensemble of 4.1G-CTD was changed by NuMA binding. 4.1G-CTD is basically a molten globule and conformations with similar topological fold have been identified in the free form 4.1G-CTD and complex ensembles (Figures 2d and 3a in [38]). However, the interaction obviously induced local structural changes in both 4.1G-CTD and NuMA, which was reflected in the changes of the secondary structural contents of both proteins in MD simulations. 4.1G-CTD and NuMA experience mutual structural adaptations upon binding. Unlike the case of coupled folding and binding, this adaptation does not lead to a unique and stable structure of complex, but a new conformational ensemble of complex (Figure 3a in [38]).

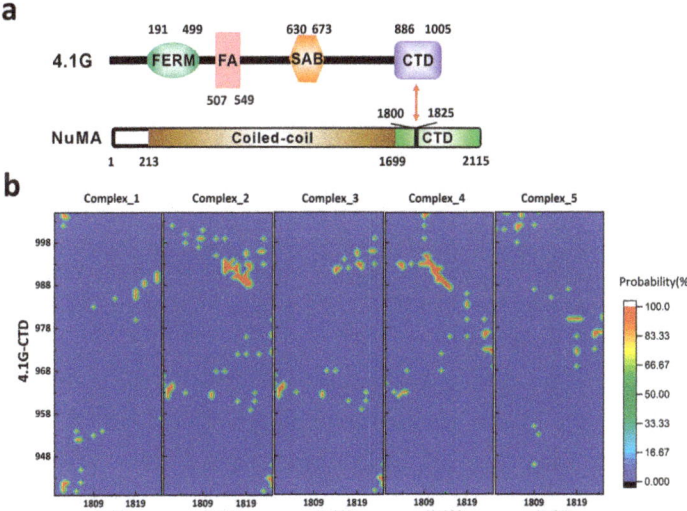

Figure 1. (a) The domain organization of 4.1G and nuclear mitotic apparatus (NuMA). (b) The contact maps between 4.1G-C-terminal domain (CTD) and NuMA in the top five clusters of 4.1G-CTD/NuMA structure ensemble based on replica exchange molecular dynamics (REMD) simulations in [38]. FERM: four.one–ezrin–radixin–moesin domain; FA: FERM adjacent domain; SAB: spectrin–actin binding domain.

3. Interaction between ProTα and H1

Another clearly characterized extremely fuzzy complex is H1 chaperone/prothymosin-α (H1/ProTα) [39]. Human linker histone H1 is positively charged and largely unstructured.

H1 chaperone/prothymosin-α is a completely unstructured protein with high content of negative charges. It has been shown that the two proteins will form a highly dynamic fuzzy complex with extremely high binding affinity (Figure 2c in [39]), although a more recent study gave a much lower binding affinity (Figure 1 in [43]). Nuclear magnetic resonance and circular dichroism (CD) experiments demonstrate that the interaction does not induce any structure formation, neither locally nor globally (Figure 1 in [39]). Single-molecule FRET combined with fluorescence correlation spectroscopy measurements have shown that the long-range distance dynamics in isolated ProTα and H1 are retained in the complex. Interestingly, the different time-scales of the dynamics (chain reconfiguration measured by fluorescence correlation spectroscopy (FCS) in isolated proteins are similar in the complex, indicating the coupling of the dynamics upon binding. Using restraints derived from the experiments and a coarse-grained force field, a structural ensemble of the H1/ProTα complex was constructed through simulation. The intra and intermolecular distance maps indicate that the interactions between ProTα and H1 are broadly distributed along their sequences. In other words, the binding interface is so large that there is barely any specific binding site on both proteins. This is different from the case of 4.1G/NuMA, where frequent contact sites on both proteins could be identified and verified by mutagenesis experiments [38]. Another feature of H1/ProTα complex that differs from 4.1G/NuMA is that the structure ensemble does not show distinct conformational clusters. This is typical for IDPs with highly disordered conformations that resemble statistical coils [13]. The charge/hydropathy (C/H) ratios [44] of ProTα and H1 indicate that the two proteins are IDPs more coil-like (or intrinsic coils [6]) in the two dimensional charge/hydropathy space (Figure 2). The C/H ratio of NuMA is very similar with that of H1, while the C/H ratio of 4.1G-CTD indicates that 4.1G-CTD is more like an intrinsic premolten globule [6] (Figure 2). In line with this conclusion, the structure ensemble of 4.1G-CTD/NuMA exhibits distinct conformational clusters and discrete binding sites [38]. Due to the high content of charged residues, the electrostatic interactions play a major part in the H1/ProTα complex formation. For 4.1G-CTD and NuMA, the calculated binding energy components using the molecular mechanics Poisson-Boltzmann surface area method (MM-PBSA) (Table 1) show that the energy of electrostatic interactions (ΔE_{ele}) and the electrostatic contribution to the solvation free energy (ΔG_{polar}) are both large in magnitude. On the other hand, the magnitudes of van der Waals interaction (ΔE_{vdW}) and nonelectrostatic contributions to solvation free energy ($\Delta G_{nonpolar}$) are relatively moderate. The summation of ΔE_{ele} and ΔG_{polar} is positive, i.e., unfavorable for binding, while the nonelectrostatic contributions are all negative. This rough estimation suggests that the binding of 4.1G-CTD to NuMA is not mainly driven by electrostatic interactions and nonpolar interactions have important contribute. This is consistent with the mutagenesis experiments in [38], where mutations of both charged and hydrophobic residues impaired the binding.

Table 1. Binding energy components of 4.1G-CTD/NuMA obtained from the molecular mechanics Poisson-Boltzmann surface area method (MM-PBSA) calculation using the g_mmpbsa [45] in GROMACS.

	Binding Energy Components (kJ/mol)
ΔE_{vdW}	-206.2 ± 2.2
ΔE_{ele}	-1496.4 ± 8.9
ΔG_{polar}	1653.3 ± 11.9
$\Delta G_{nonpolar}$	-36.9 ± 0.2
ΔG_{bind}	-86.0 ± 4.7

So far, 4.1G-CTD/NuMA and H1/ProTα are the only two clearly characterized extremely fuzzy complexes at high resolution, i.e., residue specific and/or atomic level information have been obtained. However, new evidence of extremely fuzzy complexes between two or more IDPs is emerging. For example, evidence for formation of extremely fuzzy complex between human α, β and γ synuclein have been recently reported [46,47].

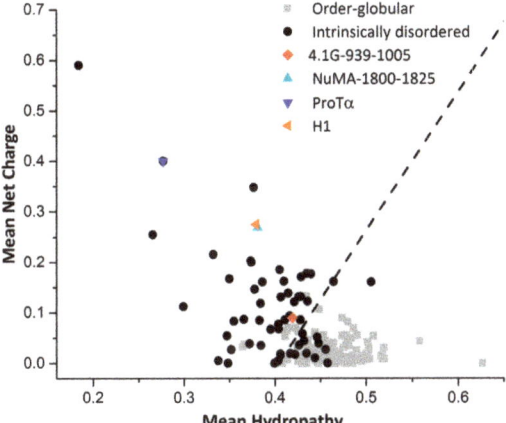

Figure 2. Charge hydropathy ratio for proteins. The dotted line represents an empirically determined charge/hydropathy relationship that distinguishes most ordered globular and intrinsically disordered proteins. The ratio was calculated using the Predictor of Natural Disordered Regions (PONDR) and the data of ordered proteins and disordered proteins were taken from PONDR website [48].

4. How Unique are Extremely Fuzzy Complexes?

The thermodynamics and kinetics of protein-protein association are far more complicated than those of small molecules [49–51]. The possible sources of the complication include the relatively weak interaction between proteins, the hydrophobic effect of water, the structural plasticity of polypeptides and the interplays among these [52]. For IDPs, these features are more prominent than structured proteins [37]. The understanding of IDP interactions is built up based on the studies of structured proteins [53–55]. Although the underlying physical principles may not be fundamentally different, the detailed mechanistic picture of IDP interaction is definitely more complicated [27,53]. So far, we do not have a clear picture of the recognition mechanism between two IDPs that form an extremely fuzzy complex [27], which may represent the complicated situation in IDP-mediated interactions. In the unbound state, both binding partners have broad conformational distributions. On each IDP, there exist multiple binding sites that could interact with multiple sites on the opposite IDP. At any given time, the two IDPs may interact through one site (monovalent), or through multiple sites simultaneously (multivalent), and the sites on two IDPs may not pair with each other in a unique way. Therefore, the number of the possible combinations of the two sets of binding sites can be quite considerable, corresponding to many different binding interfaces and an ensemble of complexes. This scenario has been pictured in the structure ensemble of 4.1G-CTD/NuMA complex derived from all-atom MD simulations [38]. Both 4.1G-CTD and NuMA have different conformations in various clusters of complexes, where variable binding modes and binding interfaces are adopted. To show this, we calculated the individual contact maps of each representative structure of the top five clusters in the ensemble of 4.1G-CTD/NuMA complex. As presented in Figure 1b, the binding patterns are all different in these five structures, including multiple binding sites and not limited to a single way. In coupled folding and binding model, there is a clear distinction between native and nonnative interactions, which are defined respectively as the interactions included and not included in the final folded complex structure. Deciphering their roles during protein recognition is crucial for understanding the binding mechanism [37]. In the case of extremely fuzzy interaction, however, the distinction between native and nonnative interactions could be obscure. The native interactions can be defined as those highly populated in the structure ensemble of the extremely fuzzy complex. However, compared with the coupled folding and binding cases, the identification of native and nonnative interactions in extremely fuzzy complexes is technically demanding. Generally, it is difficult to obtain an accurate structure ensemble of the fuzzy complex. In the case of 4.1G-CTD/NuMA, the residue pairs that show high contact probabilities (Figure 1b in this paper and Figure 3b in [38]) could be defined as native interactions, while those with negligible probabilities are nonnative. However, when inter-residue contact probabilities distribute more evenly along the sequence of the two proteins, the distinction between native and nonnative interactions is less obvious. For example, in the complex of H1/ProTα, the two IDPs seem to have a greatly extended binding interface, and the structure model derived from simulation demonstrates that almost all amino acids in the two proteins are in close contact with their binding partners and the binding is promiscuous at the same time (Figure 4b,c in [39]). In line with this picture, the association rate constant k_{on} of H1/Pro-Tα interaction is at the diffusion limit ($3.1 \pm 0.1 \times 10^9$ M^{-1} s^{-1}), suggesting that the binding process is basically barrierless. It is anticipated that for extremely fuzzy complexes similar to H1/Pro-Tα, i.e., with extended conformations and very broad binding interface, the association is basically diffusion limited.

Although the binding mechanism of extremely fuzzy complex lacks a simple picture, some established explanations for other types of IDP-mediated interactions with different degrees of fuzziness could be applicable in certain aspect. In coupled folding and binding model, it has been proposed that structure element similar to those in complex are preformed in unbound IDPs [56] and the binding process follows conformational selection mechanism. In extremely fuzzy interactions, both free form proteins and complex have broad conformational distributions. Therefore, many structures or structure elements in extremely fuzzy complex are already present in the unbound structure ensemble. The binding process could be roughly described by population shift of the structure ensemble. As in the case of 4.1G-CTD/NuMA complex, some secondary structures in isolated 4.1G-CTD are retained in the complex, and the tertiary folds of free form 4.1G-CTD does not dramatically differ from those in complex (Figures 2d and 3a in [38]). NuMA binding modulates the conformational ensemble of 4.1G-CTD as observed in the smFRET measurement and MD simulation [38]. On the other hand, the two IDPs also experience mutual modulation of their structures during the binding process. Therefore, an induced-fit mechanism is always present in the IDP-IDP interaction.

From the perspective of energy landscape [4], the binding landscape and the landscape of the final complex are all highly frustrated. Frustration is a well-defined concept in physics, and Frauenfelder et al. introduced it to protein folding theory more than two decades ago [4]. For IDPs, it means there are many local minima separated by low barriers on the energy landscape. Therefore, no single native state dominates for IDPs. For structured proteins, folding is a process with significant minimization of frustration. In the folding upon binding mechanism of IDPs, there is also a remarkable minimization of frustration. In extremely fuzzy complexes such as 4.1G-CTD/NuMA and H1/ProTα, the free energy landscape remains highly frustrated since the complex structure ensemble remains a broad conformational distribution. In addition, the promiscuous binding modes manifested in the complex structure ensembles of both 4.1G-CTD/NuMA and H1/ProTα imply that the binding landscape is also frustrated. Due to these observations, we may speculate that the overall minimization of frustration upon complex formation in extremely fuzzy interactions is limited. To examine the local effects of fuzzy interactions in terms of frustration, we calculated the frustrations of pair interactions in three 4.1G-CTD/NuMA complex structures (representative structures of the top three clusters derived from replica exchange molecular dynamics (REMD) simulations in [38]) by using the "Frustratometer" web server (http://frustratometer.qb.fcen.uba.ar/) [57] As shown in Figure 3, the highly frustrated interactions (red lines) in free form structures of 4.1G-CTD are retained in the complexes, i.e., NuMA binding does not lead to obvious local frustration reduction. This is consistent with the main feature of extremely fuzzy complex.

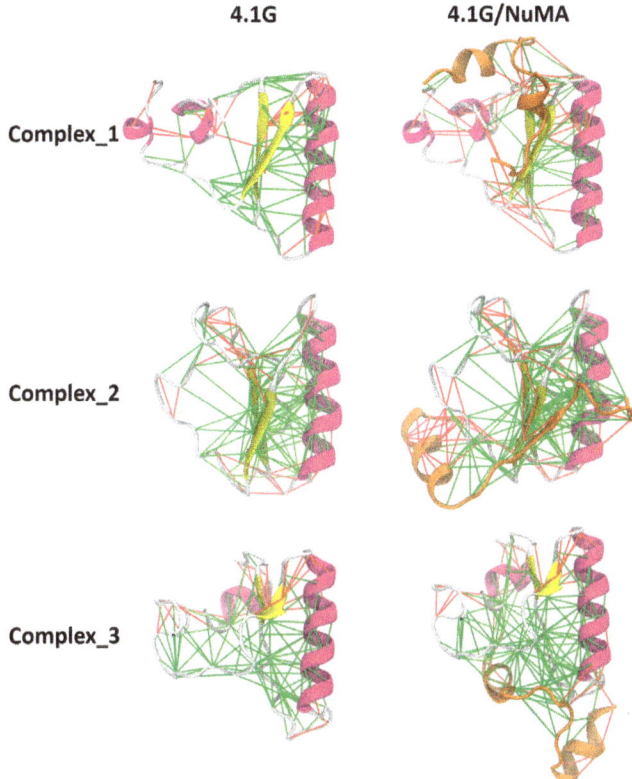

Figure 3. NuMA binding does not reduce the local frustrated interactions in 4.1G-CTD. Frustrations of pair interactions in the top three clusters of 4.1G/NuMA complex are evaluated. The green lines indicate minimally frustrated interactions, while the red lines indicate highly frustrated interactions. Representations in the left column are free form 4.1G-CTD and the ones in the right column are 4.1G/NuMA complex. NuMA peptide is colored orange and 4.1G is colored according to its secondary structure.

As mentioned above, it is difficult to define native and nonnative contacts in the binding of two IDPs. This situation is especially obvious in the case of H1/Pro-Tα. As for the 4.1G-CTD/NuMA complex, it might be possible to identify these two contact types since specific binding sites have been found. Thus, even for the two complexes representing the extremely fuzzy interactions, the detailed binding mechanisms could be different. In general, the task of achieving a holistic understanding of the mechanism for IDP-mediated interactions with various degrees of fuzziness will require the identification and evaluation of relative contributions of native and nonnative contacts, which is beyond conventional conformational selection and induced-fit models [37,58,59]. The extremely fuzzy complexes, however, pose additional challenges to this task, suggesting that the categorization of folded and not folded is no longer the essential concern [58], and the discrimination of native and nonnative contacts should be re-evaluated. Such detailed mechanistic characterization of IDPs is challenging for conventional structure biology techniques, and molecular simulation and theory is valuable complement to experiment [60–63]. On the experimental side, combination of various techniques complementary in time and space resolution is the optimal strategy. On the computational and theoretical side, molecular simulations contribute crucially to the generation of conformational ensembles [58,64]. The reliability of molecular simulation relies on further optimization of force field for disordered proteins and development of enhanced sampling methods [64]. Beyond the equilibrium conformational ensemble, exploring binding mechanism of fuzzy complex using molecular simulation requires unbiased time-evolution trajectories to obtain correct dynamic information, and many enhanced sampling techniques are not applicable. Moreover, based on accumulating data from both experimental and computational studies, development of analytical theory is expected to make testable prediction for experimental investigations of the binding mechanism of fuzzy complexes [27].

The studies of fuzzy complexes in the past two decades have provided hints on our understanding of the extreme fuzziness. The fuzzy complexes database (FuzDB) has collected dozens of fuzzy complexes characterized in detail [65]. The association mechanisms of these fuzzy complexes have been categorized into four classes: (1) conformational selection: the fuzzy regions affect the conformational equilibrium ensemble and promote the formation of secondary structure elements that is compatible for binding; (2) flexibility modulation: the fuzzy regions at the interface participate in the modulation of the binding entropy; (3) tethering: the fuzzy region increases the local concentration of the binding element in the proximity of the partner; (4) competitive binding: intramolecular interactions of the fuzzy region compete with the intermolecular interactions of the binding element [65]. These four categories, obviously, are not mutually exclusive, and many complexes could be categorized into more than one type. Therefore, the concept of fuzziness is more likely a phenomenological description of a wide spectrum of IDP complexes. In practice, the assembly mechanism of fuzzy complexes should be analyzed case by case. Finally, it is worth noting that the functional implication is important for understanding fuzziness in IDP assembly. The organizing principle of IDP fuzzy complexes has been found to manifest its uniqueness through functional roles [18]. For example, the structural heterogeneity and dynamic nature of fuzzy complexes may facilitate interactions with alternative partners simultaneously or consecutively, and posttranslational modification regulated binding etc. Intrinsically disordered proteins and fuzzy interactions are involved in important signaling pathways, and they are also attractive targets for drug design [18,66]. Designing inhibitory small molecules for IDP and dynamic binding requires new strategies, since the target is ensemble rather than a single structure. Conversely, these small molecules could be chemical probes for our understanding of IDP interaction mechanism [66].

5. Conclusions

The two extremely fuzzy complexes reported recently have given a definite answer to the question of whether fuzzy complexes can be formed by two IDPs while retaining structural dynamics. This type of fuzziness represents the dynamic extreme in the spectrum of IDP interactions, suggesting that a more general model beyond all previously proposed mechanisms is required to understand protein interactions. In the perspective of energy landscape, the whole pathway of specific protein binding may occur without marked reduction of frustration, and therefore the reconsideration of 'native' and 'nonnative' contact is necessary. Both mechanistic understanding and functional importance of the extremely fuzzy interactions are exciting aspects in IDP studies.

Funding: This work was supported by National Key Research and Development Program of China (2016YFA0501702), National Science Foundation of China (21773038, 21473034).

Conflicts of Interest: The authors declare no conflict of interest.

References

1. Anfinsen, C.B. Principles that govern the folding of protein chains. *Science* **1973**, *181*, 223–230. [CrossRef] [PubMed]
2. Linderstrøm-Lang, K.U.; Schellman, J.A. Protein Structure and Enzyme Activity. *Enzyme* **1959**, *1*, 443–510.
3. Henzler-Wildman, K.; Kern, D. Dynamic personalities of proteins. *Nature* **2007**, *450*, 964–972. [CrossRef] [PubMed]

4. Frauenfelder, H.; Sligar, S.G.; Wolynes, P.G. The energy landscapes and motions of proteins. *Science* **1991**, *254*, 1598–1603. [CrossRef] [PubMed]
5. Vendruscolo, M.; Dobson, C.M. Structural biology. Dynamic visions of enzymatic reactions. *Science* **2006**, *313*, 1586–1587. [CrossRef] [PubMed]
6. Uversky, V.N. Natively unfolded proteins: A point where biology waits for physics. *Protein Sci.* **2002**, *11*, 739–756. [CrossRef] [PubMed]
7. Tompa, P. Intrinsically unstructured proteins. *Trends Biochem. Sci.* **2002**, *27*, 527–533. [CrossRef]
8. Dyson, H.J.; Wright, P.E. Intrinsically unstructured proteins and their functions. *Nat. Rev. Mol. Cell Biol.* **2005**, *6*, 197–208. [CrossRef] [PubMed]
9. Dunker, A.K.; Garner, E.; Guilliot, S.; Romero, P.; Albrecht, K.; Hart, J.; Obradovic, Z.; Kissinger, C.; Villafranca, J.E. Protein disorder and the evolution of molecular recognition: Theory, predictions and observations. *Pac. Symp. Biocomput.* **1998**, *3*, 473–484.
10. Wright, P.E.; Dyson, H.J. Intrinsically unstructured proteins: re-assessing the protein structure-function paradigm. *J. Mol. Biol.* **1999**, *293*, 321–331. [CrossRef] [PubMed]
11. Dunker, A.K.; Lawson, J.D.; Brown, C.J.; Williams, R.M.; Romero, P.; Oh, J.S.; Oldfield, C.J.; Campen, A.M.; Ratliff, C.M.; Hipps, K.W.; et al. Intrinsically disordered protein. *J. Mol. Graph. Model.* **2001**, *19*, 26–59. [CrossRef]
12. Uversky, V.N.; Dunker, A.K. Understanding protein non-folding. *Biochim. Biophys. Acta Proteins Proteom.* **2010**, *1804*, 1231–1264. [CrossRef] [PubMed]
13. Van der Lee, R.; Buljan, M.; Lang, B.; Weatheritt, R.J.; Daughdrill, G.W.; Dunker, A.K.; Fuxreiter, M.; Gough, J.; Gsponer, J.; Jones, D.T.; et al. Classification of intrinsically disordered regions and proteins. *Chem. Rev.* **2014**, *114*, 6589–6631. [CrossRef] [PubMed]
14. Minezaki, Y.; Homma, K.; Nishikawa, K. Genome-wide survey of transcription factors in prokaryotes reveals many bacteria-specific families not found in archaea. *DNA Res.* **2005**, *12*, 269–280. [CrossRef] [PubMed]
15. Ward, J.J.; Sodhi, J.S.; McGuffin, L.J.; Buxton, B.F.; Jones, D.T. Prediction and functional analysis of native disorder in proteins from the three kingdoms of life. *J. Mol. Biol.* **2004**, *337*, 635–645. [CrossRef] [PubMed]
16. Schulenburg, C.; Hilvert, D. Protein conformational disorder and enzyme catalysis. In *Dynamics in Enzyme Catalysis*; Springer: Berlin/Heidelberg, Germany, 2013; Volume 337, pp. 41–67.
17. Uversky, V.N. Intrinsic disorder-based protein interactions and their modulators. *Curr. Pharm. Des.* **2013**, *19*, 4191–4213. [CrossRef] [PubMed]
18. Fuxreiter, M. Fuzziness in Protein Interactions-A Historical Perspective. *J. Mol. Biol.* **2018**, *430*, 2278–2287. [CrossRef] [PubMed]
19. Wright, P.E.; Dyson, H.J. Linking folding and binding. *Curr. Opin. Struct. Biol.* **2009**, *19*, 31–38. [CrossRef] [PubMed]
20. Graham, T.A.; Ferkey, D.M.; Mao, F.; Kimelman, D.; Xu, W. Tcf4 can specifically recognize beta-catenin using alternative conformations. *Nat. Struct. Biol.* **2001**, *8*, 1048–1052. [CrossRef] [PubMed]
21. Delaforge, E.; Kragelj, J.; Tengo, L.; Palencia, A.; Milles, S.; Bouvignies, G.; Salvi, N.; Blackledge, M.; Jensen, M.R. Deciphering the Dynamic Interaction Profile of an Intrinsically Disordered Protein by NMR Exchange Spectroscopy. *J. Am. Chem. Soc.* **2018**, *140*, 1148–1158. [CrossRef] [PubMed]
22. Bhattacharyya, R.P.; Remenyi, A.; Good, M.C.; Bashor, C.J.; Falick, A.M.; Lim, W.A. The Ste5 scaffold allosterically modulates signaling output of the yeast mating pathway. *Science* **2006**, *311*, 822–826. [CrossRef] [PubMed]
23. Radhakrishnan, I.; Perez-Alvarado, G.C.; Parker, D.; Dyson, H.J.; Montminy, M.R.; Wright, P.E. Solution structure of the KIX domain of CBP bound to the transactivation domain of CREB: A model for activator:coactivator interactions. *Cell* **1997**, *91*, 741–752. [CrossRef]
24. Mittag, T.; Orlicky, S.; Choy, W.Y.; Tang, X.; Lin, H.; Sicheri, F.; Kay, L.E.; Tyers, M.; Forman-Kay, J.D. Dynamic equilibrium engagement of a polyvalent ligand with a single-site receptor. *Proc. Natl. Acad. Sci. USA* **2008**, *105*, 17772–17777. [CrossRef] [PubMed]
25. Tompa, P.; Fuxreiter, M. Fuzzy complexes: polymorphism and structural disorder in protein-protein interactions. *Trends Biochem. Sci.* **2008**, *33*, 2–8. [CrossRef] [PubMed]
26. Arbesu, M.; Iruela, G.; Fuentes, H.; Teixeira, J.M.C.; Pons, M. Intramolecular Fuzzy Interactions Involving Intrinsically Disordered Domains. *Front. Mol. Biosci.* **2018**, *5*, 39. [CrossRef] [PubMed]

27. Olsen, J.G.; Teilum, K.; Kragelund, B.B. Behaviour of intrinsically disordered proteins in protein-protein complexes with an emphasis on fuzziness. *Cell. Mol. Life Sci.* **2017**, *74*, 3175–3183. [CrossRef] [PubMed]
28. Fung, H.Y.J.; Birol, M.; Rhoades, E. IDPs in macromolecular complexes: The roles of multivalent interactions in diverse assemblies. *Curr. Opin. Struct. Biol.* **2018**, *49*, 36–43. [CrossRef] [PubMed]
29. Hough, L.E.; Dutta, K.; Sparks, S.; Temel, D.B.; Kamal, A.; Tetenbaum-Novatt, J.; Rout, M.P.; Cowburn, D. The molecular mechanism of nuclear transport revealed by atomic-scale measurements. *eLife* **2015**, *4*, e10027. [CrossRef] [PubMed]
30. Milles, S.; Mercadante, D.; Aramburu, I.V.; Jensen, M.R.; Banterle, N.; Koehler, C.; Tyagi, S.; Clarke, J.; Shammas, S.L.; Blackledge, M.; et al. Plasticity of an ultrafast interaction between nucleoporins and nuclear transport receptors. *Cell* **2015**, *163*, 734–745. [CrossRef] [PubMed]
31. Muenzner, J.; Traub, L.M.; Kelly, B.T.; Graham, S.C. Cellular and viral peptides bind multiple sites on the N-terminal domain of clathrin. *Traffic* **2017**, *18*, 44–57. [CrossRef] [PubMed]
32. Zhuo, Y.; Cano, K.E.; Wang, L.; Ilangovan, U.; Hinck, A.P.; Sousa, R.; Lafer, E.M. Nuclear Magnetic Resonance Structural Mapping Reveals Promiscuous Interactions between Clathrin-Box Motif Sequences and the N-Terminal Domain of the Clathrin Heavy Chain. *Biochemistry* **2015**, *54*, 2571–2580. [CrossRef] [PubMed]
33. Zhuo, Y.; Ilangovan, U.; Schirf, V.; Demeler, B.; Sousa, R.; Hinck, A.P.; Lafer, E.M. Dynamic interactions between clathrin and locally structured elements in a disordered protein mediate clathrin lattice assembly. *J. Mol. Biol.* **2010**, *404*, 274–290. [CrossRef] [PubMed]
34. Sigalov, A.; Aivazian, D.; Stern, L. Homooligomerization of the cytoplasmic domain of the T cell receptor zeta chain and of other proteins containing the immunoreceptor tyrosine-based activation motif. *Biochemistry* **2004**, *43*, 2049–2061. [CrossRef] [PubMed]
35. Sigalov, A.B.; Zhuravleva, A.V.; Orekhov, V.Y. Binding of intrinsically disordered proteins is not necessarily accompanied by a structural transition to a folded form. *Biochimie* **2007**, *89*, 419–421. [CrossRef] [PubMed]
36. Nourse, A.; Mittag, T. The cytoplasmic domain of the T-cell receptor zeta subunit does not form disordered dimers. *J. Mol. Biol.* **2014**, *426*, 62–70. [CrossRef] [PubMed]
37. Chen, T.; Song, J.; Chan, H.S. Theoretical perspectives on nonnative interactions and intrinsic disorder in protein folding and binding. *Curr. Opin. Struct. Biol.* **2015**, *30*, 32–42. [CrossRef] [PubMed]
38. Wu, S.; Wang, D.; Liu, J.; Feng, Y.; Weng, J.; Li, Y.; Gao, X.; Liu, J.; Wang, W. The Dynamic Multisite Interactions between Two Intrinsically Disordered Proteins. *Angew. Chem. Int. Ed. Engl.* **2017**, *56*, 7515–7519. [CrossRef] [PubMed]
39. Borgia, A.; Borgia, M.B.; Bugge, K.; Kissling, V.M.; Heidarsson, P.O.; Fernandes, C.B.; Sottini, A.; Soranno, A.; Buholzer, K.J.; Nettels, D.; et al. Extreme disorder in an ultrahigh-affinity protein complex. *Nature* **2018**, *555*, 61–66. [CrossRef] [PubMed]
40. Baines, A.J.; Lu, H.C.; Bennett, P.M. The Protein 4.1 family: hub proteins in animals for organizing membrane proteins. *Biochim. Biophys. Acta* **2014**, *1838*, 605–619. [CrossRef] [PubMed]
41. Kiyomitsu, T.; Cheeseman, I.M. Cortical dynein and asymmetric membrane elongation coordinately position the spindle in anaphase. *Cell* **2013**, *154*, 391–402. [CrossRef] [PubMed]
42. Seldin, L.; Poulson, N.D.; Foote, H.P.; Lechler, T. NuMA localization, stability, and function in spindle orientation involve 4.1 and Cdk1 interactions. *Mol. Biol. Cell.* **2013**, *24*, 3651–3662. [CrossRef] [PubMed]
43. Feng, H.; Zhou, B.R.; Bai, Y. Binding Affinity and Function of the Extremely Disordered Protein Complex Containing Human Linker Histone H1.0 and Its Chaperone ProTalpha. *Biochemistry* **2018**. [CrossRef] [PubMed]
44. Uversky, V.N.; Gillespie, J.R.; Fink, A.L. Why are "natively unfolded" proteins unstructured under physiologic conditions? *Proteins* **2000**, *41*, 415–427. [CrossRef]
45. Kumari, R.; Kumar, R.; Open Source Drug Discovery Consortium; Lynn, A. g_mmpbsa—a GROMACS tool for high-throughput MM-PBSA calculations. *J. Chem. Inf. Model.* **2014**, *54*, 1951–1962. [CrossRef] [PubMed]
46. Jain, M.K.; Singh, P.; Roy, S.; Bhat, R. Comparative Analysis of the Conformation, Aggregation, Interaction, and Fibril Morphologies of Human α-, β-, and γ-Synuclein Proteins. *Biochemistry* **2018**, *57*, 3830–3848. [CrossRef] [PubMed]
47. Williams, J.K.; Yang, X.; Baum, J. Interactions between the Intrinsically Disordered Proteins beta-Synuclein and α-Synuclein. *Proteomics* **2018**, *18*, e1800109. [CrossRef] [PubMed]

48. Romero, P.; Obradovic, Z.; Li, X.; Garner, E.C.; Brown, C.J.; Dunker, A.K. Sequence complexity of disordered protein. *Proteins* **2001**, *42*, 38–48. [CrossRef]
49. Hill, T.L. Effect of rotation on the diffusion-controlled rate of ligand-protein association. *Proc. Natl. Acad. Sci. USA* **1975**, *72*, 4918–4922. [CrossRef] [PubMed]
50. Xu, G.; Weber, G. Dynamics and time-averaged chemical potential of proteins: Importance in oligomer association. *Proc. Natl. Acad. Sci. USA* **1982**, *79*, 5268–5271. [CrossRef] [PubMed]
51. Berg, O.G. Time-averaged chemical potential of proteins and the detailed-balance principle (an alternative viewpoint). *Proc. Natl. Acad. Sci. USA* **1983**, *80*, 5302–5303. [CrossRef] [PubMed]
52. Prabhu, N.; Sharp, K. Protein-solvent interactions. *Chem. Rev.* **2006**, *106*, 1616–1623. [CrossRef] [PubMed]
53. Zhou, H.-X.; Bates, P.A. Modeling protein association mechanisms and kinetics. *Curr. Opin. Struct. Biol.* **2013**, *23*, 887–893. [CrossRef] [PubMed]
54. Zhou, H.X.; Pang, X.; Lu, C. Rate constants and mechanisms of intrinsically disordered proteins binding to structured targets. *Phys. Chem. Chem. Phys.* **2012**, *14*, 10466–10476. [CrossRef] [PubMed]
55. Dogan, J.; Gianni, S.; Jemth, P. The binding mechanisms of intrinsically disordered proteins. *Phys. Chem. Chem. Phys.* **2014**, *16*, 6323–6331. [CrossRef] [PubMed]
56. Fuxreiter, M.; Simon, I.; Friedrich, P.; Tompa, P. Preformed structural elements feature in partner recognition by intrinsically unstructured proteins. *J. Mol. Biol.* **2004**, *338*, 1015–1026. [CrossRef] [PubMed]
57. Parra, R.G.; Schafer, N.P.; Radusky, L.G.; Tsai, M.Y.; Guzovsky, A.B.; Wolynes, P.G.; Ferreiro, D.U. Protein Frustratometer 2: A tool to localize energetic frustration in protein molecules, now with electrostatics. *Nucleic Acids Res.* **2016**, *44*, W356–W360. [CrossRef] [PubMed]
58. Fuxreiter, M. Fold or not to fold upon binding-does it really matter? *Curr. Opin. Struct. Biol.* **2018**, *54*, 19–25. [CrossRef] [PubMed]
59. Mollica, L.; Bessa, L.M.; Hanoulle, X.; Jensen, M.R.; Blackledge, M.; Schneider, R. Binding Mechanisms of Intrinsically Disordered Proteins: Theory, Simulation, and Experiment. *Front. Mol. Biosci.* **2016**, *3*, 52. [CrossRef] [PubMed]
60. Best, R.B. Computational and theoretical advances in studies of intrinsically disordered proteins. *Curr. Opin. Struct. Biol.* **2017**, *42*, 147–154. [CrossRef] [PubMed]
61. Levine, Z.A.; Shea, J.E. Simulations of disordered proteins and systems with conformational heterogeneity. *Curr. Opin. Struct. Biol.* **2017**, *43*, 95–103. [CrossRef] [PubMed]
62. Huang, J.; MacKerell, A.D., Jr. Force field development and simulations of intrinsically disordered proteins. *Curr. Opin. Struct. Biol.* **2018**, *48*, 40–48. [CrossRef] [PubMed]
63. Stanley, N.; Esteban-Martin, S.; De Fabritiis, G. Progress in studying intrinsically disordered proteins with atomistic simulations. *Prog. Biophys. Mol. Biol.* **2015**, *119*, 47–52. [CrossRef] [PubMed]
64. Chen, J. Towards the physical basis of how intrinsic disorder mediates protein function. *Arch. Biochem. Biophys.* **2012**, *524*, 123–131. [CrossRef] [PubMed]
65. Miskei, M.; Antal, C.; Fuxreiter, M. FuzDB: Database of fuzzy complexes, a tool to develop stochastic structure-function relationships for protein complexes and higher-order assemblies. *Nucleic Acids Res.* **2017**, *45*, D228–D235. [CrossRef] [PubMed]
66. Ruan, H.; Sun, Q.; Zhang, W.; Liu, Y.; Lai, L. Targeting intrinsically disordered proteins at the edge of chaos. *Drug Discov. Today* **2018**, *24*, 217–227. [CrossRef] [PubMed]

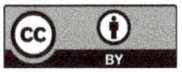

© 2019 by the authors. Licensee MDPI, Basel, Switzerland. This article is an open access article distributed under the terms and conditions of the Creative Commons Attribution (CC BY) license (http://creativecommons.org/licenses/by/4.0/).

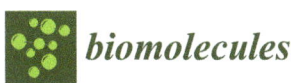

Article

Conserved Glycines Control Disorder and Function in the Cold-Regulated Protein, COR15A

Oluwakemi T. Sowemimo [1], Patrick Knox-Brown [2], Wade Borcherds [1], Tobias Rindfleisch [2], Anja Thalhammer [2,*] and Gary W. Daughdrill [1,*]

[1] Department of Cell Biology, Microbiology, and Molecular Biology, University of South Florida, Tampa, FL 33620, USA; oluwakemi@mail.usf.edu (O.T.S.); wborcher@mail.usf.edu (W.B.)
[2] Department of Physical Biochemistry, University of Potsdam, 14476 Potsdam, Germany; knoxbrown@uni-potsdam.de (P.K.-B.); rindflei@uni-potsdam.de (T.R.)
* Correspondence: thalhamm@uni-potsdam.de (A.T.); gdaughdrill@usf.edu (G.W.D.); Tel.: +49-0331-9775267 (A.T.); +1-813-974-2503 (G.W.D.)

Received: 15 January 2019; Accepted: 25 February 2019; Published: 2 March 2019

Abstract: Cold-regulated (COR) 15A is an intrinsically disordered protein (IDP) from *Arabidopsis thaliana* important for freezing tolerance. During freezing-induced cellular dehydration, COR15A transitions from a disordered to mostly α-helical structure. We tested whether mutations that increase the helicity of COR15A also increase its protective function. Conserved glycine residues were identified and mutated to alanine. Nuclear magnetic resonance (NMR) spectroscopy was used to identify residue-specific changes in helicity for wildtype (WT) COR15A and the mutants. Circular dichroism (CD) spectroscopy was used to monitor the coil–helix transition in response to increasing concentrations of trifluoroethanol (TFE) and ethylene glycol. The impact of the COR15A mutants on the stability of model membranes during a freeze–thaw cycle was investigated by fluorescence spectroscopy. The results of these experiments showed the mutants had a higher content of α-helical structure and the increased α-helicity improved membrane stabilization during freezing. Comparison of the TFE- and ethylene glycol-induced coil–helix transitions support our conclusion that increasing the transient helicity of COR15A in aqueous solution increases its ability to stabilize membranes during freezing. Altogether, our results suggest the conserved glycine residues are important for maintaining the disordered structure of COR15A but are also compatible with the formation of α-helical structure during freezing induced dehydration.

Keywords: COR15A; Late embryogenesis abundant; intrinsically disordered proteins; Trifluoroethanol; Nuclear magnetic resonance

1. Introduction

Intrinsically disordered proteins (IDPs) are proteins that lack a defined three-dimensional structure and exist in various ensembles [1,2]. Intrinsically disordered proteins are found in archaea and bacteria but are most abundant in eukaryotes [3]. The amino acid sequences of IDPs are frequently enriched with repeats of specific amino acid residues or short amino acid motifs, and they rarely form long-range intramolecular interactions [4]. Intrinsically disordered proteins contain a high number of charged and polar amino acid residues, and few hydrophobic residues, which prevents the formation of a hydrophobic core [2,5]. Cold-regulated (COR) 15A is an intrinsically disordered protein from the model plant *Arabidopsis thaliana*, that belongs to the group of late embryogenesis abundant (LEA) proteins. Late embryogenesis abundant proteins accumulate during later stages of seed development and are also found in vegetative tissues of plants [6–8]. Late embryogenesis abundant proteins have been previously categorized based on amino acid sequence similarity [8,9]. We are focusing on the archetypical LEA protein COR15A, which is one of the best characterized LEA proteins to date [7,10,11]. During dehydration, either directly administered by modulation of the relative humidity or modelled by increasing solution osmolarity, the intrinsically disordered COR15A accumulates α-helical structure [10,12]. Homology modelling suggests COR15A forms two α-helices connected by a flexible linker in response to water deprivation, that are reversible upon rehydration [10].

Previous work established that overexpression of COR15A which localizes to the chloroplast stroma, increases the tolerance of plant leaves to freezing temperatures and that silencing COR15A and its close homolog COR15B leads to a decrease in freezing tolerance [13]. Late embryogenesis abundant proteins hypothetically function by stabilizing enzymes and membranes [13,14]. In vitro enzyme activity studies have shown that recombinant COR15A stabilizes isolated lactate dehydrogenase by preventing aggregation but has no effect on enzymes that are not prone to aggregation [14–18]. However, in vivo studies suggest that COR15A is not involved in the stabilization of chloroplast-localized enzymes during freezing, but instead stabilizes the chloroplast and plasma membranes [11,14]. Such a membrane-stabilizing function after a freeze–thaw cycle was also reported in vitro, using recombinant COR15A and large unilamellar vesicles (LUVs) modelling the lipid composition of inner chloroplast membrane [14]. Hypothetically, COR15A stabilizes the chloroplast membrane by preventing the lamellar-to-hexagonal phase II transitions as a result of freeze-induced dehydration and by increasing membrane fluidity [14,19]. Interestingly, COR15A interacts with lipids in a partially folded state [12,14,20]. Although COR15A has been studied extensively, there have been no nuclear magnetic resonance experiments performed to examine the atomic level structure and dynamics of COR15A. In this report, the structure and dynamics of COR15A wildtype (WT) and the two mutants predicted to increase helicity were examined in the presence and absence of trifluoroethanol (TFE), and the impact of these mutants on the stability of model membranes after a freeze–thaw cycle was investigated by fluorescence spectroscopy. We further investigated the helix–coil transition of COR15A WT and the mutants in increasing concentrations of TFE and the osmolyte ethylene glycol (EG). TFE is an alcohol based co-solvent that induces/stabilizes helical structure in peptides [21]. If the amino acid sequence of COR15A evolved to be disordered under hydrating conditions and becomes helical under dehydrating conditions, there should be conserved residues that control this behavior. We demonstrate that the α-helicity of COR15A can be increased as a result of specific amino acid substitutions, and this increased α-helicity positively affected its membrane stabilizing function during freezing.

Sequence alignments of various COR15A homologs and AGADIR predictions were used to determine amino acid residues that were likely to impact the α-helical folding state and capacity of COR15A [22,23]. Heteronuclear single quantum coherence (^{1}H-^{15}N HSQC), HNCACB, HNCO and CBCACONH NMR experiments were used to examine structural differences between COR15A WT and the mutants in the absence and presence of TFE [1,24,25].

2. Materials and Methods

2.1. Sequence Selection and Alignment

A BLAST search was performed using the non-redundant protein sequences(nr) database with mature COR15A excluding the N-terminal chloroplast localization signal. The alignments were carried out with the Geneious software version 10.0.8 (Biomatters Ltd.) [26] using the Geneious aligner algorithm set to use the Blosum62 matrix with gap open penalty of 12 and extension penalty of 3, and 2 refinement iterations [26]. The accession numbers of the protein sequences are NP_181782, AY587559.1, JF718274.1, EF532304.1, EF526218.1, EU285582.1, FJ594771.1. The sequence alignments of various COR15A homologs were used to determine amino acid residues that were likely to impact the α-helical folding state and capacity of COR15A.

2.2. Plasmids and Cell Lines

The codon optimized *cor15a* gene (Invitrogen, Thermofisher Scientific, Carlsbard, CA, USA) was cloned either into a pProEX HTb plasmid or a pET-28a plasmid, which carry a TEV or thrombin cleavage sequence between 6xHIS tag and inserted gene, respectively. Both encode the WT protein sequence. MAAKGDGNILDDLNEATKKASDFVTDKTKEALADGEKAKDYVVEKNSETADTLGKEAE KAAAYVEEKGKEAANKAAEFAEGKAGEAKDATK. Site directed mutagenesis was performed on the wildtype construct without the chloroplast localization signal to obtain the single mutant G68A using the QuikChange Site-Directed Mutagenesis kit (Agilent, Savage, MD, USA). The gene encoding the 4GtoA mutant was synthesized by Invitrogen, Thermofisher Scientific, then sub-cloned into a pET-28a vector and transformed into BL21-DE3 cells from *E. coli* for protein expression. The correct full-length peptide has 140 amino acids of which the signal peptide constitutes the N-terminal 49 amino acids. Thus, the mature COR15A without signal peptide after cleavage of the 6xHIS-tag consists of 91 + 2 amino acids. The latter two are relics from the cleavage sequence between 6xHIS-tag and COR15A sequence.

2.3. Protein Production and Purification

2.3.1. Protein Production and Purification for Nuclear Magnetic Resonance Experiments

Uniformly ^{15}N-labeled and ^{15}N- and ^{13}C-labeled samples of COR15A WT and mutants (residues 1–91) were expressed in BL21-DE3 cells grown in M9 medium. They were incubated at 37 °C for about 3 h, then transferred to a 15 °C incubator for 15 min and induced at an OD_{600} of 0.6 with 1 mM isopropyl β-D-1-thiogalactopyranoside (IPTG) and left to grow for 24 h, after which they were centrifuged at 11,280 g for 5 min at 4 °C and pellets were frozen at −80 °C. The pellets were resuspended in nickel load buffer (50 mM NaH_2PO_4, 300 mM NaCl, 10 mM imidazole, 0.02% sodium azide, pH 8.0) and lysed with a French press pressure cell using a minimum pressure of 20,000 psi. The lysate was centrifuged at 38,720 g for 1 h. The supernatant was loaded onto a column containing Nickel-NTA resin. The column was washed with nickel load buffer then eluted with nickel elution buffer (50 mM NaH_2PO_{4r}, 300 mM NaCl, 250 mM imidazole, 0.02% sodium azide, pH 8.0). Fractions containing the fusion protein were confirmed using sodium dodecyl sulfate polyacrylamide gel electrophoresis (SDS-PAGE) and dialyzed into gel filtration buffer (50 mM NaH_2PO_4, 300 mM NaCl, 1 mM EDTA, 0.02% NaN_3, pH 7.0) using dialysis tubing with a cutoff of 3.5 kDa. The histidine tag was cleaved using Thrombin CleanCleave Kit (Sigma-Aldrich, St. Louis, MO, USA. The samples were then loaded onto a GE HiLoad 16/60 Superdex 75 column. The column was equilibrated, and the protein eluted with gel filtration buffer at a flow rate of 1 ml/min. Protein purity was verified using SDS-PAGE analysis after the size exclusion.

2.3.2. Protein Production and Purification for Fluorescence Spectroscopy and Circular Dichroism Experiments

The gene containing pProEX Htb vectors were expressed in *E. coli* BL21(DE3) growing in LB medium for 8 h at 37 °C. After cell harvest, cells were resuspended in solubilization buffer (20 mM NaH_2PO_4 pH 7.0, 500 mM NaCl), lysed by sonication (Bandelin, SONOPULS) or French press and incubated at 100 °C in a water bath for 10 min. After centrifugation, the supernatant containing heat soluble proteins was purified by affinity chromatography using a Ni^{2+}-NTA Sepharose 6 Fast Flow (GE Healthcare, Little Chalfont, UK). COR15A was eluted from the column with solubilization buffer containing 250 mM imidazole. The N-terminal histidine tag was removed by a custom-made TEV protease, due to a TEV-cleavage site within this vector, during overnight dialysis against 10 mM Tris/HCl, pH 8.0; 150 mM NaCl; 1 mM DTT; 0.1 mM EDTA at 4 °C (MWCO 3.5 kDa, Spectrum labs, Los Angeles, CA, USA). Purification was finalized by a second affinity chromatography and a subsequent size exclusion chromatography using a Sepharose 75 26/60 column attached to an ÄKTA system (GE Healthcare, Little Chalfont, UK). Protein solutions were dialyzed against 10 mM TES, 50 mM NaCl and 0.1 mM EDTA, pH 7.4 at 4 C (MWCO 3.5 kDa, Spectrum labs, Los Angeles, CA, USA) or 10 mM NaH_2PO_4 and concentrated using an Amicon ultrafiltration cell (Merck Millipore, Darmstadt, Germany) with an MWCO of 3.5 kDa. Protein purity was evaluated by SDS-PAGE and dynamic light scattering. Protein identity was checked by Western Blot analysis using an anti-(His)6 epitope-tag antibody (Dianova GmbH, Hamburg, Germany) and was visualized by an alkaline phosphatase reaction by a secondary antibody (Sigma-Aldrich, Taufenkirchen, Germany).

2.4. Nuclear Magnetic Resonance Spectroscopy

The concentration of the WT and mutant proteins used for the NMR experiments were 400–500 µM. Protein concentration was measured using an ND1000 nanodrop. The extinction coefficient of COR15A is 2980 M^{-1} cm^{-1}, so we tend to use the 280 nm absorbance data from more concentrated samples to estimate concentration. The lower detection limit of the Nanodrop U/V spectrophotometer used is 0.03 AU. For the NMR experiments, we usually work in the range of 100 µM and above, which gives an absorbance value of about 0.15AU, which is well above the sensitivity limit of the detector. All the protein samples used are diluted from concentrated protein stock solutions, and this method of measuring concentration is used consistently in all three proteins. The reliability of the COR15A protein concentrations calculated using UV absorbance was confirmed using BCA. The NMR experiments on the samples were carried out at 25 °C on the Varian VNMRS 800 MHz spectrometer equipped with a triple resonance pulse field Z-axis gradient cold probe. To make the amide ^1H and ^{15}N as well as $^{13}C_\alpha$ and $^{13}C_\beta$ resonance assignments, sensitivity enhanced ^1H-^{15}N HSQC and three-dimensional HNCACB and HNCO experiments were performed on the uniformly ^{15}N-labeled and ^{15}N- and ^{13}C-labeled samples of COR15AWT and mutants in 90% H_2O, 10% D_2O, 50 mM NaCl, NaH_2PO_4, 50 mM NaCl, 1 mM EDTA, 0.02% NaN_3, pH 6.8 for the samples without TFE. The samples with TFE were in 70% H_2O, 20%TFE, 10% D_2O, 50 mM NaCl, NaH_2PO_4, 50 mM NaCl, 1 mM EDTA, 0.02% NaN_3, pH 6.8. For the HNCACB and HNCO experiment, data were acquired in ^1H, ^{13}C, and ^{15}N dimensions using 9689.9228 (t_3) X 14075.1787 (t_2) X 1944.3904 (t_1) Hz sweep widths, and 1024 (t_3) X 128 (t_2) X 32 (t_1), respectively. For the HSQC experiments, the sweep width 9689.9228 (t_2) X 1944.3524 (t_1), and the increments were 1024 (t_2) and 128 (t_1). The NMR spectra were undertaken with a NMRFx Processor and analyzed using NMRViewJ (One Moon Scientific, Inc., Westfield, NJ, USA).

The data from the 2D and 3D NMR experiments were analyzed using the neighbor-corrected intrinsically disordered protein (NCIDP) random coil values and the Vendruscolo δ2D software [24,25]. The random coil values were included in the calculation of the alpha carbon secondary chemical shifts, while the δ2D software was used for the calculation of the % helix values [24,25].

2.5. Circular Dichroism Spectroscopy

Circular dichroism (CD) measurements were performed in a Jasco J-815 spectrometer (Jasco, Japan) equipped with a thermostatted, Peltier-controlled cell holder. Four spectra were recorded and averaged using quartz cuvettes with a path length of 1 mm (Hellma, Germany) at protein concentrations of 0.10 g/L in 10 mM NaH_2PO_4 pH 7.4 in the absence of co-solvent and with increasing concentrations of ethylene glycol (EG) or trifluoroethanol (TFE). All spectra were corrected for buffer contributions and converted to mean residue ellipticities [θ_{MRW}] using mean residue weights of 104.1 g/mol, 104.3 g/mol and 104.8 g/mol for COR15A WT, G68A and 4GtoA, respectively. Instrument calibration was done with 1S-(+)-10-camphorsulphonic acid. The ratio of α-helix was estimated using θ_{MRW} at 222 nm [27].

2.6. Carboxy Fluorescein (CF) Leakage Assay

All lipids were purchased from Avanti Polar Lipids (Alabaster, AL, USA) and dissolved in chloroform prior to mixing in the respective ratio to model the lipid composition of inner chloroplast membranes (40% monogalactosyldiacylglycerol; 30% digalactosyldiacylglycerol; 15% sulfoquinovosyldiacylglycerol; 15% egg phosphatidylglycerol) referred to as ICMM [14]. A total of 10 mg lipids was dried in a glass tube under a stream of N_2 at 60 °C and subsequently under vacuum overnight to remove the solvent completely. Dry lipids were rehydrated in 100 mM carboxy fluorescein (CF); 10 mM TES, 50 mM NaCl and 0.1 mM EDTA, pH 7.4 as described previously [28,29]. The mixture was vortexed for 5 s and resuspended multiple times over an interval of 15 min to resolve all the lipids, followed by extrusion through two layers of polycarbonate membranes with 100 nm pore size in a handheld extruder (Avanti Polar Lipids, Alabaster, AL, USA) for the formation of large unilamellar vesicles (LUVs). Liposomes were loaded onto a S75 13/300 size exclusion column connected to the Fast protein liquid chromatography (FPLC) ÄKTA system (GE Healthcare, Freiburg, Germany) to remove free CF. Fractions containing liposomes were detected at 280 nm using the absorption of CF in the ultraviolet (UV) region. The hydrodynamic radius of the liposomes was measured by dynamic light scattering at a scattering angle of 90° with a custom-built apparatus, equipped with a 0.5 W diode-pumped continuous-wave laser (Cobolt Samba 532 nm, Cobolt AB, Solna, Sweden), a high quantum yield avalanche photo diode and an ALV 7002/USB 25 correlator (ALV-GmbH, Langen, Germany) at 23 °C. Hydrodynamic radii of liposomes were calculated from fits of the accumulated autocorrelation functions using the CONTIN algorithm implemented in a custom-made MatLab script (The Math-Works, Natick, MA, USA) [30].

Carboxy Fluorescein containing ICMM LUVs were mixed in equal volumes of respective protein solutions in final molar protein to lipid ratios ranging from 1:50 to 1:200 in polymerase chain reaction (PCR) tubes. Prior to this, protein concentrations were determined by ultraviolet/visible (UV/VIS) spectroscopy using the sequence-specific extinction coefficient at 280 nm of 2560 M^{-1} cm^{-1} valid for all three proteins [31]. Samples were rapidly frozen in an ethylene glycol bath precooled to -20 °C for 2 h [32]. The frozen samples were thawed at 23 °C and transferred to 96 well fluorescent plates. CF leakage was determined with a VIROSKAN FLASH plate reader (Thermo Scientific, Waltham, MA, USA) using an excitation wavelength of 492 nm and an emission wavelength of 517 nm before and after disrupting the liposomes with Triton X-100 (Merck, Darmstadt, Germany). CF leakage from the liposomes was calculated as described previously and normalized to control ICMM LUVs which had not been subjected to a freeze–thaw cycle set as 0% leakage [33]. All proteins were tested for a significance level of $p < 0.001$ compared to ICMM LUVs without protein (w/o) or to COR15A WT, respectively in a one-way analysis of variance (ANOVA).

3. Results and Discussion

3.1. Sequence Alignments of COR15A

To identify COR15A homologs, a BLAST search using the non-redundant sequence database was performed [34]. Seven COR15A homologs were identified. The sequence alignments were then performed using Geneious and the sequence similarity of the homologs is shown in the multiple protein sequence alignment (Figure 1). One feature that stood out in the alignment was the presence of several highly conserved glycine residues. We thought the conserved glycines were interesting because they are not frequently found in α-helices [35].

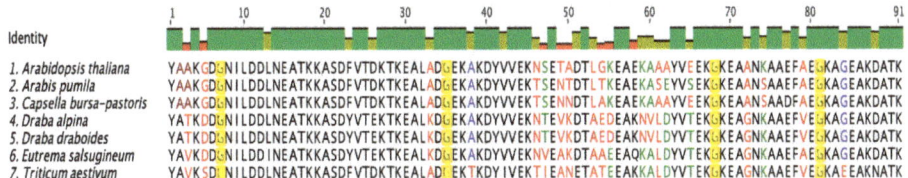

Figure 1. Sequence alignment of cold-regulated (COR) 15A homologs in various plant species. To examine the structure of the *Arabidopsis thaliana* COR15A sequence, alignments were performed using sequences of various species of plants that express this protein. The black letters indicate 100% sequence similarity, the blue letters indicate 80–99%, the green letters indicate 60–79%, and the red letters indicate less than 60% similarity. The residues highlighted in yellow are the glycine residues that are conserved in the examined homologs.

The *Arabidopsis thaliana* COR15A protein sequence has 7 glycine residues distributed at the N- and C- termini. Using sequence alignments, the four glycine residues that are conserved in the COR15A sequence across all seven plant species were identified (Figure 1). Glycine residues as structure breakers are known to be predominant in disordered proteins, thus presenting a first indication that the glycine residues are important in regulating the disordered character of COR15A [3,4]. To assess the potential effect of mutating each glycine residue on the structure of COR15A in *Arabidopsis thaliana*, % helicity predictions were performed using AGADIR [22,23].

3.2. Structural Characterization of COR15A

Using AGADIR, each of the seven glycine residues in the *Arabidopsis thaliana* COR15A WT sequence was substituted with an alanine residue to test how this affected the % helix prediction in the wildtype protein (data not shown) [22,23]. The glycine residues were substituted one at a time, then multiple glycine exchanges were also tested. Based on the sequence alignments and AGADIR predictions, we designed alanine substitutions at position 68 (G68A) and positions 54, 68, 81, and 84 (4GtoA), because they gave the highest predicted increase in helical content compared to WT (Figure 2). Even though glycines at positions 54 and 84 were not very conserved we mutated them because of the predicted increase in helicity. We analyzed a number of other sequences using AGADIR. The % helicity predictions for five of the six of the COR15A homologs were lower than *Arabidopsis thaliana*. We also looked at sequences that were expected to increase the number of salt bridges which are thought to be important for stabilizing the dehydrated structure of COR15A [10]. None of the salt bridge mutants increased % helicity prediction.

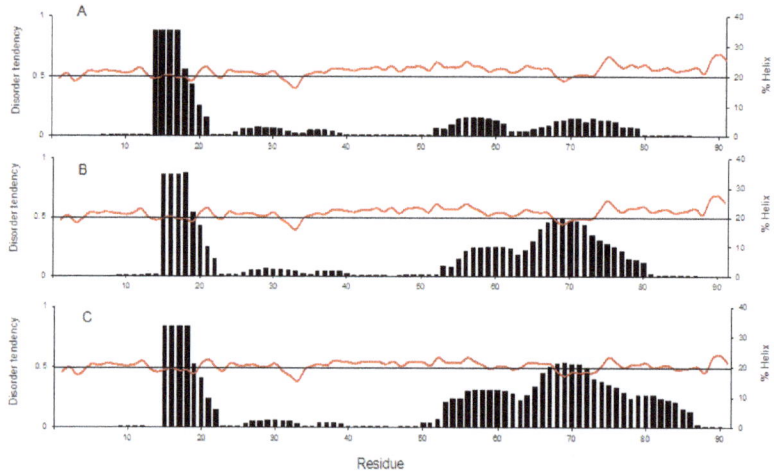

Figure 2. AGADIR % helix and IUPred disorder predictions for individual residues in COR15A wildtype (WT) and mutants. The AGADIR predictions are represented by the black bars, while the IUPred predictions are represented by the red line. (**A**) COR15A WT, (**B**) single mutant G68A, (**C**) quadruple mutant 4GtoA. The primary vertical axis represents disorder tendency as predicted by IUPred, while the secondary vertical axis shows the % helix as predicted by AGADIR. The horizontal axis represents the residue number/position.

AGADIR predicted the presence of two α-helical segments in all three protein sequences, with one segment located in the N-terminal half and the other in the C-terminal half, connected by a linker region (Figure 2A–C). The predicted helicity for the segment closer to the N-terminus is about the same in all three proteins with an average α-helicity of 24% from residues 1–22 (Figure 2A–C). The predicted average α-helicity in the C-terminal segment, residues 53–79, increases from 4% in WT to 11% in the single mutant and 14% in the quadruple mutant. In the IUPred disorder prediction, values above 0.5 predict disorder [36,37]. In Figure 2A–C, the pattern of disorder predicted for the WT and mutant proteins is similar, but there is a reduction in predicted disorder going from the WT (Figure 2A) via G68A (Figure 2B) to 4GtoA (Figure 2C) in the C-terminal half of the sequence. The % α-helix prediction for COR15A WT is in line with the well-known disordered character of the protein in the hydrated state. In Figure 2A–C, it can also be observed that the IUPred disorder prediction for COR15A does not stray far from 0.5, which is an indication that COR15A is on the verge of disorder over the full length of the sequence. Based on our analysis of the AGADIR and IUPred predictions, NMR-labelled recombinant COR15A WT and mutant proteins were expressed and purified [38].

We performed ^{1}H-^{15}N (HSQC) heteronuclear single quantum coherence NMR experiments for COR15A WT and the two mutants in the absence of TFE (Figure 3). The spectra for all three ^{1}H-^{15}N HSQC experiments were overlaid using NMRViewJ in order to compare the chemical shift distribution of each residue in the proton and nitrogen dimensions. The distribution of chemical shifts in the nitrogen dimension is dependent on the specific amino acid. In these spectra, it does not indicate any significant structural changes, but we observe disappearance of resonances in the specific regions where glycines are detected (~108 ppm), and the appearance of resonances in the region of the spectra where alanines are detected (~123 ppm) [3].

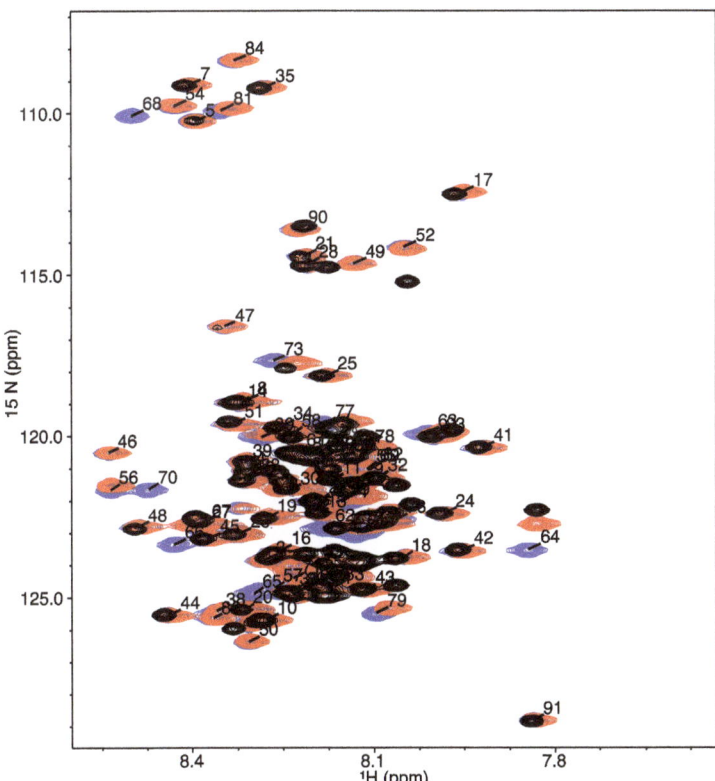

Figure 3. ^{1}H-^{15}N heteronuclear single quantum coherence nuclear magnetic resonance (HSQC NMR) spectra for COR15A WT and mutants in the absence of trifluoroethanol (TFE). The blue peaks depict the WT protein, the red peaks indicate the single mutant G68A and the quadruple 4GtoA mutant is represented by the black peaks. The peaks are labelled with the residue-specific assignments for the WT protein.

We previously reported that COR15A folds into predominantly a α-helical structure in response to dehydration and desiccation, and α-helical structure can be induced by either full desiccation or the addition of 20% TFE [10,12,39]. We also performed ^{1}H-^{15}N HSQC experiments using osmolytes like ethylene glycol and the cosolvent TFE. Analysis of the HSQC spectra of COR15A in 10 M ethylene glycol showed resonance broadening and associated intensity loss (data not shown) due to the effect of increasing viscosity on rotational tumbling of COR15A. In contrast, resonance line shapes and intensities for COR15A in the presence of up to 20% TFE were in a good range for NMR.

The ^{1}H-^{15}N HSQC spectra of COR15A WT and mutants were overlaid using NMRViewJ, to compare the residue-specific chemical shift dispersion in 20% TFE (Figure 4) as was previously done in the absence of TFE (Figure 3). The distribution pattern of the chemical shifts in the ^{15}N and ^{1}H dimension indicates structural changes in the backbone structure of the protein, which was not observed in the absence of TFE. This is most apparent in the G68A mutation in the single and the quadruple mutant, which display the largest peak shifts (Figure 4).

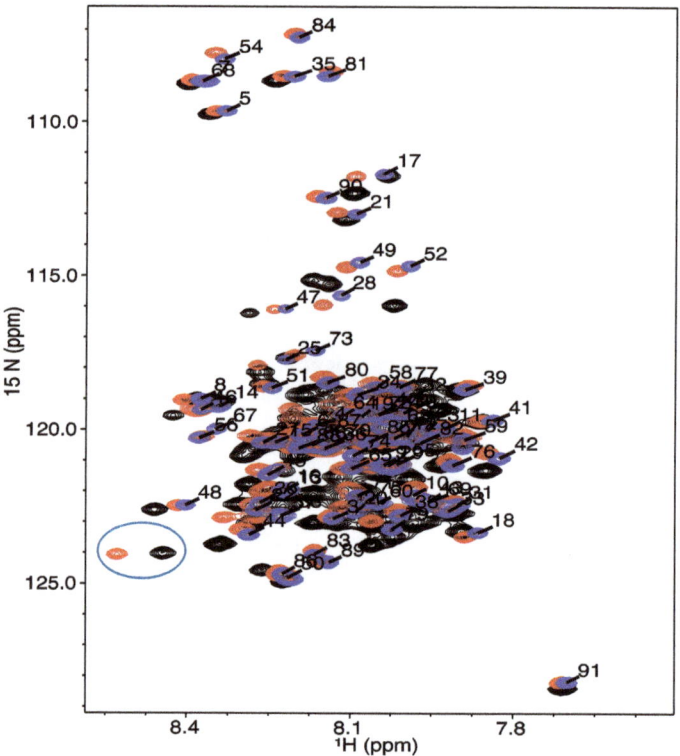

Figure 4. ^{1}H-^{15}N HSQC NMR spectra for COR15A WT and mutants in the presence of 20% TFE. The blue peaks depict the WT protein, the red peaks indicate the single mutant G68A and the quadruple 4GtoA mutant is represented by the black peaks. The peaks are labelled with the residue-specific assignments for the WT protein and the two circled unlabeled peaks at the bottom left represent the G68A residue in the single and quadruple mutant.

To further characterize the structural changes that may be occurring in the WT and mutant proteins, backbone resonance assignments were made using data from ^{1}H-^{15}N HSQC, HNCACB, HNCO and CBCACONH experiments. Using the resonance assignments, the alpha carbon secondary chemical shifts and residue specific % helicity values were calculated and plotted (Figures 5 and 6).

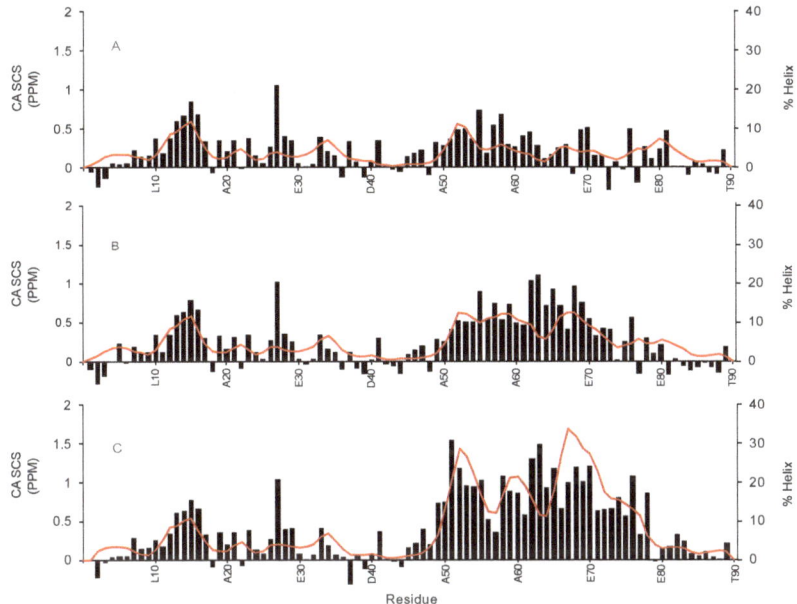

Figure 5. Residue-specific alpha carbon secondary chemical shift and % helix plot for COR15A WT and mutants in 0% TFE. Alpha carbon secondary chemical shifts (black bars) and % helix values (red line) measured using NMR experiments for COR15A WT and mutants in the absence of TFE are shown. The NMR experiments used include ^{1}H-^{15}N HSQC, HNCACB and HNCO. The alpha carbon secondary chemical shifts are on the primary vertical axis and the measured % helix values are on the secondary vertical axis, while the residue number/position for every 10 residues is on the horizontal axis. (**A**): COR15A WT, (**B**): single mutant G68A, which has the glycine at residue 68 mutated to an alanine, (**C**): quadruple mutant 4GtoA, with glycine residues at positions 54, 68, 81 and 84 mutated to alanine residues.

Figure 5 shows the alpha carbon secondary chemical shifts and the % helix values calculated from all the backbone NMR chemical shifts using δ2D, in 0% TFE, for COR15A WT and the G68A and 4GtoA mutants [24]. % helix, as labeled on the y-axis of Figures 5 and 6 is equal to the δ2D values multiplied by 100. The plots (Figure 5) indicate that the first 10 residues from the N- and C- termini of all three proteins have very little α-helical structure. The average α-helical content of the N-terminal α-helix (residues 10–31) is 4.6% in all three proteins, which is about a quarter of the % α-helix value predicted by AGADIR. The C- terminal α-helix, ranging from residues 50–84, increases from 4.6% in WT to 7.9% in G68A to 16.4% in 4GtoA. The two mutants show increased α-helicity, which is restricted to the C-terminal segment (Figure 5A–C). The overall α-helical content in 0% TFE of the WT protein (3.7%) is similar to that calculated using the Chen algorithm (3.5%), but less than that obtained from CDpro (5.5%), using data from previously performed circular dichroism experiments [10,27,40]. Furthermore, the overall average α-helical content of the three proteins as calculated using NMR data are less than the values predicted using AGADIR. The values calculated from the NMR data for WT is 3.7%, the single mutant is 5% and the quadruple mutant is 8.3%, while those calculated from the AGADIR predictions are 4.4% WT, 6.8% G68A and 8% 4GtoA. The α-carbon secondary chemical shifts for the three proteins at the N-terminus are about the same, and it is approximately 0.33 ppm, but at the C-terminus, it increases from 0.3 ppm in WT to 0.5 ppm in G68A to 0.8 ppm in 4GtoA. The increase in the α-carbon secondary chemical shifts in the N-terminal segments of the three proteins indicates an increase in α-helical content from WT to the single and quadruple mutants. The analysis of the secondary chemical shift values for COR15A WT and mutants was also performed for the 20% TFE samples to compare the changes in the α-helical content of the proteins in the hydrated state (Figure 5A–C) and the dehydrated state which is mimicked by the addition of 20% TFE (Figure 6A–C) [21,25].

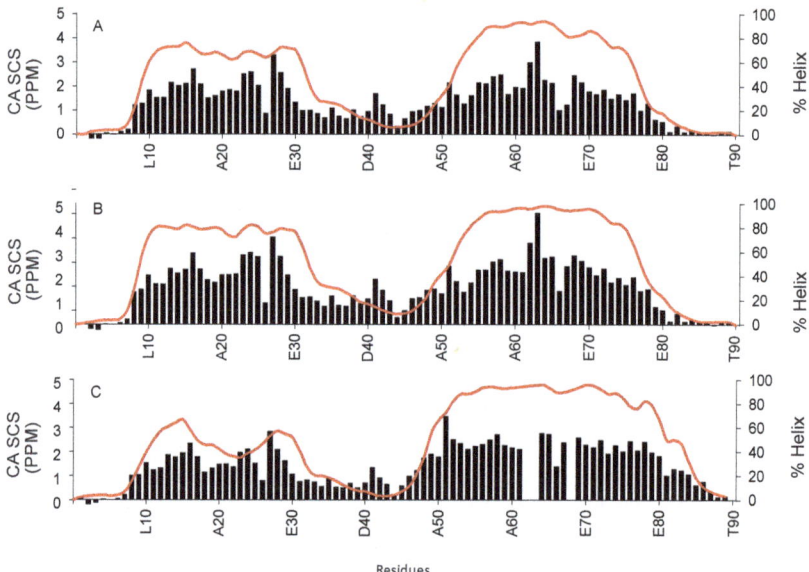

Figure 6. Residue-specific alpha carbon secondary chemical shift and % helix plot for COR15A WT and mutants in the presence of 20% TFE. Alpha carbon secondary chemical shifts (black bars) and % helix values (red line) measured using δ2D data for COR15A WT and mutants in the presence of 20% TFE. The alpha carbon secondary chemical shifts are on the primary vertical axis and the measured % helix values are on the secondary vertical axis, while the residue number/position for every 10 residues is on the horizontal axis. (**A**): COR15A WT, (**B**): single glycine mutant G68A, (**C**): quadruple mutant 4GtoA, with glycine residues at positions 54, 68, 81 and 84 mutated to alanine residues.

In 20% TFE, both α-helical segments in the N- and C-terminal half of COR15A WT and mutants are altered. There is a significant increase in α-helical content compared to the samples without TFE (Figure 5A–C). The middle region is proposed to maintain its disordered nature even in the presence of TFE, thus acting as an unstructured linker and the α-helical population of the residues present is similarly low in all three proteins (Figure 6A–C). The N-terminal α-helical population increases from 67.6% in WT (Figure 6A) to 77.6% in the single mutant (Figure 6B). However, in the quadruple mutant 4GtoA, the α-helical content of the N-terminal segment is decreased to 48.1% (Figure 6C). This decrease in the α-helical population in the N- terminal segment (residues 10–31) is also apparent in the α-carbon secondary chemical shifts, where the average WT value is 1.97 ppm, G68A is 2.19 ppm and 4GtoA is 1.63 ppm, even though there are no mutations in the N-terminal segment. The C-terminal α-helical segment from residues 50–84 has a higher average of α-helical content compared to the N-terminal segment in all three proteins, and the 4GtoA mutant also has the lowest values in the N-terminal segment. Additionally, the C-terminal α-helix is extended towards the C-terminus exclusively in the 4GtoA mutant, which harbors all 4 glycine to alanine mutations in the C-terminal segment (Figure 6C), compared to the single mutant with one mutation in the C-terminal segment and the WT (Figure 6A,B). The C-terminal α-helix, which includes residues 50–84, increases from 65.2% in WT to 72.3% in the single mutant to 82.8% in the quadruple mutant. The overall α-helical content of the WT protein in 20% TFE from the NMR experiments (~47.5%) is similar to that calculated using the Chen algorithm

(49.7%), but less than that obtained from CDpro (56.4%), using data from previously performed circular dichroism experiments [10,27,40]. The α-carbon secondary chemical shifts at the C-terminus, increases from 1.66 ppm in WT to 1.95 ppm in G68A to 2.19 ppm in 4GtoA. The increase in the α-carbon secondary chemical shifts in the C-terminal segments of the three proteins indicates an increase in α-helical content from WT to the single and quadruple mutants.

Since we could not collect high-quality NMR spectra of COR15A in ethylene glycol, we used CD to confirm the levels of helicity induced by TFE were consistent with those induced by ethylene glycol, which is important since we argue that the TFE-induced structure may be similar to what is observed during freezing induced dehydration.

Far-UV CD spectroscopy was used to investigate secondary structure transitions of COR15A WT and mutants in response to increasing concentrations of the co-solvents TFE and ethylene glycol (EG) (Figure 7). Both mutants are more α-helical in buffer and in high concentrations of TFE, in agreement with the NMR data. The osmolyte EG presents a useful model system for the severely reduced water availability in a cellular environment during freezing, which COR15A encounters under physiological conditions. The concentration range of EG used in our analysis corresponds to osmolarities plant cells encounter in physiological freezing temperatures down to about −30 °C [41]. Interestingly, all three proteins show comparable CD spectra in 30% TFE and 12 M EG, indicating that a similar coil–helix transition of COR15A and the mutants can be induced by both co-solvents and thus underlining the relevance of the NMR data acquired in TFE. The coil–helix transitions seem to be mostly complete at 30% TFE for COR15A WT and G68A. We were not able to record CD spectra of 4GtoA in sufficiently high TFE concentrations to reach a stable post-transition stage due to protein aggregation, so we cannot state a similar finding for 4GtoA. It is obvious from the CD spectra and the derived α-helicity that the latter must be slightly overrated, which is most likely due to an underestimation of protein concentration. This is a general problem for IDPs due to the underrepresentation of aromatic amino acids [42]. Thus, the α-helix ratios cannot be directly compared to those derived from NMR analyses. However, as all three proteins present an identical molar extinction coefficient at 280 nm, a direct comparison of the ellipticities and the derived α-helicity among the proteins is valid. Both mutants are noticeably more α-helical than the WT in the absence of co-solvent and throughout the complete co-solvent induced transition. As the transitions in most cases lack well-defined pre- and post-transition baselines, the co-solvent concentration in the transition midpoints cannot be determined exactly but only estimated to be similar for all three proteins. Differences between the mutants are obvious. G68A is more α-helical than 4GtoA over the whole range of TFE concentrations and at EG concentrations above 10 M, thus corroborating and strengthening the NMR data in 20% TFE. Interestingly, the α-helicity of 4GtoA and G68A are similar in the absence of co-solvent. However, upon increasing TFE and EG concentrations, G68A becomes considerably more α-helical than 4GtoA, evidencing a higher overall folding propensity. In contrast, the overall folding propensity of 4GtoA is similar to the WT.

Taken together, the structure of COR15A in 20% TFE closely resembles that obtained from homology modelling in a vacuum, both describing a mainly α-helical molecule, made of two α-helical regions connected by a flexible linker [10]. Interestingly, there are distinct differences between the mutants in 20% TFE, when looking at changes in the α-helicity of the N-terminal segment. In the single G68A mutant, the overall α-helicity of the N-terminal segment is increased. In contrast, the mutation of four C-terminal glycine residues reduces the α-helical content of the N-terminal segment. These findings point towards the apparent presence of long-range interactions between the two α-helices, indicating a mutual stabilization. This is apparently increased by the single GtoA mutation and decreased by the mutation of the four glycine residues. Considering the amphipathic nature of the modeled α-helices, such a mutual stabilization is likely achieved by hydrophobic interaction [10]. In such a scenario, the mutated glycine residues may be crucial for a proper orientation of the hydrophobic α-helical segments towards each other, which would be compromised by the GtoA mutations.

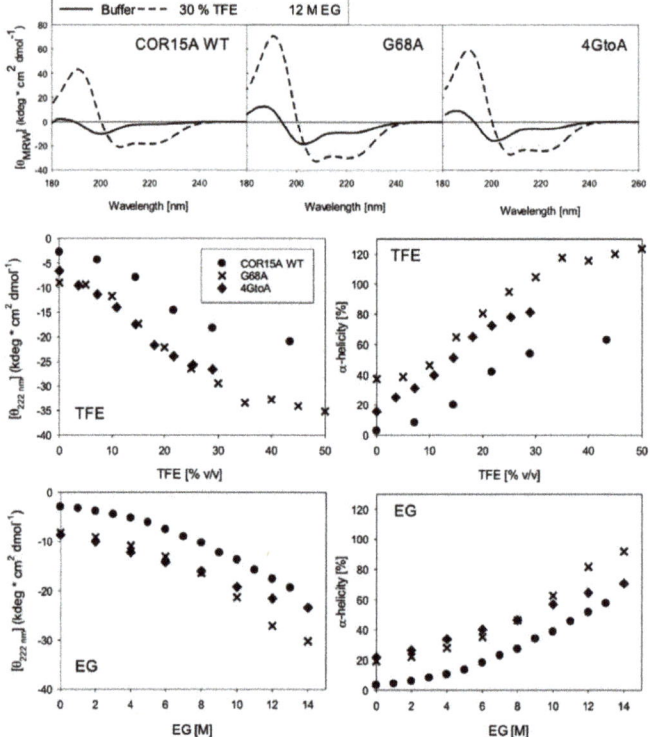

Figure 7. Far-ultraviolet (UV) circular dichroism (CD) spectra in buffer, 20 (v/v) % TFE and 12 M Ethylene Glycol for COR15A WT, G68A and 4GtoA (**A**). The mutants have more α-helical spectra than the WT in buffer alone, and in the presence of high concentrations of both co-solvents. Coil-helix transitions of COR15A WT and both mutants in TFE (**B**) and EG (**C**), specified by θ$_{MRW}$ at 222 nm (left panels) and derived α-helix ratios (right panels).

3.3. Functional Characterization of COR15A

Previous research has indicated that the interaction of COR15A with galactolipids of inner chloroplast membranes may be the mechanism by which COR15A increases *Arabidopsis* freezing tolerance [19]. To test the effectiveness of the COR15A mutants compared to the WT protein in stabilizing these membranes during a freeze-thaw cycle, leakage of the fluorescent dye carboxy fluorescein from LUVs mimicking the lipid composition of these membranes was measured in the presence and absence of recombinant proteins in different protein: lipid molar ratios.

Liposomes without any protein added were strongly compromised after freezing and subsequent thawing (Figure 8), with dye leakage of about 90%, which is directly proportional to LUV damage. Similar to previously reported results, COR15A WT significantly stabilized the LUVs in a concentration-dependent manner during a freeze–thaw cycle, with dye leakage between 30–50% [16]. The degree of liposome damage in the presence of the two mutants is less than in the presence of the WT protein. The quadruple mutant 4GtoA showed a small but still significantly better LUV stabilization than COR15A WT ($p < 0.001$) in protein:lipid molar ratios above 1:50. G68A stabilized the LUVs significantly better ($p < 0.001$) than COR15A WT in all tested protein:lipid ratios. This is an interesting finding when combined with the higher overall α-helicity of G68A compared to 4GtoA in high co-solvent concentrations, assuming that COR15A associates with and consequently stabilizes membranes in a folded state as induced by the investigated co-solvents. This finding supports the hypothesis that actually COR15A functionality is directly related to α-helicity. Previous reports suggested that COR15A might form oligomeric structures in the fully hydrated state, as shown by crosslinking experiments [16]. If it actually does so under conditions of reduced water availability, as experienced during freezing, has not been investigated. Thus, we cannot rule out the possibility that COR15A oligomer formation might be impacted in the mutants, thus influencing functionality. In contrast to COR15A WT, the protective effect of the mutants was independent of the lipid:protein ratio, indicating that a lower amount of mutant protein is sufficient to tap their stabilization potential. The reference protein RNase A had a minor, nevertheless significant protective effect on liposome stability, whereas Bovine serum albumin, as a known membrane stabilizer, significantly better protected the LUVs from dye leakage in a concentration dependent manner, compared to COR15A WT. These data corroborate the previous finding of COR15A associating with membranes exclusively in a folded state [12,43]. The folding state seemingly does not only influence membrane association but consequently also membrane stabilization. So, what is the apparent advantage of COR15A in being intrinsically disordered? The coil-helix transition of COR15A is strictly modulated by the osmolarity of the cellular environment, which increases with decreasing freezing temperature [41]. The major finding we report here is that increased α-helicity of COR15A directly translates into increased functionality. This presents crucial progress in understanding the structure–function relationship of COR15A specifically and should be investigated regarding other LEA proteins in the future with respect to the long-term perspective of manufacturing plants with improved desiccation, dehydration or freezing tolerance.

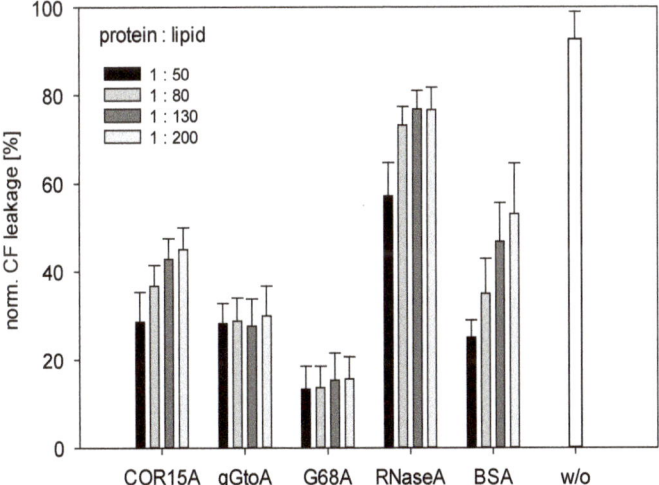

Figure 8. α-helical mutants reduce carboxy fluorescein (CF) leakage from vesicles. Carboxy flourescein leakage of inner chloroplast membranes (ICMM) large unilamellar vesicles (LUVs) after freezing and subsequent thawing was performed using the fluorescence signal detected by λ_{ex} = 492nm and λ_{em} = 517nm. The protein:lipid molar ratios used were 1:50, 1:80, 1:130, 1:200, and these are shown in different shades. All proteins showed a significance level $p < 0.001$ compared to ICMM LUVs without protein (w/o). Error bars refer to the standard derivation of triplicates from up to three experiments.

4. Conclusions

This study examines the importance of conserved glycine residues on maintaining the disordered structure of COR15A using sequence alignments. The role of increasing helicity on the membrane-stabilizing function of COR15A. The sequence alignments in Figure 1 show that glycine residues at positions 7, 35, 68, and 81 in the COR15A sequence are conserved across several plant species. In addition, the glycine residue at position 84 is mostly conserved and that at position 54 is not. AGADIR predicted that the glycine residue at position 68 had a stronger impact on COR15A disorder than the remaining glycine residues. It also predicted that the glycine residues at positions 54, 68, 81 and 84 in the C-terminal segment of the protein had a stronger impact on the preservation of COR15A disorder compared to the glycine residues in the N-terminal segment. Based on these indications, we made a single glycine to alanine mutation at position 68 and a quadruple mutant at residues 54, 68, 81 and 84. The mutant proteins and COR15A were subject to a detailed structural and functional analysis.

In previous work by Thalhammer and colleagues, a homology model was published for the dehydrated state of COR15A. In this model, COR15A forms a structure with N- and C-terminal helices separated by a long loop [10]. The length and flexibility of the long loop may control interactions between the N- and C-terminal helix. In 0% TFE (Figure 5A–C), the N-terminal helix (residues 10–31) has an average helicity of 4.6% and is not affected by C-terminal mutations. However, the helicity of the C-terminal helix (residues 50–84) increases from WT (4.6%) to G68A (7.9%) to 4GtoA (16.4%). The 20% TFE samples, show a different trend. The helical content of the N-terminal helix increases from WT (67.6%) to G68A (77.6%), but in 4GtoA (48.1%), the helical content decreases. However, in the C-terminal helix, there is an increase in helical content from WT (65.2%) to G68A (72.3%) to 4GtoA (81.6%). Based on this analysis, we think it is possible that the observed decrease in the helical content of 4GtoA in 20% TFE, may be due to a decrease in the interaction of the two helical segments in 20% TFE due to the G54A mutation.

The NMR and CD studies performed on the WT and mutant proteins showed that in the absence of TFE, COR15A WT had lower α-helicity compared to both mutants. As expected, in the presence of the α-helix-inducing agent TFE, α-helicity was increased in all proteins. While both mutants had higher α-helicity than the WT, the single mutant had higher α-helicity than the quadruple mutant in the N-terminal α-helix. Functionally, higher α-helicity resulted in increased liposome stabilization in response to freezing (Figure 8). This effect was greater for the G68A mutant, which showed the highest overall α-helical content in high TFE and EG concentrations. This finding is consistent with our current understanding of membrane association of COR15A via α-helical segments [10,11,14]. The functionality of COR15A is modulated by the folding state of the protein and more helical variants appear to provide greater protection to the membrane. The impact of this observation is significant, considering the possibility of increasing plant responses to dehydrative stress simply by shifting the coil–helix equilibrium towards the more folded conformation.

Author Contributions: Conceptualization, G.W.D., A.T. and W.B.; methodology, G.W.D., A.T., W.B., T.R., P.K.-B. and O.T.S.; validation, G.W.D., A.T., W.B., P.K.-B. and O.T.S.; formal analysis, G.W.D., A.T., W.B., P.K.-B. and O.T.S.; investigation, G.W.D., A.T., W.B., P.K.-B., O.T.S. and T.R.; resources, G.D. and A.T.; data curation, G.W.D., A.T., W.B., P.K.-B. and O.T.S.; writing—original draft preparation, G.W.D., A.T., P.K.-B. and O.T.S.; writing—review and editing, G.W.D., A.T., W.B., P.K.-B. and O.T.S.; visualization, G.W.D., A.T., W.B., P.K.-B. and O.T.S.; supervision, G.W.D. and A.T.; project administration, G.W.D.; funding acquisition, G.D., A.T.

Funding: G.W.D. is supported by the National Institutes of Health (2R01CA14124406-A1 and 1R01GM115556-01A1) and A.T. is supported by a KoUP grant from the University of Potsdam.

Conflicts of Interest: The authors declare no conflict of interest.

References

1. Uversky, V.N. Intrinsically disordered proteins and their environment: Effects of strong denaturants, temperature, pH, counter ions, membranes, binding partners, osmolytes, and macromolecular crowding. *Protein J.* **2009**, *28*, 305–325. [CrossRef] [PubMed]
2. Uversky, V.N.; Dunker, A.K. Understanding protein non-folding. *Biochim. Biophys. Acta* **2010**, *1804*, 1231–1264. [CrossRef] [PubMed]
3. Dunker, A.K.; Obradovic, Z.; Romero, P.; Garner, E.C.; Brown, C.J. Intrinsic protein disorder in complete genomes. *Genome Inform.* **2000**, *11*, 161–171. [PubMed]

4. Brown, C.J.; Johnson, A.K.; Dunker, A.K.; Daughdrill, G.W. Evolution and disorder. *Curr. Opin. Struct. Biol.* **2011**, *21*, 441–446. [CrossRef] [PubMed]
5. van der Lee, R.; Buljan, M.; Lang, B.; Weatheritt, R.J.; Daughdrill, G.W.; Dunker, A.K.; Fuxreiter, M.; Gough, J.; Gsponer, J.; Jones, D.T.; et al. Classification of intrinsically disordered regions and proteins. *Chem. Rev.* **2014**, *114*, 6589–6631. [CrossRef] [PubMed]
6. Battaglia, M.; Covarrubias, A.A. Late Embryogenesis abundant (LEA) proteins in legumes. *Front. Plant Sci.* **2013**, *4*, 190. [CrossRef] [PubMed]
7. Hundertmark, M.; Hincha, D.K. LEA (late embryogenesis abundant) proteins and their encoding genes in Arabidopsis thaliana. *BMC Genomics* **2008**, *9*, 118. [CrossRef] [PubMed]
8. Hincha, D.K.; Thalhammer, A. LEA proteins: IDPs with versatile functions in cellular dehydration tolerance. *Biochem. Soc. Trans.* **2012**, *40*, 1000–1003. [CrossRef] [PubMed]
9. Bies-Etheve, N.; Gaubier-Comella, P.; Debures, A.; Lasserre, E.; Jobet, E.; Raynal, M.; Cooke, R.; Delseny, M. Inventory, evolution and expression profiling diversity of the LEA (late embryogenesis abundant) protein gene family in *Arabidopsis thaliana*. *Plant Mol. Biol.* **2008**, *67*, 107–124. [CrossRef] [PubMed]
10. Navarro-Retamal, C.; Bremer, A.; Alzate-Morales, J.; Caballero, J.; Hincha, D.K.; Gonzalez, W.; Thalhammer, A. Molecular dynamics simulations and CD spectroscopy reveal hydration-induced unfolding of the intrinsically disordered LEA proteins COR15A and COR15B from Arabidopsis thaliana. *Phys. Chem. Chem. Phys.* **2016**, *18*, 25806–25816. [CrossRef] [PubMed]
11. Thalhammer, A.; Hundertmark, M.; Popova, A.V.; Seckler, R.; Hincha, D.K. Interaction of two intrinsically disordered plant stress proteins (COR15A and COR15B) with lipid membranes in the dry state. *Biochim. Biophys. Acta* **2010**, *1798*, 1812–1820. [CrossRef] [PubMed]
12. Bremer, A.; Kent, B.; Hauss, T.; Thalhammer, A.; Yepuri, N.R.; Darwish, T.A.; Garvey, C.J.; Bryant, G.; Hincha, D.K. Intrinsically disordered stress protein COR15A resides at the membrane surface during dehydration. *Biophys. J.* **2017**, *113*, 572–579. [CrossRef] [PubMed]
13. Artus, N.N.; Uemura, M.; Steponkus, P.L.; Gilmour, S.J.; Lin, C.; Thomashow, M.F. Constitutive expression of the cold-regulated arabidopsis thaliana COR15A gene affects both chloroplast and protoplast freezing tolerance. *Proc. Natl. Acad. Sci. USA* **1996**, *93*, 13404–13409. [CrossRef] [PubMed]
14. Thalhammer, A.; Bryant, G.; Sulpice, R.; Hincha, D.K. Disordered cold regulated 15 proteins protect chloroplast membranes during freezing through binding and folding, but do not stabilize chloroplast enzymes in vivo. *Plant Physiol.* **2014**, *166*, 190–201. [CrossRef] [PubMed]
15. Lin, C.; Thomashow, M.F. A cold-regulated arabidopsis gene encodes a polypeptide having potent cryoprotective activity. *Biochem. Biophys. Res. Commun.* **1992**, *183*, 1103–1108. [CrossRef]
16. Nakayama, K.; Okawa, K.; Kakizaki, T.; Honma, T.; Itoh, H.; Inaba, T. Arabidopsis COR15am is a chloroplast stromal protein that has cryoprotective activity and forms oligomers. *Plant Physiol.* **2007**, *144*, 513–523. [CrossRef] [PubMed]
17. Nakayama, K.; Okawa, K.; Kakizaki, T.; Inaba, T. Evaluation of the protective activities of a late embryogenesis abundant (LEA) related protein, COR15am, during various stresses in vitro. *Biosci. Biotechnol. Biochem.* **2008**, *72*, 1642–1645. [CrossRef] [PubMed]
18. Popova, A.V.; Hundertmark, M.; Seckler, R.; Hincha, D.K. Structural transitions in the intrinsically disordered plant dehydration stress protein LEA7 upon drying are modulated by the presence of membranes. *Biochim. Biophys. Acta* **2011**, *1808*, 1879–1887. [CrossRef] [PubMed]
19. Steponkus, P.L.; Uemura, M.; Joseph, R.A.; Gilmour, S.J.; Thomashow, M.F. Mode of action of the COR15A gene on the freezing tolerance of arabidopsis thaliana. *Proc. Natl. Acad. Sci. USA* **1998**, *95*, 14570–14575. [CrossRef] [PubMed]
20. Navarro-Retamal, C.; Bremer, A.; Ingolfsson, H.I.; Alzate-Morales, J.; Caballero, J.; Thalhammer, A.; Gonzalez, W.; Hincha, D.K. Folding and lipid composition determine membrane interaction of the disordered protein COR15A. *Biophys. J.* **2018**, *115*, 968–980. [CrossRef] [PubMed]
21. Buck, M. Trifluoroethanol and colleagues: Cosolvents come of age. Recent studies with peptides and proteins. *Q. Rev. Biophys.* **1998**, *31*, 297–355. [CrossRef] [PubMed]
22. Lacroix, E.; Viguera, A.R.; Serrano, L. Elucidating the folding problem of alpha-helices: Local motifs, long-range electrostatics, ionic-strength dependence and prediction of NMR parameters. *J. Mol. Biol.* **1998**, *284*, 173–191. [CrossRef] [PubMed]

23. Munoz, V.; Serrano, L. Development of the multiple sequence approximation within the AGADIR model of alpha-helix formation: Comparison with Zimm-Bragg and Lifson-Roig formalisms. *Biopolymers* **1997**, *41*, 495–509. [CrossRef]
24. Camilloni, C.; De Simone, A.; Vranken, W.F.; Vendruscolo, M. Determination of secondary structure populations in disordered states of proteins using nuclear magnetic resonance chemical shifts. *Biochemistry* **2012**, *51*, 2224–2231. [CrossRef] [PubMed]
25. Tamiola, K.; Acar, B.; Mulder, F.A. Sequence-specific random coil chemical shifts of intrinsically disordered proteins. *J. Am. Chem. Soc.* **2010**, *132*, 18000–18003. [CrossRef] [PubMed]
26. Kearse, M.; Moir, R.; Wilson, A.; Stones-Havas, S.; Cheung, M.; Sturrock, S.; Buxton, S.; Cooper, A.; Markowitz, S.; Duran, C.; et al. Geneious basic: An integrated and extendable desktop software platform for the organization and analysis of sequence data. *Bioinformatics* **2012**, *28*, 1647–1649. [CrossRef] [PubMed]
27. Chen, Y.H.; Yang, J.T.; Martinez, H.M. Determination of the secondary structures of proteins by circular dichroism and optical rotatory dispersion. *Biochemistry* **1972**, *11*, 4120–4131. [CrossRef] [PubMed]
28. Hincha, D.K. Release of two peripheral proteins from chloroplast thylakoid membranes in the presence of a hofmeister series of chaotropic anions. *Arch. Biochem. Biophys.* **1998**, *358*, 385–390. [CrossRef] [PubMed]
29. Oliver, A.E.; Hincha, D.K.; Crowe, L.M.; Crowe, J.H. Interactions of arbutin with dry and hydrated bilayers. *Biochim. Biophys. Acta* **1998**, *1370*, 87–97. [CrossRef]
30. Provencher, S.W. Contin: A general purpose constrained regularization program for inverting noisy linear algebraic and integral equations. *Comput. Phys. Commun.* **1982**, *27*, 229–242. [CrossRef]
31. Eftink, M.R. Fluorescence techniques for studying protein structure. *Methods Biochem. Anal.* **1991**, *35*, 127–205. [PubMed]
32. Hincha, D.K. Effects of calcium-induced aggregation on the physical stability of liposomes containing plant glycolipids. *Biochim. Biophys. Acta* **2003**, *1611*, 180–186. [CrossRef]
33. Hincha, D.K.; Zuther, E.; Hellwege, E.M.; Heyer, A.G. Specific effects of fructo- and gluco-oligosaccharides in the preservation of liposomes during drying. *Glycobiology* **2002**, *12*, 103–110. [CrossRef] [PubMed]
34. Coordinators, N.R. Database resources of the national center for biotechnology information. *Nucleic Acids Res.* **2018**, *46*, D8–D13. [CrossRef] [PubMed]
35. Lopez-Llano, J.; Campos, L.A.; Sancho, J. Alpha-helix stabilization by alanine relative to glycine: Roles of polar and apolar solvent exposures and of backbone entropy. *Proteins* **2006**, *64*, 769–778. [CrossRef] [PubMed]
36. Dosztanyi, Z. Prediction of protein disorder based on iupred. *Protein Sci.* **2018**, *27*, 331–340. [CrossRef] [PubMed]
37. Dosztanyi, Z.; Csizmok, V.; Tompa, P.; Simon, I. Iupred: Web server for the prediction of intrinsically unstructured regions of proteins based on estimated energy content. *Bioinformatics* **2005**, *21*, 3433–3434. [CrossRef] [PubMed]
38. Vise, P.D.; Baral, B.; Latos, A.J.; Daughdrill, G.W. NMR chemical shift and relaxation measurements provide evidence for the coupled folding and binding of the p53 transactivation domain. *Nucl. Acids Res.* **2005**, *33*, 2061–2077. [CrossRef] [PubMed]
39. Bremer, A.; Wolff, M.; Thalhammer, A.; Hincha, D.K. Folding of intrinsically disordered plant LEA proteins is driven by glycerol-induced crowding and the presence of membranes. *FEBS J.* **2017**, *284*, 919–936. [CrossRef] [PubMed]
40. Sreerama, N.; Woody, R. Estimation of protein secondary structure from circular dichroism spectra: Comparison of CONTIN, SELCON, and CDSSTR methods with an expanded reference set. *Anal. Biochem.* **2000**, *287*, 252–260. [CrossRef] [PubMed]
41. Bakaltcheva, I.; Schmitt, J.M.; Hincha, D.K. Time- and temperature-dependent solute loading of isolated thylakoids during freezing. *Cryobiology* **1992**, *29*, 607–615. [CrossRef]

42. Contreras-Martos, S.; Nguyen, H.H.; Nguyen, P.N.; Hristozova, N.; Macossay-Castillo, M.; Kovacs, D.; Bekesi, A.; Oemig, J.S.; Maes, D.; Pauwels, K.; et al. Quantification of intrinsically disordered proteins: A problem not fully appreciated. *Front. Mol. Biosci.* **2018**, *5*, 83. [CrossRef] [PubMed]
43. Colmenero-Flores, J.M.; Moreno, L.P.; Smith, C.E.; Covarrubias, A.A. Pvlea-18, a member of a new late-embryogenesis-abundant protein family that accumulates during water stress and in the growing regions of well-irrigated bean seedlings. *Plant Physiol.* **1999**, *120*, 93–104. [CrossRef] [PubMed]

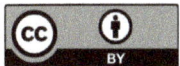

© 2019 by the authors. Licensee MDPI, Basel, Switzerland. This article is an open access article distributed under the terms and conditions of the Creative Commons Attribution (CC BY) license (http://creativecommons.org/licenses/by/4.0/).

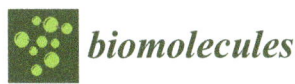

Article

p53 Phosphomimetics Preserve Transient Secondary Structure but Reduce Binding to Mdm2 and MdmX

Robin Levy [1,2], Emily Gregory [1,2], Wade Borcherds [1,2] and Gary Daughdrill [1,2,*]

[1] Department of Cell Biology, Microbiology, and Molecular Biology, University of South Florida, Tampa, FL 33620, USA; robinlevy@mail.usf.edu (R.L.); egregorylott@mail.usf.edu (E.G.); wborcher@mail.usf.edu (W.B.)
[2] Center for Drug Discovery and Innovation, University of South Florida, Tampa, FL 33612, USA
* Correspondence: gdaughdrill@usf.edu; Tel.: +1-813-974-2503

Academic Editors: Prakash Kulkarni and Vladimir N. Uversky
Received: 23 January 2019; Accepted: 28 February 2019; Published: 2 March 2019

Abstract: The disordered p53 transactivation domain (p53TAD) contains specific levels of transient helical secondary structure that are necessary for its binding to the negative regulators, mouse double minute 2 (Mdm2) and MdmX. The interactions of p53 with Mdm2 and MdmX are also modulated by posttranslational modifications (PTMs) of p53TAD including phosphorylation at S15, T18 and S20 that inhibits p53-Mdm2 binding. It is unclear whether the levels of transient secondary structure in p53TAD are changed by phosphorylation or other PTMs. We used phosphomimetic mutants to determine if adding a negative charge at positions 15 and 18 has any effect on the transient secondary structure of p53TAD and protein-protein binding. Using a combination of biophysical and structural methods, we investigated the effects of single and multisite phosphomimetics on the transient secondary structure of p53TAD and its interaction with Mdm2, MdmX, and the KIX domain. The phosphomimetics reduced Mdm2 and MdmX binding affinity by 3–5-fold, but resulted in minimal changes in transient secondary structure, suggesting that the destabilizing effect of phosphorylation on the p53TAD-Mdm2 interaction is primarily electrostatic. Phosphomimetics had no effect on the p53-KIX interaction, suggesting that increased binding of phosphorylated p53 to KIX may be influenced by decreased competition with its negative regulators.

Keywords: tumor protein p53; mouse double minute 2; mouse double minute 4; Kinase-inducible domain interacting domain; phosphorylation; phosphomimetics; nuclear magnetic resonance; intrinsically disordered proteins; transient secondary structure

---

1. Introduction

Loss of function mutations in the p53 pathway frequently arise during cancer development [1–3]. Approximately half of all human tumors express p53 mutants with reduced DNA-binding affinity which reduces or eliminates transactivation [3,4]. The tumor suppressor protein p53 is a well-known intrinsically disordered protein (IDP) whose disorder is a major component of its functionality [5,6]. An IDP is a protein that lacks a fixed or ordered structure. IDPs are structurally very different from ordered proteins and tend to have distinct properties in terms of function, sequence, interactions, evolution and regulation [7–9]. Many IDPs like p53 form transient secondary structures and undergo coupled folding and binding when they are bound to their targets [10–12]. Intrinsically disordered proteins cover a range of different states from fully unstructured to partially structured [8,13,14]. Modulation of the degree of transient secondary structure affects p53's interactions with its binding partners [15]. Posttranslational modifications (PTMs) also regulate the activity of IDPs [16,17]. In normal cells, p53 is present at low concentrations due to its interaction with the E3 ubiquitin ligase Mdm2; however, under stress conditions, p53 is phosphorylated, leading to its dissociation from Mdm2, migration to the nucleus, and the transcriptional activation of its target genes [18]. Cells with mutant or deleted p53 are unable to respond to stress appropriately, and this leads to mutations and the development of cancer [19].

Mouse double minute 2 (Mdm2), also known as E3 ubiquitin-protein ligase Mdm2 proto-oncogene, and its homolog Mmd4, also known as MdmX, are negative regulators of p53 [20–22]. Mdm2 is overexpressed in several human tumor types, such as soft tissue sarcomas as well as breast tumors [23]. p53 levels are suppressed by the Mdm2/MdmX heterodimer which promotes the polyubiquitination of p53 leading to its degradation [24,25]. Mouse double minute 2 and p53 are involved in an auto-regulatory feed-back loop where p53 stimulates the expression of Mdm2; Mdm2, in turn, inhibits p53 activity because it stimulates its degradation [26,27]. Even though MdmX lacks ubiquitin E3 ligase activity it is able to directly bind to and inhibit p53 activity independently of Mdm2 [24,28,29]. Cellular stress such as DNA damage activates kinases that phosphorylate p53 at residues S15, T18 and S20, which stabilize and activate p53 by inhibiting Mdm2 binding [30–32]. In vitro, p53 phosphorylation affects its interaction with Mdm2, where phosphorylation of S15 and S20 residues individually result in a 2 and 1.5-fold reduction, respectively [33]. Phosphorylation of T18 leads to a 19–22-fold reduction in binding affinity of p53TAD to Mdm2, and one study has described an equivalent effect of phosphorylated T18 on Mdm2 and MdmX binding to p53 [10,33,34]. Dually phosphorylated p53 at S15/T18 results in a binding reduction equivalent to that of T18 alone, suggesting that T18 phosphorylation is the driver of reduced binding affinity of p53 to Mdm2, though the T18 site of p53 cannot be phosphorylated until the S15 site is phosphorylated first [30,33,35–38]. The phosphorylation of T18 creates additional charge-charge repulsion, creating an energetically unfavorable environment for p53 and Mdm2 binding, however, the contribution of phosphorylated p53's structural changes to Mdm2 binding has not been assessed [30,35–38].

Phosphorylation of p53TAD upon cellular stress leads to increased transcription of its target genes and increased association with its coactivator, CREB binding protein (CBP)/p300 [39]. The CBP protein is a transcriptional coactivator and histone acetyltransferase that facilitates transcription initiation of p53 target genes and stabilizes p53 by acetylating its lysines that would otherwise be ubiquitinated by Mdm2 [40,41]. It contains four domains capable of binding p53TAD, and it has been proposed that all four domains may bind tetrameric p53 in the nucleus to facilitate transcription initiation [42]. Whereas Mdm2 and MdmX interact with p53's TAD1 region, which spans approximately residues 1–40, the KIX, TAZ1, TAZ2, and IBiD domains of CBP interacts with both TAD1 and TAD2 of p53, approximately residues 41–60 [10]. Thus, CBP competes with Mdm2 and MdmX for binding to p53, though it has also been shown that CBP and Mdm2 may form a ternary complex with p53 in vitro [10]. Phosphorylation of the TAD1 region of p53 increases binding affinity with the KIX, TAZ1, and TAZ2 domains of CBP, though possibly by different mechanisms [33,43]. In this study we focus on the kinase-inducible domain interacting domain (KIX), for which the bound state of p53 has not been determined. Phosphorylation of S15 or T18 is reported to result in a 1.7–4-fold increase in binding affinity with KIX, but an increase of 3–11-fold for the same residues when binding to TAZ2. S15/T18 phosphorylation, however, has been reported to result in 16 and 8-fold changes in binding affinity for KIX and TAZ2, respectively [43]. Likewise, where binding of p53 to the KIX domain is controlled by a combination of conformational selection and electrostatic attraction, for example, TAZ2 interaction with the phosphorylated T18 is likely driven by electrostatic attraction [44–46].

During phosphorylation the phosphate group contains a double negative charge that affects protein conformation mainly due to the electrostatic effects that occur between the phosphate and surrounding charged atoms of the protein [47,48]. These conformational changes can be local and/or long-range, affect protein-protein interactions, and increase or decrease levels of disorder [48]. Posttranslational modifications-mediated folding of the IDP 4E-BP2 allows it to regulate translation initiation [17]. Multisite phosphorylation stabilizes 4E-BP2 and decreases affinity to its binding partner eIF4E by a factor of 4000 compared to single-site phosphorylation which only decreases affinity by 100-fold [17]. Phosphorylation of T51 conforms PAGE4 into a more compact structure that still maintains a flexible state for long range interactions. Phosphorylation of PAGE4 also increases c-Jun transactivation but decreases the affinity of PAGE4 to c-Jun, which is believed to occur due to the compact structure of PAGE4 [49]. This attenuation of binding due to phosphorylation is common between many IDPs, which are known to form transient secondary structures and undergo coupled folding and binding when they are bound to their targets [9–11]. The first transactivation domain of p53 forms a short helix when bound to Mdm2 and MdmX anchored via the hydrophobic residues F19, W23, L26, and TAD2 forms a short helix when bound to the TAZ2 domain of CBP anchored around the hydrophobic residues I50, W53 and F54 [43,50]. Electrostatic interactions control the stability of the helix [51]. Such helices will have a macroscopic helical dipole with a partial positive charge at the N-terminus and a partial negative charge at the C-terminus, which could stabilize the helix dipole [52,53].

To study the effects of phosphorylation on protein structure and function phosphomimetic mutations have been used extensively. Phosphomimetic mutations are amino acid substitutions (Ser/Thr to Asp or Glu and Tyr to Glu) that mimic the effect of a phosphorylated residue [54–56]. There are no natural amino acid side chains that provide the combination of negative charge with a tetrahedral center. However, there are numerous studies showing partial phenotypes when aspartic acid is substituted for phospho-serine or glutamic acid is substituted for phospho-threonine [39,57]. In our phosphomimic mutants, the TAD1 helix, which corresponds to residues 19–25, has one or two additional negative charges added towards the N-terminus. The addition of negative charge might be thought to stabilize the helix as seen between antiparallel alpha helices where the close proximity of opposing charges stabilizes each [53]. However, computational studies have predicted that p53 T18 phosphorylation would destabilize the helix by causing a long-range interaction with the K24 residue of p53, interfering with the D21 interaction with K24 [50]. Relatedly, phosphorylation of S20 is predicted to increase helical propensity by stabilizing the D21-K24 interaction [51].

In this present study, we obtain insights into the role of phosphorylation in modulating interactions of p53 with Mdm2, MdmX, and CBP/KIX and the effect of phosphorylation on transient secondary structure. We assessed the effects of single- and double-site phosphomimetic mutations of p53TAD upon binding to the N-terminal domain of Mdm2, MdmX, and the KIX domain of CBP. Due to the location of S15 and T18 in a region of p53TAD containing transient helical secondary structure and the importance of their phosphorylation for regulation, we engineered p53TAD phosphomimetics, S15D and S15D/T18E, to determine if the phosphomimicry of p53TAD at these sites affects protein-protein binding and changes the levels of transient helical secondary structure. Our data shows that multisite phosphomimicry reduces the binding affinity of p53TAD to Mdm2 and MdmX. In contrast to earlier published results on p53 phosphorylation, single and multisite phosphomimetics of p53TAD have equivalent, small effects on binding with KIX [33,43,46]. We observe little, if any, change to the transient secondary structure of p53TAD.

2. Materials and Methods

2.1. Purification of Mdm2, MdmX, KIX, and Labeled p53TAD Constructs

All cell growth experiments were performed in M9 media. In order to make ^{15}N-labeled or ^{15}N- and ^{13}C-labeled samples 1 g/L of ^{15}N-labeled ammonium chloride and/or 0.2% (w/v) ^{13}C-labeled glucose were added in the place of nitrogen and carbon sources (Cambridge Isotopes, Andover, MA, USA).

Samples of human Mdm2 and MdmX, corresponding to residues 17–125 and 23–111, respectively, were expressed using pGEX-6p-2 vectors in BL21 (DE3) *Escherichia coli* cells grown in M9 medium. These cultures were induced at an OD$_{600}$ of 0.6 with 1 mM Isopropyl-β-D-thiogalactopyranoside and grown for 18 h at 15 °C. Cultures were centrifuged at 11,000× g and frozen at −80 °C. Pellets were resuspended in glutathione S-transferase (GST) binding buffer (25 mM Tris Base, 25 mM Tris-HCl, 300 mM NaCl, 2.5 mM ethylenediaminetetraacetic acid (EDTA), 0.02% NaN$_3$, 2 mM dithiothreitol (DTT), pH 7.4) containing protease inhibitors (Thermo Fisher, Rockford, IL, USA) per 2 L of culture and lysed with a French Press pressure cell using a minimum pressure of 20,000 pounds per square inch (psi). The lysate was centrifuged at 38,720× g for 1 h. The supernatant was filtered and then applied to a column containing 25 mL Glutathione Sepharose 4 Fast Flow resin. Protein fractions were eluted with three column volumes of 25 mM Tris Base, 25 mM Tris-HCl, 300 mM NaCl, 2.5 mM EDTA, 0.02% NaN$_3$, 2 mM DTT, pH 7.4 and 10 mM reduced glutathione. Fractions were analyzed using polyacrylamide gel electrophoresis (PAGE) and those fractions containing the protein were combined and dialyzed into 25 mM Tris Base, 25 mM Tris-HCl, 300 mM NaCl, 2.5 mM EDTA, 0.02% NaN$_3$, 2 mM DTT, pH 7.4, and the GST tag was cleaved using a 1:100 ratio of Human Rhinovirus 3C (HRV3C) protease. Samples were then applied to a column containing 25 mL Glutathione Sepharose 4 Fast Flow resin. Fractions were analyzed using PAGE and those fractions containing the protein were combined and dialyzed into gel filtration buffer (50 mM NaH$_2$PO$_4$, 300 mM NaCl, 1 mM EDTA and 0.02% NaN$_3$, pH 7.0) containing 2 mM DTT. The constructs were then loaded onto a GE HiLoad 16/60 Superdex 75 column. The column was equilibrated and the protein eluted with gel filtration buffer at a flow rate of 1.5 mL/min. Protein purity was verified using PAGE analysis.

The KIX (586–672) construct was expressed as N-terminal fusions with a 7-His tag. The plasmid was transformed into BL21 (DE3) *Escherichia coli* cells from New England Biolabs (Ipswich, MA, USA) for expression using the heat-shock method then plated on agar plates that contained kanamycin for expression. Single colonies from this transformation were used to inoculate 50 mL cultures of M9 media that were grown overnight. The overnight cultures were then re-inoculated into 2 L of M9 media at an OD600 of 0.04. These cultures were induced at an OD600 of 0.6 with 1 mM Isopropyl-β-D-thiogalactopyranoside and grown for 22 h at 15 °C. Cultures were centrifuged at 11.000× g and frozen at −80 °C. After expression, pellet was suspended in 25 mL of lysis buffer (50 mM NaH$_2$PO$_4$, 300 mM NaCl, 10 mM Imidazole, 0.02% NaN$_3$, pH 8.0) containing protease inhibitors (Thermo Fisher, Rockford, IL, USA) per 2 L of culture and lysed with a French Press pressure cell using a minimum pressure of 20,000 psi. The soluble fraction was isolated by centrifugation at 38,720 g for 1 h. The supernatant was filtered and added to a column containing 30 mL of Ni-NTA Superflow resin (Qiagen, Hilden, Germany). All buffers used on the NiNTA column were run at a flow rate of 3 mL/min. The column was washed with two column volumes of lysis buffer and the p53 eluted with three column volumes of elution buffer (50 mM NaH$_2$PO$_4$, 300 mM NaCl, 250 mM imidazole, 0.02% NaN$_3$, pH 8.0). Fractions were analyzed using PAGE and those fractions containing the protein were combined and dialyzed into gel filtration buffer (50 mM NaH$_2$PO$_4$, 300 mM NaCl, 1 mM EDTA and 0.02% NaN$_3$, pH 7.0) using 3500 Da MWCO dialysis tubing (FisherBrand, Pittsburg, PA, USA). The p53 protein was then concentrated in an Amicon Ultra-15 3K centrifugal filter device and the HIS-tag was removed by cleaving for 3 h at room temperature for the p53TAD WT (p53TAD) and overnight at room temperature for the other constructs with the Sigma-Aldrich Thrombin CleanCleave Kit (RECOMT) (St. Louis, MO, USA). The completion of the cleavage reaction was verified using PAGE. The cleaved p53 constructs were dialyzed in lysis buffer and then further purified by chromatography on Ni-NTA resin. Fractions were analyzed using PAGE and those fractions containing the protein were combined and dialyzed into gel filtration buffer and the constructs were then loaded onto a GE HiLoad 16/60 Superdex 75 column. The column was equilibrated and the protein eluted with gel filtration buffer at a flow rate of 1.5 mL/min. Protein purity was verified using PAGE analysis.

Constructs for S15D (residues 1–73), and S15D/T18E (residues 1–73) were generated by Polymerase chain reaction (PCR) site-directed mutagenesis QuickChange II (Agilent Technologies, Santa Clara, CA, USA) using the following primers for S15D d(GTCGAGCCCCCTCTGGATCAGGAAACATTTTC) and d(GAAAATGTTTCCTGATCCAGAGGGGGCTCGAC) and for S15D/T18E d(CGAGCCCCCTCTGGA TCAGGAAGAATTTTCAGACCTATGG) and d(CCATAGGTCTGAAAATTCTTCCTGATCCAGAGG GGGCTCG). All p53TAD constructs were expressed as N-terminal fusions with a 7-HIS tag. The samples were then cleaved with Fisher Bioreagents OPTIMIZED (Rockford, IL, USA) Dpn1, then were transformed into XL1-Blue cells from Agilent Technologies using agar plates that contained kanamycin. The plasmids from the bacterial colonies were isolated using the Thermo Scientific GeneJET Plasmid Miniprep kit.

The plasmid samples were sequenced at Eurofins Genomics and then transformed into BL21 (DE3) *Escherichia coli* cells from New England Biolabs using the heat-shock method then plated on agar plates that contained kanamycin for expression. Single colonies from this transformation were used to inoculate 60 mL cultures of M9 media that were grown overnight. The overnight cultures were then re-inoculated into 2 L of M9 media at an OD_{600} of 0.04. These cultures were induced at an OD_{600} of 0.6 with 1 mM Isopropyl-β-D-thiogalactopyranoside and grown for 5 h at 37 °C. Cultures were centrifuged at 11,000× g and frozen at −80°C. After expression, pellets containing unlabeled and double-labeled (^{15}N, ^{13}C) p53TAD peptides were suspended in 25 mL of lysis buffer (50 mM NaH_2PO_4, 300 mM NaCl, 10 mM Imidazole, 0.02% NaN_3, pH 8.0) containing protease inhibitors (Sigma Aldrich) per 2 L of culture and lysed with a French Press pressure cell using a minimum pressure of 20,000 psi. The soluble fraction was isolated by centrifugation at 38,720 g for 1 h. The supernatant was filtered and added to a column containing 30 mL of Ni-NTA Superflow resin (Qiagen, Hilden, Germany). All buffers used on the NiNTA column were run at a flow rate of 3 mL/min. The column was washed with two column volumes of lysis buffer and the p53 eluted with three column volumes of elution buffer (50 mM NaH_2PO_4, 300 mM NaCl, 250 mM imidazole, 0.02% NaN_3, pH 8.0). Fractions were analyzed using PAGE and those fractions containing the protein were combined and dialyzed into gel filtration buffer (50 mM NaH_2PO_4, 300 mM NaCl, 1 mM EDTA and 0.02% NaN_3, pH 7.0) using 3500Da MWCO dialysis tubing (FisherBrand, Pittsburg, PA, USA). The p53 protein was then concentrated in an Amicon Ultra-15 3K centrifugal filter device and the HIS-tag was removed by cleaving for 4 h at room temperature for the p53TAD and overnight at room temperature for the other constructs with the Sigma-Aldrich Thrombin CleanCleave Kit (RECOMT) (St. Louis, MO, USA). The completion of the cleavage reaction was verified using PAGE. The cleaved p53 constructs were dialyzed in lysis buffer and then further purified by chromatography on Ni-NTA resin. Fractions were analyzed using PAGE and those fractions containing the protein were combined and dialyzed into gel filtration buffer and the constructs were then loaded onto a GE HiLoad 16/60 Superdex 75 column. The column was equilibrated and the protein eluted with gel filtration buffer at a flow rate of 1.5 mL/min. Protein purity was verified using PAGE analysis.

2.2. Isothermal Titration Calorimetry

Isothermal titration calorimetry (ITC) experiments were performed using a GE MicroCal VP-ITC instrument. Proteins were dialyzed against 50 mM NaH_2PO_4, 150 mM NaCl, 1 mM EDTA, 0.02% NaN_3, 8 mM β-mercaptoethanol, pH 6.8. Binding experiments involving KIX were dialyzed against 50 mM Tris, 50 mM NaCl, pH 7.0. Experiments were performed at 25 °C. The typical concentration of p53 constructs (syringe) ranged from 50–500 µM and for Mdm2, MdmX and KIX (cell) 5–50 µM. Peptide concentrations were determined by absorbance at 280 nm. A typical ITC experiment consisted of one injection of 5 µL, followed by 29 injections of 10 µL up to a 2.5-fold molar excess of titrant. Data were analyzed with the Origin70 ITC software from MicroCal. Averages and standard deviations from three different ITC experiments are shown. Integrated ITC data were fit with single-site binding models and the stoichiometry ranged from 0.8 to 1.2. Errors in K_d were calculated from triplicate measurements.

2.3. Nuclear Magnetic Resonance Spectroscopy

Nuclear magnetic resonance (NMR) experiments for p53TAD and the phosphomimetics were performed using uniformly ^{15}N- and ^{13}C-labeled samples at 50 µM, at 25 °C on a Varian VNMRS 800 MHz spectrometer equipped with a triple-resonance pulse field Z-axis gradient cold probe. To make the amide ^{1}H and ^{15}N as well as ^{13}Cα, ^{13}Cβ, and ^{13}CO resonance assignments, sensitivity-enhanced ^{1}H–^{15}N heteronuclear single quantum coherence (HSQC) and three-dimensional HNCACB and HNCO experiments were performed on the uniformly ^{15}N- and ^{13}C-labeled samples in 90% H_2O/8% D_2O, 50 mM NaH_2PO_4, 50 mM NaCl, 1 mM EDTA, and 0.02% NaN_3, pH 6.8. For the HNCO the Varian VNMRS 600 MHz spectrometer with a triple resonance pulse field Z-axis gradient cold probe was used. The sweep widths were 9689.9 (t_3) Hz × 3770.1 (t_2) Hz × 1944.5 (t_1) Hz, and complex data points were 1024 (t_3) Hz × 64 (t_2) Hz × 32 (t_1) Hz. For p53TAD the HSQC and the HNCACB were performed on the 600 MHz spectrometer. The sweep widths and complex points for the HSQC were 7225.4 (t_2) Hz × 1500 (t_1) Hz and 1024 (t_2) Hz × 128 (t_1) Hz, respectively. The HNCACB experiment, data were acquired in the ^{1}H, ^{13}C, and ^{15}N dimensions using 7225.4 (t_3) Hz × 12063.8 (t_2) Hz × 1500 (t_1) Hz sweep widths and 1024 (t_3) Hz × 128 (t_2) Hz × 32 (t_1) Hz complex data points. For S15D the HSQC was performed on the 600 MHz spectrometer and the HNCACB was performed on the 800 MHz spectrometer. The sweep widths and complex points for the HSQC were 7266 (t_2) Hz × 1943.2 (t_1) Hz and 1024 (t_2) Hz × 128 (t_1) Hz, respectively. The HNCACB experiment, data were acquired in the ^{1}H, ^{13}C, and ^{15}N dimensions using 9689.9 (t_3) Hz × 14074.9 (t_2) Hz × 1944.3 (t_1) Hz sweep widths and 1024 (t_3) Hz × 128 (t_2) Hz × 32 (t_1) Hz complex data points. For S15D/T18E the HSQC and the HNCACB were performed on the 800 MHz spectrometer. The sweep widths and complex points for the HSQC were 9689.9 (t_2) Hz × 1944.4 (t_1) Hz and 1024 (t_2) Hz × 128 (t_1) Hz, respectively. The HNCACB experiment, data were acquired in the ^{1}H, ^{13}C, and ^{15}N dimensions using 9689.9 (t_3) Hz × 14074.9 (t_2) Hz × 1944.3 (t_1) Hz sweep widths and 1024 (t_3) Hz × 128 (t_2) Hz × 32 (t_1) Hz complex data points. All NMR spectra were processed with NMRFxProcessor and analyzed using NMRView J software (Standford, CA, USA) [58,59]. Secondary chemical shift values were calculated by subtracting the residue specific random coil chemical shifts in the prediction of temperature, neighbor and pH-corrected chemical shifts for intrinsically disordered proteins (POTENCI) from the measured chemical shifts [60]. Secondary structure populations were calculated with δ2D using the measured proton, nitrogen, and α, β, and carbonyl carbon chemical shifts [61]. The overall helicity was calculated as the mean of the per residue δ2D helical population estimates.

3. Results and Discussion

We attempted in vitro phosphorylation experiments with NMR labeled p53TAD using DNA-PK and CK1γ2 kinases to determine changes to transient secondary structure but were unable to get 100% phosphorylation at either S15 or T18 compared to that of previous studies (Figure S1) [62]. Therefore, we chose to use phosphomimetic mutations. The phosphorylation of p53 makes it more negatively charged. In studying protein phosphoreguation, it has become common to mutate phosphorylation sites to phosphomimetic residues to attempt to study the constitutively phosphorylated state of the protein [33,55,56,63–67]. We designed p53TAD phosphomimetics (residues 1–73) by mutating S15 to Asp and S15/T18 to Asp/Glu, which will be referred to as S15D and S15D/T18E, respectively. We used NMR spectroscopy to measure any changes in the transient secondary structure of p53TAD wild type (p53TAD) and mutants. An overlay of the ^{1}H-^{15}N heteronuclear single quantum coherence (HSQC) spectra of p53TAD and the phosphomimetics is shown in Figure 1. The labeled peaks show the resonance assignments of p53TAD residues (black peaks). There is hardly any shift in the majority of the residues for the S15D (red peaks) and S15D/T18E (blue peaks) mutants compared to p53TAD. We do see a significant shift at residues that are close to the mutated sites of S15 and T18 suggesting that any structural effects from the mutation(s) will be local.

Secondary chemical shift values were calculated using the prediction of temperature, neighbor and pH-corrected chemical shifts for intrinsically disordered proteins (POTENCI) software (Figure 2). This software calculates residue specific random coil chemical shifts from an amino acid sequence and these values are subtracted from the NMR measured chemical shift values to give the corrected secondary chemical shift values [60]. Positive alpha carbon secondary chemical shifts are indicative of alpha helix formation [68,69]. All of the measured chemical shifts (NH, N, CA, CB, and CO) were used to calculate the distribution of transient secondary structure using the δ2D software [61]. The negative charge produced during phosphorylation affects protein conformation mainly due to the electrostatic effects and these changes can be local and long-range, effect protein-protein interactions, and increase or decrease levels of disorder [47,48]. A short helix compromising residues 19–25 has one or two additional negative charges added towards the N-terminus in our phosphomimetic mutants which might stabilize the helix due to the close proximity of opposing charges. We observed small differences in the transient helical secondary structure between p53TAD, S15D and S15D/T18E

(Figure 2). However, of the changes that were present most were within the Mdm2/MdmX binding site. There was a slight increase in helicity for the mutants, with p53TAD having 36.4% helicity at its highest point and S15D and S15D/T18E having 39.8% and 39.9% helicity at their highest points, respectively, as indicated by the δ2d plots (Figure 2 red line). The reported accuracy of δ2D is 2%. The changes in the secondary chemical shifts, though minimal, were also observed within the Mdm2/MdmX binding site (Figure 2 black bars).

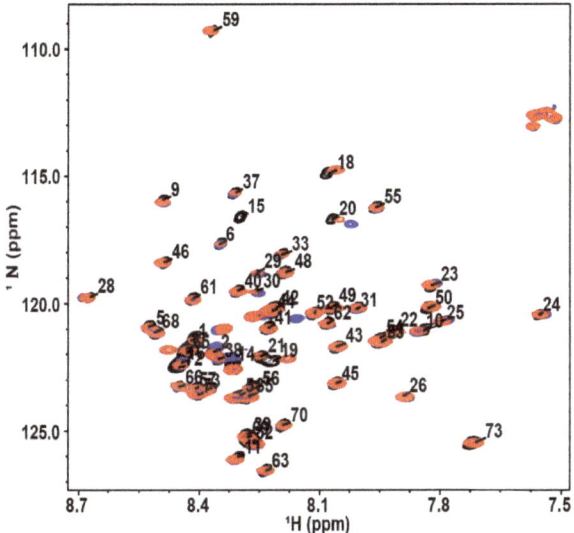

Figure 1. p53TAD and phosphomimics. ^{1}H-^{15}N HSQC spectra overlay of ^{15}N-labeled p53TAD (black), ^{15}N-labeled S15D mutant (red), ^{15}N-labeled S15D/T18E mutant (blue).

Next, we used isothermal titration calorimetry (ITC) to determine the effect of the phosphomimetic mutations on p53TAD binding to Mdm2 (residues 17–125), MdmX (residues 23–111), excluding the N-terminal "lid" and KIX (residues 586–672) (Figure 3) [70–72]. Compared to qualitative methods of measuring protein-protein binding (e.g., immunoprecipitation, western blot, GST pull-down) ITC is a widely used technique for quantitative studies of an extensive variety of biomolecular interactions [73–77]. It is mostly used to observe the binding between molecules like protein and DNA by measuring the binding affinity, enthalpy and stoichiometry of interacting molecules [73]. Isothermal titration calorimetry measures the heat that is either expelled or consumed by the interaction of the molecules present and modern ITC instruments make it possible to measure the differences in heat as small as 0.1 µcal (0.4 µJ) [78]. It can simultaneously determine multiple binding parameters in a single experiment and does not require the modification of binding partners with fluorescent tags or through immobilization; ITC measures the affinity of binding partners in their native states. Isothermal titration calorimetry experiments were performed by titrating the p53TAD phosphomimetics into Mdm2, MdmX, and KIX. The ITC experiments were performed in triplicate and the values averaged (Table 1). Data were analyzed with the Origin70 ITC software from MicroCal and the integrated ITC data were fit with single-site binding models and the stoichiometry ranged from 0.8 to 1.2. A standard deviation was calculated for K_d using data from triplicate measurements. Our results showed that p53TAD and S15D bound Mdm2/MdmX with similar affinities, whereas S15D/T18E displayed a 2.5–4.5-fold reduction with Mdm2 and a 5-fold reduction with MdmX (Figure 3A,B). Binding affinity of p53 to KIX was similar between p53TAD and all the phosphomimetics. Binding of p53TAD to KIX was endothermic with similar values for S15D (Figure 3C and Table 1). However, S15D/T18E was exothermic (Figure 3C and Table 1). Interestingly, the phosphomimetics had no effect on the transient helical secondary structure of p53TAD. Taken together, the results argue that binding affinity between phosphorylated and unphosphorylated p53 to Mdm2/MdmX is primarily controlled by electrostatics and the binding to KIX is unchanged.

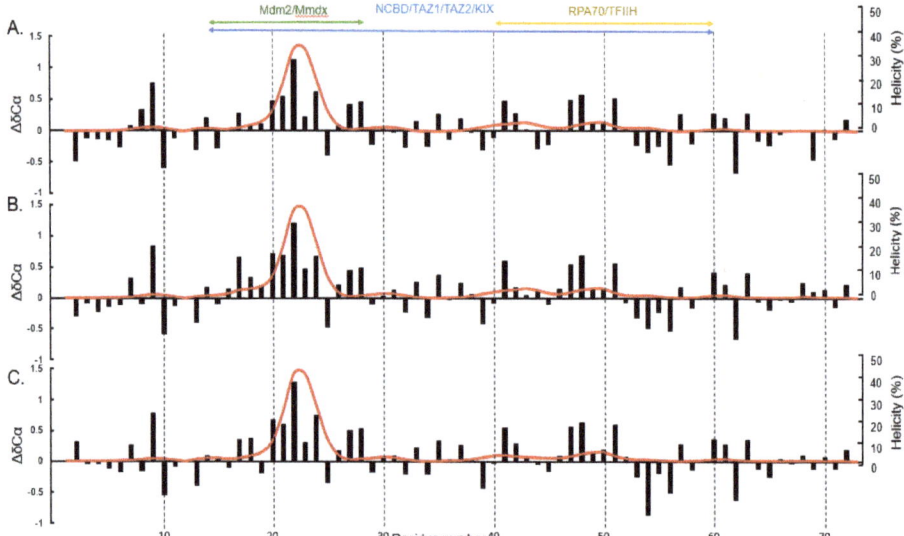

Figure 2. Residue specific secondary structure of p53TAD and phosphomimetics. Secondary chemical shift plots and δ2D plot for p53TAD and phosphomimetics determined from nuclear magnetic resonance (NMR) spectroscopy. (**A**) p53TAD (**B**) S15D (**C**) S15D/T18E. α-carbon secondary chemical shift (ΔδCα, black bars) and helical δ2D plots (red line) for the p53TAD and phosphomimetics as determined by NMR spectroscopy. Colored bars indicate binding sites for respective protein partners. The α-carbon chemical shifts for p53TAD was collected on a 600 MHz NMR at a digital resolution of 0.31 ppm. The alpha carbon chemical shifts for S15D and S15D/T18E was collected on an 800 MHz NMR at a digital resolution of 0.27 ppm.

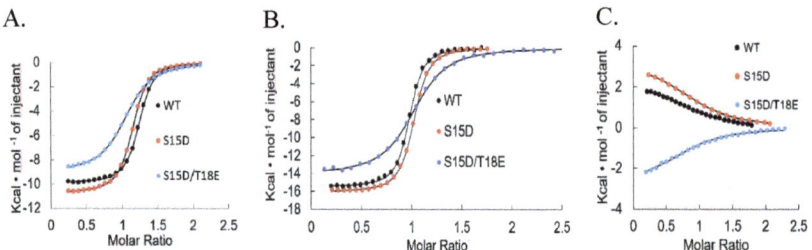

Figure 3. Binding Isotherms of Mdm2, MdmX and KIX with p53TAD and mutants. Isothermal calorimetry titrations of (**A**). Mdm2 and p53TAD and mutants (**B**). MdmX and p53TAD and mutants and (**C**). KIX and p53TAD and mutants. WT: wild type.

Table 1. Isothermal titration calorimetry (ITC) values for interactions between Mdm2, MdmX and KIX with p53TAD and mutants.

		p53TAD	S15D	S15D/T18E
Mdm2	K_d (nM)	219.5 ± 0.012	392.5 ± 0.015	1.001 ± 0.016
	ΔG (Kcal/mol)	-9.1	-8.75 ± 0.071	-8.2
	ΔH (Kcal/mol)	-9.721 ± 0.202	-11.335 ± 0.827	-8.173 ± 1.203
	$T\Delta S$ (Kcaal/mol/deg)	-0.634 ± 0.236	-2.499 ± 0.977	-0.964 ± 0.188
MdmX	K_d (nM)	29 ± 0.004	30 ± 0.002	108 ± 12.5
	ΔG (Kcal/mol)	-10.3 ± 0.100	-10.27 ± 0.058	-9.5 ± 0.07
	ΔH (Kcal/mol)	-16.260 ± 0.913	-16.99 ± 1.405	-14.27 ± 0.19
	$T\Delta S$ (Kcal/mol/deg)	-5.960 ± 0.988	-6.794 ± 1.55	-4.75 ± 0.16
KIX	K_d (nM)	$11,000 \pm 2.700$	8200 ± 1870	8380 ± 969
	ΔG (Kcal/mol)	-6.77 ± 0.157	-6.95 ± 0.127	-6.92 ± 0.056
	ΔH (Kcal/mol)	2.606 ± 0.308	2.926 ± 0.416	-2.822 ± 0.079
	$T\Delta S$ (Kcal/mol/deg)	9.377 ± 0.165	9.874 ± 0.308	3.963 ± 0.270

4. Conclusions

Using phosphomimetic mutations we investigated the effect of phosphorylation on the binding of p53 with Mdm2, MdmX, and CBP/KIX and the transient secondary structure of p53TAD. By increasing negative charge of neighboring residues at the positive end (N-terminus) of the helix formed by p53 in the bound state with Mdm2, we expected a stabilization of the helical dipole in accordance with what is seen in antiparallel helix interactions [53]. Conversely, simulations suggest that phosphorylation of T18 has a destabilizing effect on the helix in the bound state [30]. Our results show that neither an increase nor decrease in transient helicity occurs for S15D or S15D/T18E.

Binding affinities of the p53TAD phosphomimetics for the Mdm2, MdmX and KIX were determined using ITC (Figure 3). For both Mdm2 and MdmX, S15D showed similar binding to p53TAD. S15D/T18E showed a decrease in binding to Mdm2 and MdmX with binding being 4.5 times and 5 times weaker than p53TAD, respectively (Table 1). Many studies have shown that phosphorylation of S15 and T18 play a critical role in preventing the interaction with Mdm2 [32,35,79]. There has been some disagreement regarding the impact of phosphorylation on binding; there is a good consistency for unphosphorylated peptides (residues 10–57) binding to Mdm2 but there is some variation in the binding affinity of phosphorylated peptides that does not appear to correlate with different techniques or sizes of the peptides being used [10,43,80,81]. Though we do not see much structural change with the phosphomimetics, we do see binding results consistent with other studies that phosphorylated p53 at the same residues. Previous studies showed a 10–20-fold reduction in binding of p53 to Mdm2 due to p53 phosphorylation as compared to our results where we see a 3–5-fold reduction [10,43,80–82]. The results of our binding experiments with phosphomimetics are consistent with previous findings suggesting that the phosphorylation of T18 is the driving force for inhibiting Mdm2/MdmX binding [30,50,80–83]. Furthermore, there has not yet been a quantitative study of the effect of p53 phosphorylation on MdmX binding. Our results suggest that p53 phosphorylation may in some cases have an equivalent effect on MdmX as on Mdm2.

Binding affinity of p53 to KIX was not significantly altered between p53TAD and the phosphomimetics. We found p53TAD binds to KIX with a K_d of 11 µM, similar to values found in previous studies [10,33,46]. In contrast to previous studies on p53 phosphorylation, however, these phosphomimetic mutations increased binding affinity for KIX by only 1.3-fold. Phosphorylation of p53 at S15 has been shown to result in a 1.7–4-fold increase and S15/T18 phosphorylation results in a 16-fold increase in binding affinity to KIX in vitro [10,33,43,84]. The increase in binding affinity of phosphorylated p53 to the domains of CBP has been attributed to an increase in electrostatic attraction independent of site-specific affinity; however, it is unclear if this trend applies to KIX, which has been suggested to have a relatively weak response to phosphorylation of p53 compared to other CBP/p300 domains [43]. Our results show that an increase in negative charge of p53TAD alone is not sufficient to significantly increase binding affinity for KIX [33]. Instead, it seems that the increase in binding affinity to KIX by p53 phosphorylation may occur by way of a structural change that is not fully replicated in the phosphomimetics produced here. We postulate that the phosphomimetics of p53 created here represent an intermediate phenotype between that of phosphorylated and unphosphorylated p53 and may be useful for future cell and molecular biology studies.

Supplementary Materials: The following are available online at http://www.mdpi.com/2218-273X/9/3/83/s1, Figure S1: Partial phosphorylation yields no chemical shifts in the primary MDM2 binding region.

Author Contributions: Conceptualization, G.D., W.B. and R.L.; methodology, G.D., W.B. and R.L.; validation, G.D., W.B., R.L., and E.G.; formal analysis, G.D., W.B., R.L. and E.G.; investigation, W.D., R.L. and E.G.; resources, G.D., W.B., R.L. and E.G.; data curation, W.B. and R.L.; writing—original draft preparation, G.D., R.L.; writing—review and editing, D.G., W.B., R.L. and E.G.; visualization, G.D., W.B., R.L. and E.G.; supervision, G.D. and W.B.; project administration, G.D.; funding acquisition, G.D.

Funding: G.D. is supported by the National Institutes of Health (2R01CA14124406-A1 and 1R01GM115556-01A1).

Conflicts of Interest: The authors declare no conflict of interest.

References

1. Blagosklonny, M.V. P53: An ubiquitous target of anticancer drugs. *Int. J. Cancer* **2002**, *98*, 161–166. [CrossRef] [PubMed]
2. Chene, P. Targeting p53 in cancer. *Curr. Med. Chem. Anticancer Agents* **2001**, *1*, 151–161. [CrossRef] [PubMed]
3. Hainaut, P.; Hollstein, M. P53 and human cancer: The first ten thousand mutations. *Adv. Cancer Res.* **2000**, *77*, 81–137. [PubMed]
4. Sigal, A.; Rotter, V. Oncogenic mutations of the p53 tumor suppressor: The demons of the guardian of the genome. *Cancer Res.* **2000**, *60*, 6788–6793. [PubMed]
5. Dunker, A.K.; Brown, C.J.; Lawson, J.D.; Iakoucheva, L.M.; Obradovic, Z. Intrinsic disorder and protein function. *Biochemistry* **2002**, *41*, 6573–6582. [CrossRef] [PubMed]
6. Matas, D.; Sigal, A.; Stambolsky, P.; Milyavsky, M.; Weisz, L.; Schwartz, D.; Goldfinger, N.; Rotter, V. Integrity of the n-terminal transcription domain of p53 is required for mutant p53 interference with drug-induced apoptosis. *EMBO J.* **2001**, *20*, 4163–4172. [CrossRef] [PubMed]
7. Dunker, A.K.; Silman, I.; Uversky, V.N.; Sussman, J.L. Function and structure of inherently disordered proteins. *Curr. Opin. Struct. Biol.* **2008**, *18*, 756–764. [CrossRef] [PubMed]
8. Uversky, V.N. Intrinsically disordered proteins and novel strategies for drug discovery. *Expert Opin. Drug Discov.* **2012**, *7*, 475–488. [CrossRef] [PubMed]
9. van der Lee, R.; Buljan, M.; Lang, B.; Weatheritt, R.J.; Daughdrill, G.W.; Dunker, A.K.; Fuxreiter, M.; Gough, J.; Gsponer, J.; Jones, D.T.; et al. Classification of intrinsically disordered regions and proteins. *Chem. Rev.* **2014**, *114*, 6589–6631. [CrossRef] [PubMed]
10. Ferreon, J.C.; Lee, C.W.; Arai, M.; Martinez-Yamout, M.A.; Dyson, H.J.; Wright, P.E. Cooperative regulation of p53 by modulation of ternary complex formation with cbp/p300 and hdm2. *Proc. Natl. Acad. Sci. USA* **2009**, *106*, 6591. [CrossRef] [PubMed]
11. Oda, K.; Arakawa, H.; Tanaka, T.; Matsuda, K.; Tanikawa, C.; Mori, T.; Nishimori, H.; Tamai, K.; Tokino, T.; Nakamura, Y.; et al. P53aip1, a potential mediator of p53-dependent apoptosis, and its regulation by Ser-46-phosphorylated p53. *Cell* **2000**, *102*, 849–862. [CrossRef]
12. Scoumanne, A.; Harms, K.L.; Chen, X. Structural basis for gene activation by p53 family members. *Cancer Biol. Ther.* **2005**, *4*, 1178–1185. [CrossRef] [PubMed]
13. Lee, S.H.; Kim, D.H.; Han, J.J.; Cha, E.J.; Lim, J.E.; Cho, Y.J.; Lee, C.; Han, K.H. Understanding pre-structured motifs (presmos) in intrinsically unfolded proteins. *Curr. Protein Pept. Sci.* **2012**, *13*, 34–54. [CrossRef] [PubMed]
14. Oldfield, C.J.; Dunker, A.K. Intrinsically disordered proteins and intrinsically disordered protein regions. *Annu. Rev. Biochem.* **2014**, *83*, 553–584. [CrossRef] [PubMed]
15. Crabtree, M.D.; Borcherds, W.; Poosapati, A.; Shammas, S.L.; Daughdrill, G.W.; Clarke, J. Conserved helix-flanking prolines modulate intrinsically disordered protein:Target affinity by altering the lifetime of the bound complex. *Biochemistry* **2017**, *56*, 2379–2384. [CrossRef] [PubMed]

16. Bah, A.; Forman-Kay, J.D. Modulation of intrinsically disordered protein function by post-translational modifications. *J. Biol. Chem.* **2016**, *291*, 6696–6705. [CrossRef] [PubMed]
17. Bah, A.; Vernon, R.M.; Siddiqui, Z.; Krzeminski, M.; Muhandiram, R.; Zhao, C.; Sonenberg, N.; Kay, L.E.; Forman-Kay, J.D. Folding of an intrinsically disordered protein by phosphorylation as a regulatory switch. *Nature* **2015**, *519*, 106–109. [CrossRef] [PubMed]
18. Oren, M. Regulation of the p53 tumor suppressor protein. *J. Biol. Chem.* **1999**, *274*, 36031–36034. [CrossRef] [PubMed]
19. Donehower, L.A.; Harvey, M.; Slagle, B.L.; McArthur, M.J.; Montgomery, C.A., Jr.; Butel, J.S.; Bradley, A. Mice deficient for p53 are developmentally normal but susceptible to spontaneous tumours. *Nature* **1992**, *356*, 215–221. [CrossRef] [PubMed]
20. Oliner, J.D.; Kinzler, K.W.; Meltzer, P.S.; George, D.L.; Vogelstein, B. Amplification of a gene encoding a p53-associated protein in human sarcomas. *Nature* **1992**, *358*, 80–83. [CrossRef] [PubMed]
21. Badciong, J.C.; Haas, A.L. Mdmx is a ring finger ubiquitin ligase capable of synergistically enhancing Mdm2 ubiquitination. *J. Biol. Chem.* **2002**, *277*, 49668–49675. [CrossRef] [PubMed]
22. Picksley, S.M.; Lane, D.P. The p53-Mdm2 autoregulatory feedback loop: A paradigm for the regulation of growth control by p53? *Bioessays* **1993**, *15*, 689–690. [CrossRef] [PubMed]
23. Wienken, M.; Dickmanns, A.; Nemajerova, A.; Kramer, D.; Najafova, Z.; Weiss, M.; Karpiuk, O.; Kassem, M.; Zhang, Y.; Lozano, G.; et al. Mdm2 associates with polycomb repressor complex 2 and enhances stemness-promoting chromatin modifications independent of p53. *Mol. Cell* **2016**, *61*, 68–83. [CrossRef] [PubMed]
24. Shvarts, A.; Steegenga, W.T.; Riteco, N.; van Laar, T.; Dekker, P.; Bazuine, M.; van Ham, R.C.; van der Houven van Oordt, W.; Hateboer, G.; van der Eb, A.J.; et al. Mdmx: A novel p53-binding protein with some functional properties of Mdm2. *EMBO J.* **1996**, *15*, 5349–5357. [CrossRef] [PubMed]
25. Stad, R.; Little, N.A.; Xirodimas, D.P.; Frenk, R.; van der Eb, A.J.; Lane, D.P.; Saville, M.K.; Jochemsen, A.G. Mdmx stabilizes p53 and Mdm2 via two distinct mechanisms. *EMBO Rep.* **2001**, *2*, 1029–1034. [CrossRef] [PubMed]
26. Haupt, Y.; Maya, R.; Kazaz, A.; Oren, M. Mdm2 promotes the rapid degradation of p53. *Nature* **1997**, *387*, 296–299. [CrossRef] [PubMed]
27. Kubbutat, M.H.; Jones, S.N.; Vousden, K.H. Regulation of p53 stability by Mdm2. *Nature* **1997**, *387*, 299–303. [CrossRef] [PubMed]
28. Francoz, S.; Froment, P.; Bogaerts, S.; De Clercq, S.; Maetens, M.; Doumont, G.; Bellefroid, E.; Marine, J.C. Mdm4 and Mdm2 cooperate to inhibit p53 activity in proliferating and quiescent cells *in vivo*. *Proc. Natl. Acad. Sci. USA* **2006**, *103*, 3232–3237. [CrossRef] [PubMed]
29. Xiong, S.; Van Pelt, C.S.; Elizondo-Fraire, A.C.; Liu, G.; Lozano, G. Synergistic roles of Mdm2 and Mdm4 for p53 inhibition in central nervous system development. *Proc. Natl. Acad. Sci. USA* **2006**, *103*, 3226–3231. [CrossRef] [PubMed]
30. Jabbur, J.R.; Tabor, A.D.; Cheng, X.; Wang, H.; Uesugi, M.; Lozano, G.; Zhang, W. Mdm-2 binding and TAF$_{II}$31 recruitment is regulated by hydrogen bond disruption between the p53 residues Thr18 and Asp21. *Oncogene* **2002**, *21*, 7100–7113. [CrossRef] [PubMed]
31. Serrano, M.A.; Li, Z.; Dangeti, M.; Musich, P.R.; Patrick, S.; Roginskaya, M.; Cartwright, B.; Zou, Y. DNA-PK, ATM and ATR collaboratively regulate p53-RPA interaction to facilitate homologous recombination DNA repair. *Oncogene* **2013**, *32*, 2452–2462. [CrossRef] [PubMed]
32. Shieh, S.Y.; Ikeda, M.; Taya, Y.; Prives, C. DNA damage-induced phosphorylation of p53 alleviates inhibition by Mdm2. *Cell* **1997**, *91*, 325–334. [CrossRef]
33. Lee, C.W.; Ferreon, J.C.; Ferreon, A.C.; Arai, M.; Wright, P.E. Graded enhancement of p53 binding to CREB-binding protein (CBP) by multisite phosphorylation. *Proc. Natl. Acad. Sci. USA* **2010**, *107*, 19290–19295. [CrossRef] [PubMed]
34. Bottger, V.; Bottger, A.; Garcia-Echeverria, C.; Ramos, Y.F.; van der Eb, A.J.; Jochemsen, A.G.; Lane, D.P. Comparative study of the p53-Mdm2 and p53-Mmdmx interfaces. *Oncogene* **1999**, *18*, 189–199. [CrossRef] [PubMed]
35. Baresova, P.; Musilova, J.; Pitha, P.M.; Lubyova, B. P53 tumor suppressor protein stability and transcriptional activity are targeted by Kaposi's Sarcoma-associated herpesvirus-encoded viral interferon regulatory factor 3. *Mol. Cell. Biol.* **2014**, *34*, 386–399. [CrossRef] [PubMed]

36. Dumaz, N.; Milne, D.M.; Meek, D.W. Protein kinase CK1 is a p53-threonine 18 kinase which requires prior phosphorylation of serine 15. *FEBS Lett.* **1999**, *463*, 312–316. [CrossRef]
37. Saito, S.; Yamaguchi, H.; Higashimoto, Y.; Chao, C.; Xu, Y.; Fornace, A.J., Jr.; Appella, E.; Anderson, C.W. Phosphorylation site interdependence of human p53 post-translational modifications in response to stress. *J. Biol. Chem.* **2003**, *278*, 37536–37544. [CrossRef] [PubMed]
38. McKinney, K.; Prives, C. Efficient specific DNA binding by p53 requires both its central and C-terminal domains as revealed by studies with high-mobility group 1 protein. *Mol. Cell. Biol.* **2002**, *22*, 6797–6808. [CrossRef] [PubMed]
39. Dumaz, N.; Meek, D.W. Serine15 phosphorylation stimulates p53 transactivation but does not directly influence interaction with HDM2. *EMBO J.* **1999**, *18*, 7002–7010. [CrossRef] [PubMed]
40. Grossman, S.R.; Perez, M.; Kung, A.L.; Joseph, M.; Mansur, C.; Xiao, Z.X.; Kumar, S.; Howley, P.M.; Livingston, D.M. P300/Mdm2 complexes participate in Mdm2-mediated p53 degradation. *Mol. Cell* **1998**, *2*, 405–415. [CrossRef]
41. Kruse, J.P.; Gu, W. Modes of p53 regulation. *Cell* **2009**, *137*, 609–622. [CrossRef] [PubMed]
42. Teufel, D.P.; Freund, S.M.; Bycroft, M.; Fersht, A.R. Four domains of p300 each bind tightly to a sequence spanning both transactivation subdomains of p53. *Proc. Natl. Acad. Sci. USA* **2007**, *104*, 7009–7014. [CrossRef] [PubMed]
43. Teufel, D.P.; Bycroft, M.; Fersht, A.R. Regulation by phosphorylation of the relative affinities of the N-terminal transactivation domains of p53 for p300 domains and Mdm2. *Oncogene* **2009**, *28*, 2112–2118. [CrossRef] [PubMed]
44. Feng, H.; Jenkins, L.M.; Durell, S.R.; Hayashi, R.; Mazur, S.J.; Cherry, S.; Tropea, J.E.; Miller, M.; Wlodawer, A.; Appella, E.; et al. Structural basis for p300 Taz2-p53 TAD1 binding and modulation by phosphorylation. *Structure* **2009**, *17*, 202–210. [CrossRef] [PubMed]
45. Huang, Y.; Gao, M.; Yang, F.; Zhang, L.; Su, Z. Deciphering the promiscuous interactions between intrinsically disordered transactivation domains and the KIX domain. *Proteins* **2017**, *85*, 2088–2095. [CrossRef] [PubMed]
46. Lee, C.W.; Arai, M.; Martinez-Yamout, M.A.; Dyson, H.J.; Wright, P.E. Mapping the interactions of the p53 transactivation domain with the KIX domain of CBP. *Biochemistry* **2009**, *48*, 2115–2124. [CrossRef] [PubMed]
47. Stock, J.; Da Re, S. Signal transduction: Response regulators on and off. *Curr. Biol.* **2000**, *10*, R420–R424. [CrossRef]
48. Johnson, L.N.; Lewis, R.J. Structural basis for control by phosphorylation. *Chem. Rev.* **2001**, *101*, 2209–2242. [CrossRef] [PubMed]
49. He, Y.; Chen, Y.; Mooney, S.M.; Rajagopalan, K.; Bhargava, A.; Sacho, E.; Weninger, K.; Bryan, P.N.; Kulkarni, P.; Orban, J. Phosphorylation-induced conformational ensemble switching in an intrinsically disordered cancer/testis antigen. *J. Biol. Chem.* **2015**, *290*, 25090–25102. [CrossRef] [PubMed]
50. Kussie, P.H.; Gorina, S.; Marechal, V.; Elenbaas, B.; Moreau, J.; Levine, A.J.; Pavletich, N.P. Structure of the mdm2 oncoprotein bound to the p53 tumor suppressor transactivation domain. *Science* **1996**, *274*, 948–953. [CrossRef] [PubMed]
51. Mavinahalli, J.N.; Madhumalar, A.; Beuerman, R.W.; Lane, D.P.; Verma, C. Differences in the transactivation domains of p53 family members: A computational study. *BMC Genom.* **2010**, *11* (Suppl. 1), S5. [CrossRef] [PubMed]
52. Hol, W.G. The role of the α-helix dipole in protein function and structure. *Prog. Biophys. Mol. Biol.* **1985**, *45*, 149–195. [CrossRef]
53. Sheridan, R.P.; Levy, R.M.; Salemme, F.R. α-helix dipole model and electrostatic stabilization of 4-α-helical proteins. *Proc. Natl. Acad. Sci. USA* **1982**, *79*, 4545–4549. [CrossRef] [PubMed]
54. Guerra-Castellano, A.; Diaz-Moreno, I.; Velazquez-Campoy, A.; De la Rosa, M.A.; Diaz-Quintana, A. Structural and functional characterization of phosphomimetic mutants of cytochrome c at Threonine 28 and Serine 47. *Biochim. Biophys. Acta* **2016**, *1857*, 387–395. [CrossRef] [PubMed]
55. Luwang, J.W.; Natesh, R. Phosphomimetic mutation destabilizes the central core domain of human p53. *IUBMB Life* **2018**, *70*, 1023–1031. [CrossRef] [PubMed]
56. Pecina, P.; Borisenko, G.G.; Belikova, N.A.; Tyurina, Y.Y.; Pecinova, A.; Lee, I.; Samhan-Arias, A.K.; Przyklenk, K.; Kagan, V.E.; Huttemann, M. Phosphomimetic substitution of cytochrome C Tyrosine 48 decreases respiration and binding to cardiolipin and abolishes ability to trigger downstream caspase activation. *Biochemistry* **2010**, *49*, 6705–6714. [CrossRef] [PubMed]

57. Loughery, J.; Cox, M.; Smith, L.M.; Meek, D.W. Critical role for p53-serine 15 phosphorylation in stimulating transactivation at p53-responsive promoters. *Nucleic Acids Res.* **2014**, *42*, 7666–7680. [CrossRef] [PubMed]
58. Johnson, B.A. Using nmrview to visualize and analyze the NMR spectra of macromolecules. *Methods Mol. Biol.* **2004**, *278*, 313–352. [PubMed]
59. Johnson, B.A.; Blevins, R.A. NMR view: A computer program for the visualization and analysis of NMR data. *J. Biomol. NMR* **1994**, *4*, 603–614. [CrossRef] [PubMed]
60. Nielsen, J.T.; Mulder, F.A.A. Potenci: Prediction of temperature, neighbor and pH-corrected chemical shifts for intrinsically disordered proteins. *J. Biomol. NMR* **2018**, *70*, 141–165. [CrossRef] [PubMed]
61. Camilloni, C.; De Simone, A.; Vranken, W.F.; Vendruscolo, M. Determination of secondary structure populations in disordered states of proteins using nuclear magnetic resonance chemical shifts. *Biochemistry* **2012**, *51*, 2224–2231. [CrossRef] [PubMed]
62. Theillet, F.X.; Rose, H.M.; Liokatis, S.; Binolfi, A.; Thongwichian, R.; Stuiver, M.; Selenko, P. Site-specific nmr mapping and time-resolved monitoring of serine and threonine phosphorylation in reconstituted kinase reactions and mammalian cell extracts. *Nat. Protoc.* **2013**, *8*, 1416–1432. [CrossRef] [PubMed]
63. Gokirmak, T.; Denison, F.C.; Laughner, B.J.; Paul, A.L.; Ferl, R.J. Phosphomimetic mutation of a conserved serine residue in arabidopsis thaliana 14-3-3omega suggests a regulatory role of phosphorylation in dimerization and target interactions. *Plant Physiol. Biochem.* **2015**, *97*, 296–303. [CrossRef] [PubMed]
64. Cheng, Q.; Chen, L.; Li, Z.; Lane, W.S.; Chen, J. ATM activates p53 by regulating Mdm2 oligomerization and E3 processivity. *EMBO J.* **2009**, *28*, 3857–3867. [CrossRef] [PubMed]
65. Cheng, Q.; Cross, B.; Li, B.; Chen, L.; Li, Z.; Chen, J. Regulation of Mdm2 E3 ligase activity by phosphorylation after DNA damage. *Mol. Cell. Biol.* **2011**, *31*, 4951–4963. [CrossRef] [PubMed]
66. Nakamizo, A.; Amano, T.; Zhang, W.; Zhang, X.Q.; Ramdas, L.; Liu, T.J.; Bekele, B.N.; Shono, T.; Sasaki, T.; Benedict, W.F.; et al. Phosphorylation of Thr18 and Ser20 of p53 in AD-p53-induced apoptosis. *Neuro Oncol.* **2008**, *10*, 275–291. [CrossRef] [PubMed]
67. Sato, Y.; Kamura, T.; Shirata, N.; Murata, T.; Kudoh, A.; Iwahori, S.; Nakayama, S.; Isomura, H.; Nishiyama, Y.; Tsurumi, T. Degradation of phosphorylated p53 by viral protein-ECS E3 ligase complex. *PLoS Pathog.* **2009**, *5*, e1000530. [CrossRef] [PubMed]
68. Jane Dyson, H.; Ewright, P. Insights into the structure and dynamics of unfolded proteins from nuclear magnetic resonance. In *Advances in Protein Chemistry*; Academic Press: Cambridge, MA, USA, 2002; Volume 62, pp. 311–340.
69. Borcherds, W.M.; Daughdrill, G.W. Using nmr chemical shifts to determine residue-specific secondary structure populations for intrinsically disordered proteins. *Methods Enzymol.* **2018**, *611*, 101–136. [PubMed]
70. Bista, M.; Wolf, S.; Khoury, K.; Kowalska, K.; Huang, Y.; Wrona, E.; Arciniega, M.; Popowicz, G.M.; Holak, T.A.; Domling, A. Transient protein states in designing inhibitors of the Mdm2-p53 interaction. *Structure* **2013**, *21*, 2143–2151. [CrossRef] [PubMed]
71. Chan, J.V.; Ping Koh, D.X.; Liu, Y.; Joseph, T.L.; Lane, D.P.; Verma, C.S.; Tan, Y.S. Role of the N-terminal lid in regulating the interaction of phosphorylated Mmdmx with p53. *Oncotarget* **2017**, *8*, 112825–112840. [CrossRef] [PubMed]
72. McCoy, M.A.; Gesell, J.J.; Senior, M.M.; Wyss, D.F. Flexible lid to the p53-binding domain of human Mdm2: Implications for p53 regulation. *Proc. Natl. Acad. Sci. USA* **2003**, *100*, 1645–1648. [CrossRef] [PubMed]
73. Pierce, M.M.; Raman, C.S.; Nall, B.T. Isothermal titration calorimetry of protein-protein interactions. *Methods* **1999**, *19*, 213–221. [CrossRef] [PubMed]
74. Rajarathnam, K.; Rosgen, J. Isothermal titration calorimetry of membrane proteins—Progress and challenges. *Biochim. Biophys. Acta* **2014**, *1838*, 69–77. [CrossRef] [PubMed]
75. Borcherds, W.; Theillet, F.-X.; Katzer, A.; Finzel, A.; Mishall, K.M.; Powell, A.T.; Wu, H.; Manieri, W.; Dieterich, C.; Selenko, P.; et al. Disorder and residual helicity alter p53-Mdm2 binding affinity and signaling in cells. *Nat. Chem. Biol.* **2014**, *10*, 1000. [CrossRef] [PubMed]
76. Fraser, J.A.; Madhumalar, A.; Blackburn, E.; Bramham, J.; Walkinshaw, M.D.; Verma, C.; Hupp, T.R. A novel p53 phosphorylation site within the Mdm2 ubiquitination signal: II. A model in which phosphorylation at ser269 induces a mutant conformation to p53. *J. Biol. Chem.* **2010**, *285*, 37773–37786. [CrossRef] [PubMed]
77. Lu, M.; Breyssens, H.; Salter, V.; Zhong, S.; Hu, Y.; Baer, C.; Ratnayaka, I.; Sullivan, A.; Brown, N.R.; Endicott, J.; et al. Restoring p53 function in human melanoma cells by inhibiting MDM2 and cyclin B1/CDK1-phosphorylated nuclear iASPP. *Cancer Cell* **2016**, *30*, 822–823. [CrossRef] [PubMed]

78. Freyer, M.W.; Lewis, E.A. Isothermal titration calorimetry: Experimental design, data analysis, and probing macromolecule/ligand binding and kinetic interactions. *Methods Cell Biol.* **2008**, *84*, 79–113. [PubMed]
79. Pise-Masison, C.A.; Radonovich, M.; Sakaguchi, K.; Appella, E.; Brady, J.N. Phosphorylation of p53: A novel pathway for p53 inactivation in human T-cell lymphotropic virus type 1-transformed cells. *J. Virol.* **1998**, *72*, 6348–6355. [PubMed]
80. Sakaguchi, K.; Saito, S.; Higashimoto, Y.; Roy, S.; Anderson, C.W.; Appella, E. Damage-mediated phosphorylation of human p53 threonine 18 through a cascade mediated by a casein 1-like kinase. Effect on Mdm2 binding. *J. Biol. Chem.* **2000**, *275*, 9278–9283. [CrossRef] [PubMed]
81. Schon, O.; Friedler, A.; Bycroft, M.; Freund, S.M.; Fersht, A.R. Molecular mechanism of the interaction between Mdm2 and p53. *J. Mol. Biol.* **2002**, *323*, 491–501. [CrossRef]
82. Yadahalli, S.; Neira, J.L.; Johnson, C.M.; Tan, Y.S.; Rowling, P.J.E.; Chattopadhyay, A.; Verma, C.S.; Itzhaki, L.S. Kinetic and thermodynamic effects of phosphorylation on p53 binding to Mdm2. *Sci. Rep.* **2019**, *9*, 693. [CrossRef] [PubMed]
83. Vega, F.M.; Sevilla, A.; Lazo, P.A. P53 stabilization and accumulation induced by human vaccinia-related kinase 1. *Mol. Cell. Biol.* **2004**, *24*, 10366–10380. [CrossRef] [PubMed]
84. Dornan, D.; Hupp, T.R. Inhibition of p53-dependent transcription by BOX-I phospho-peptide mimetics that bind to p300. *EMBO Rep.* **2001**, *2*, 139–144. [CrossRef] [PubMed]

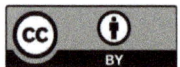

© 2019 by the authors. Licensee MDPI, Basel, Switzerland. This article is an open access article distributed under the terms and conditions of the Creative Commons Attribution (CC BY) license (http://creativecommons.org/licenses/by/4.0/).

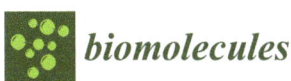

Article

Functional Segments on Intrinsically Disordered Regions in Disease-Related Proteins

Hiroto Anbo, Masaya Sato, Atsushi Okoshi and Satoshi Fukuchi *

Department of Life Science and Informatics, Faculty of Engineering, Maebashi Institute of Technology, 460-1, Kamisadori, Maebashi, Gunma 371-0816, Japan; koume8@icloud.com (H.A.); mail_address107@icloud.com (M.S.); m1461008@maebashi-it.ac.jp (A.O.)
* Correspondence: sfukuchi@maebashi-it.ac.jp

Received: 22 January 2019; Accepted: 25 February 2019; Published: 5 March 2019

Abstract: One of the unique characteristics of intrinsically disordered proteins (IPDs) is the existence of functional segments in intrinsically disordered regions (IDRs). A typical function of these segments is binding to partner molecules, such as proteins and DNAs. These segments play important roles in signaling pathways and transcriptional regulation. We conducted bioinformatics analysis to search these functional segments based on IDR predictions and database annotations. We found more than a thousand potential functional IDR segments in disease-related proteins. Large fractions of proteins related to cancers, congenital disorders, digestive system diseases, and reproductive system diseases have these functional IDRs. Some proteins in nervous system diseases have long functional segments in IDRs. The detailed analysis of some of these regions showed that the functional segments are located on experimentally verified IDRs. The proteins with functional IDR segments generally tend to come and go between the cytoplasm and the nucleus. Proteins involved in multiple diseases tend to have more protein-protein interactors, suggesting that hub proteins in the protein-protein interaction networks can have multiple impacts on human diseases.

Keywords: intrinsically disordered regions; functional segments; disease-related proteins; protein-protein interaction; subcellular location

---

1. Introduction

Intrinsically disordered proteins (IDPs) are proteins that do not adopt unique three-dimensional structures under physiological conditions [1–3]. They are fully or partially disordered and are abundant among eukaryotic proteins [4–6]. One of the unique features of IDPs is their ability to bind to binding partners. The regions performing such binding are generally short segments ranging from several residues to tens of residues and can adopt local two-dimensional structures in association with this binding. This has been referred to as the coupled folding and binding mechanism. These interactions are transient, specific, and low-affinity. Through this mechanism, intrinsically disordered regions (IDRs) play crucial roles in many biological processes, such as signal transduction and transcriptional regulation [1–3,7].

The importance of IDPs in human diseases has been reported [8,9]. Intrinsically disordered proteins are found in high concentrations in plaques and brain deposits in neurodegenerative patients, and mutations in IDRs can increase aggregation propensity. Intrinsically disordered proteins such as α-synuclein, the amyloid β peptide, and huntingtin have been directly linked to diseases such as Alzheimer's, Parkinson's, and Huntington's diseases [10–16]. It has been shown that many IDPs participate in cell signaling and cancer-associated proteins [7]. Breast cancer type 1 susceptibility protein (BRCA1) is one of the most typical IDPs, with a long central region of 1480 residues shown to be disordered by nuclear magnetic resonance (NMR) and circular dichroism (CD) spectroscopy [17]. This long IDR has many binding segments for proteins such as p53, retinoblastoma protein, and the oncogenes c-Myc and JunB. p53 Is a transcription factor that has IDRs in its N- and C-terminus. These IDRs have binding sites for many partner proteins. Among these, the interaction between p53 and E3 ubiquitin-protein ligase Mdm2 (MDM2) has been given much attention in cancer research, as p53 can induce apoptosis to suppress tumor progression [18,19]. Bioinformatics work has also shown that IDRs are rich in proteins involved in cancer, neurodegenerative diseases, cardiovascular diseases, and diabetes [9,20]. Intrinsically disordered proteins have gained attention as drug targets. Inhibitors targeting IDR and globular domain interactions have been developed for the interaction between Bcl-xL and BAK [21,22], MDM2 and p53 [23], interleukin (IL)-2 receptor α and IL-2 [24,25], XIAP and Smac [26,27], and CBP and β-catenin [28].

As shown above, protein–protein interactions (PPIs) occurring on IDRs have high potential as drug targets. The IDP databases, IDEAL [29,30] and DisProt [31], have 913 and 803 proteins, and IDEAL has collected 559 protein-binding segments on IDRs called "protean segments (ProSs)" in the database. Protean segments are defined as sequences with experimental evidence of being both disordered in an isolated state and ordered in a binding state. In contrast, several tools for predicting such binding regions have been developed to suggest that there are more than 100,000 protein-binding segments in the human proteome [32]. Considering this prediction, our knowledge on IDR-mediated interactions is still limited because the number of ProSs with experimental evidence of ordered and disordered states is only about 600. However, we have a lot of PPI data accumulating and several computer programs to predict IDRs. The performance of IDR predictions has reached a standard for practical use, and PPI annotations found in predicted IDRs can be considered protein-binding segments in IDRs. In this study, we combined the annotations of the UniProt database and IDR predictions to find these possible protein-binding regions on IDRs and analyzed these regions in the context of human disease.

2. Materials and Methods

We selected human proteins from the Swiss-Prot section of the UniProt XML file [33] from UniProt release 2018_07. We extracted the feature (FT) section information. A single FT section has a feature type, a description, and a location, and all of them were extracted. The IDEAL database provides binding segments in IDRs as "ProSs". Protean segments are mostly short segments consisting of less than 30 amino acid residues to which more than 80% of ProSs belong. Thus, we selected for feature information shorter than 30 residues. Next, we picked binding-associated features from the selected features. By manually surveying feature descriptions, the features "region of interest" and "mutagenesis site" are found to contain binding-related features. Adding to these two features, "short sequence motif" also contains functional segments in IDRs. Out of the selected features of "region of interest", the features having the terms "interact", "bind", or "motif" in their description were selected. Of the "mutagenesis site" features, those with "interact" or "bind" were selected. From the selected features of "mutagenesis site", those having "no" or "not" were discarded. We wrote some in-house scripts to find the selected features located in IDRs. A feature region found in an IDR was defined as a possible ProS, hereafter referred to as a pProS.

We used three predictors for IDR prediction. MobiDB [31] provided predicted IDRs for several proteome datasets. We downloaded the human proteome dataset and used MobiDB-lite [34] predictions for predicted IDRs. MobiDB-lite uses eight different predictors, three variants of ESpritz (DisProt, NMR, X-ray), two variants of IUpred (long, short), two variants of DisEMBL (465, hot loops), and GlobPlot. MobiDB-lite uses the results of these predictors to combine them into a consensus result, where at least five out of eight methods must define a residue as disordered. Thus, the predicted IDRs reflect different types of predictions at one time. DISOPRED3 [35] is an extension of the previous program, DISOPRED2, to improve predictions of long IDRs. In order to achieve this goal, DISOPRED3 uses a neural network-based predictors trained on a dataset rich in long IDRs. The training was done on a position-specific scoring matrix (PSSM) generated by PSI-BLAST. This program is one of the benchmark IDR predictors, which was one of the top ranked predictors in CASP10 [36]. DICHOT is the predictor combining the homology-based domain assignments and the support vector machine learning. First, it conducts a PSI-BLAST search against the Protein Data Bank (PDB) to mask structural regions, and then the unmasked regions are judged by using the support vector machine-based predictor trained on a multiple alignment of homologs. This predictor divides an entire amino acid chain into structural domains and IDRs, which is unique compared to other predictors. We selected regions where any of the two predictors predicted an IDR.

Human disease information was obtained from the KEGG database [37]. KEGG has a collection of disease entries called KEGG DISEASE. KEGG DISEASE provides Search Disease, which is a mapping tool against disease genes accumulated in KEGG DISEASE entries. Thus, the Search Disease tool provides information on which disease a protein is involved in. The mapped disease-related proteins were divided into pProS-containing proteins and non-pProS proteins, according to the existence or absence of pProSs.

We used the UniProt annotations of subcellular locations for protein localizations. We counted terms that appeared in the annotations by the disease-related proteins and all human proteins. We defined those proteins as only having the annotation of nucleus as nuclear protein, those proteins only having that of cytoplasm as cytoplasm protein, those only having that of membrane as membrane protein, and those having both of the annotations of cytoplasm and nucleus as cytoplasm and nuclear protein. The annotations of other locations were discarded because of shortages of appearance. The disease-related proteins were further divided into pProS-containing proteins and non-pProS proteins, and the ratios of each of the terms were obtained for the disease-related proteins and all human proteins. The logarithms of the ratios of two ratios were used in analysis.

The brief outline of the procedure can be found in Supplementary Figure S1.

3. Results

The UniProt database has 20,410 human proteins, and 3378 proteins (16.6%) were assigned human diseases by the Search Disease tool, as shown in Table 1. In the human UniProt and the disease-related proteins, 29,145 and 18,450 regions of the feature annotation shorter than 30 residues were found, respectively. From these regions, we selected the feature annotations of "region of interest", "mutagenesis site", and "short sequence motif" to pick up pProSs. Out of 3378 disease related proteins, 402 proteins (11.9%) had pProSs. Out of 18,450 feature annotations found in the disease related proteins, 8.3%, 3.4%, and 24.4% were found in the predicted IDRs for "region of interest", "mutagenesis site", and "short sequence motif", respectively. Thus, the regions of these annotations are defined as pProSs in this study.

Table 1. Statistics of the UniProt annotations.

	All Proteins	Disease-Related	pProS	pProS (%)
No. proteins	20,410	3378	402	11.9
No. annotations shorter than 30 residues	29,145	18,450	1124	6.1
"Region of interest"	4646	2656	220	8.3
"Mutagenesis site"	21,269	14,056	479	3.4
"Short sequence motif"	3230	1740	425	24.4

pProS: Possible protean segment.

We illustrate how these annotations occur in IDRs in Figure 1. In this study, some of the proteins are stored in the IDEAL database [38]. In such cases, we denoted IDEAL identifiers for reference. p53 is one of the typical IDPs and has relatively short IDRs in the N- and C-terminus in addition to between the DNA-binding domain and the tetramerization domain (IDEAL: IID00015). p53 has three annotations from residues 15 to 25, one annotation from residues 48 to 56, one annotation from 305 to 321, four annotations from 359 to 363, and one annotation from 370 to 372 and 368 to 387. Among them, "TAD I", "TAD II", "bipartite nuclear localization signal" and "[KR]-[STA]-K motif" are from "short sequence motif", "interaction with USP7" and "basic" are from "region of interest", and "loss of interactions with MDM2", "loss of interaction with PPP2R5C, PPP2CA and PPP2R1A", and "abolishes binding to USP7" are from "mutagenesis site". As shown in Figure 1, some of these annotations overlap each other. We counted these overlapped annotations separately in the statistics in this study because they can be different annotations even if their regions are overlapped. For example, although "TAD I" overlaps "loss of interaction with MDM2" and "loss of interaction with PPP2R5C, PPP2CA and PPP2R1A", they describe different phenomena. Thus, we would like readers to note that the statistics in this study contain such multiple counts in some cases.

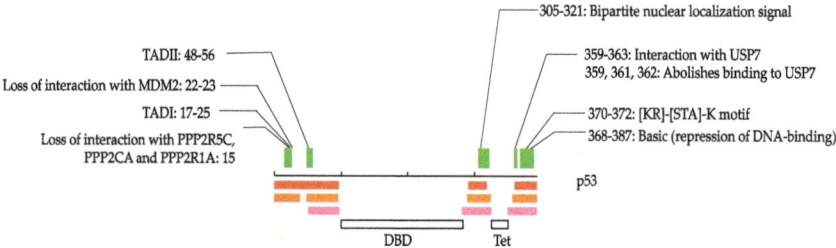

Figure 1. An example of possible protean segment (pProS) definition, illustrated by p53. The black line in the middle represents the amino acid chain, and the intrinsically disordered regions (IDR) predictions are presented below. Pink, orange, and red represent the results by MobiDB-lite, DISOPRED3, and DICHOT, respectively. Regions where any of the two methods predict IDR are defined as IDRs. The green bars represent pProSs, and the annotations defining pProS are shown above with residue numbers of the annotations. DBD: DNA-binding domain; Tet: Tetramerization domain.

Most of the annotations we picked in this analysis occur at one time in the dataset. As seen in the example of p53, the annotations of interest in this study are in forms such as "interaction with protein A" or "loss of interaction with protein B", etc., which can be assigned on a single or a small numbers of proteins binding onto a specific protein. However, some of the annotations appeared multiple times. These frequently appearing annotations in pProSs are listed in Supplementary Table S1. They contain targeting sequences, such as a nuclear localization signal (NLS). Retinoblastoma-associated protein has an NLS from residues 858 to 881. This region has been described as disordered in the isolated state [39], though the binding structure with importin has been solved (IDEAL: IID00017) [40]. Another class of frequently found annotations is segments binding upon promiscuously interacting domains, such as the SH3 domain and the PDZ domain. The SH3 domain mediates PPIs via a short ambiguous peptide motif to assemble cell regulatory systems [41] and is annotated as ProS in the IDEAL database (IDEAL: IIDE00256). The PDZ domain is a scaffold protein that forms protein complexes in signaling pathways or cell trafficking [42]. The binding segment is disordered in an isolated state (IDEAL: IID9005) [43]. We also frequently found the LXXLL motif, which exists in co-repressors or co-activators of nuclear receptors. The LXXLL motif in peroxisome proliferator-activated receptor gamma co-activator 1 α has been reported as disordered, and the binding structure with steroid hormone receptor has been elucidated (IDEAL: IID00103) [44,45].

The disease-related proteins are classified into 15 categories by KEGG DISEASE, which are: cancers (Can); cardiovascular diseases (Car); congenital disorders of metabolism (Dme); congenital malformations (Mal); digestive system diseases (Dig); endocrine and metabolic diseases (End); immune system diseases (Imm); musculoskeletal diseases (Mus); nervous system diseases (Ner); other congenital disorders (Oco); reproductive system diseases (Rep); respiratory diseases (Res); skin diseases (Ski); urinary system diseases (Uri); and other diseases (Oth). These categories have subcategories into which these diseases are classified. The details of the disease classifications can be found on the web page for KEGG DISEASE [46].

We classified disease-related proteins into the disease categories and showed the statistics in Table 2. The rank of the numbers of unique pProSs is as follows, in descending order: "congenital malformations"; "nervous system diseases"; "cancers"; and "cardiovascular diseases". The numbers depend on the number of proteins in each of the categories, as seen in Table 2. However, the category possessing many proteins does not necessarily contain many pProSs. For example, the "congenital disorders of metabolism" contains 687 proteins, though only 40 pProSs were identified. The values of protein coverage represent the ratio of the numbers of pProS-containing proteins to the numbers of proteins in a category. "cancers" shows the top coverage, followed by "congenital disorders," "digestive system diseases," and "reproductive system diseases." The average values of annotations represent the values of the number of pProSs in a category divided by the number of pProS-containing proteins, wherein most of the values are greater than 2. As shown in Figure 1, some annotations are found in different regions, and some annotations overlap each other. The average annotation values here contain both cases. The annotations of "mutagenesis site" tend to overlap with other annotations, where 70% of them coincide with other annotations. This overlap of "mutagenesis site" may enlarge the average annotation values. The total amount of proteins with pProS over all disease categories differs from the number of pProS-containing proteins shown in Table 1. This is because some proteins were assigned to multiple diseases.

Table 2. Statistics of pProS by the disease category.

Category	No. Unique pProSs	No. Proteins with pProS	No. Proteins	Protein Coverage (%)	Average Annotations
Cancers	147	57	204	27.9	2.6
Cardiovascular diseases	93	41	335	12.2	2.3
Congenital disorders of metabolism	53	40	687	5.8	1.3
Congenital malformations	242	111	832	13.3	2.2
Digestive system diseases	32	15	79	19.0	2.1
Endocrine and metabolic diseases	63	30	213	14.1	2.1
Immune system diseases	56	31	256	12.1	1.8
Musculoskeletal diseases	69	26	149	17.4	2.7
Nervous system diseases	199	95	795	11.9	2.1
Other congenital disorders	39	20	91	22.0	2.0
Reproductive system diseases	21	12	63	19.0	1.8
Respiratory diseases	1	1	55	1.8	1.0
Skin diseases	22	14	104	13.5	1.6
Urinary system diseases	33	9	66	13.6	3.7
Other diseases	68	30	194	15.5	2.3

Figure 2 shows the IDR ratios by the disease categories. The IDR ratio of all disease proteins (27.0%) is similar to that of the UniProt human proteins (28.7%, the dashed line in Figure 2). However, the IDR fractions of each category differ, where "cancers," "congenital malformations", "other congenital disorders", "reproductive system diseases", and "other diseases" are over-represented. These IDR-rich categories also have high fractions of IDRs in the pProS-containing proteins. Although the IDR fractions of pProS-containing proteins correlate with the protein coverage (Table 2), a high fraction of IDRs does not necessarily mean high protein coverage. For example, although "urinary diseases" shows a very high IDR fraction in their pProS-containing proteins, the protein coverage is not high. This means that the pProS-containing proteins in this category contain high fractions of IDR, but a number of non-pProS-containing proteins also belong to this category. On the other hand, "musculoskeletal diseases" has low IDR fractions in both pProS-containing proteins and all proteins. However, the protein coverage is relatively high, suggesting that many proteins with relatively short IDR fractions have functional regions in such IDRs. Iakoucheva et al. [7] showed that cancer related proteins have high fractions of IDRs, and the result of the present analysis confirms this trend. Moreover, the current results suggest that cancer-related proteins have a lot of pProSs compared to the proteins in the other categories.

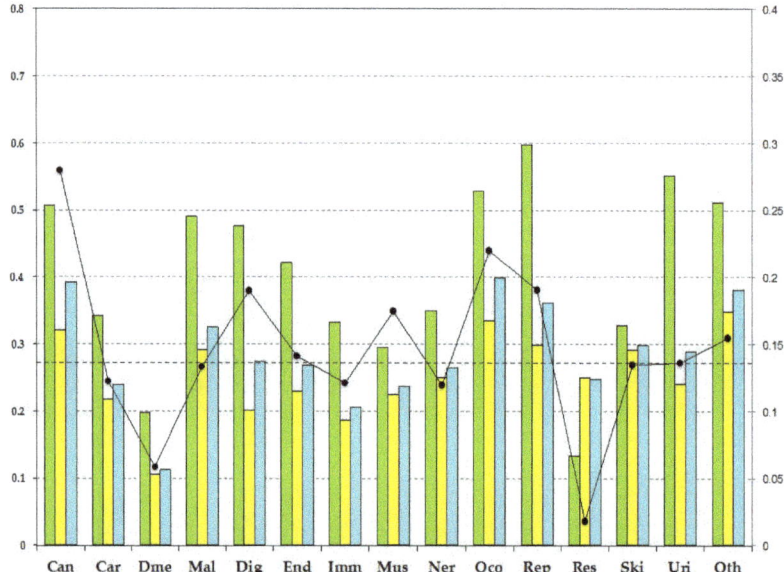

Figure 2. The IDR ratios by disease category. The green, yellow, and blue bars represent the IDR fractions of the pProS-containing proteins, the non-pProS proteins, and the total proteins in each of the disease categories, respectively. The measure on the left axis represents the IDR fractions. The black line with dots represents the protein coverage found in Table 2. The measure on the right axis represents the protein coverage. The dashed line represents the IDR ratio of the human proteome. Can: Cancers; Car: Cardiovascular diseases; Dme: Congenital disorders of metabolism; Mal: Congenital malformations; Dig: Digestive system diseases; End: Endocrine and metabolic diseases; Imm: Immune system diseases; Mus: Musculoskeletal diseases; Ner: Nervous system diseases; Oco: Other congenital disorders; Rep: Reproductive system diseases; Res: Respiratory diseases; Ski: Skin diseases; Uri: Urinary system diseases; Oth: Other diseases.

Table 3 shows the top-ranked proteins in terms of the numbers of pProS residues. Although we counted overlapped annotations separately in Table 2, we counted "pPros residues" without redundancy. For example, when there are annotations of "from 360 to 365" and "from 360 to 362", we counted six for this region. "Cancers" and p53 appear again, and the proteins belonging to "nervous system diseases" are listed frequently. As shown in Figure 2, "cancers" has the largest IDR fraction and the top ranked protein coverage. Thus, it is natural for the proteins in "cancers" to contain proteins with a large fraction of pProS residues. On the other hand, "nervous system diseases" has an IDR fraction smaller than that of the UniProt human proteins, and the protein coverage is low. Therefore, the proteins in "nervous system diseases" do not generally contain a large fraction of IDR and pProS. However, some of them have long pProSs, even in relatively short IDRs. On the other hand, "nervous system diseases" has an IDR fraction smaller than that of the UniProt human proteins. Raychaudhuri et al. reported similar results, where in the nervous system disease related proteins, Huntington's and Alzheimer's disease proteins have large fractions of IDRs, and Parkinson's disease proteins do not [20], suggesting the similarity of the average IDR fraction of these nervous disease proteins to that of UniProt human proteins. Therefore, the proteins in "nervous system diseases" do not generally contain a large fraction of IDR and pProS. However, some of them have long pProSs, even in relatively short IDRs. The example of "nervous system diseases" suggests that even if the IDR fraction and protein coverage of pProS-containing proteins are low, some proteins in a disease category can have considerable lengths of pProSs.

Table 3. The list of the proteins with long pProSs.

Protein Name	UniProt Accession	pProS Residues	No. Disease	Disease Category	Disease
DNA excision repair protein ERCC-6	Q03468	63	4	Ner Ner Mal Ski	Age-related macular degeneration Cockayne syndrome Disorders of nucleotide excision repair Ultra violet-sensitive syndrome
Cellular tumor antigen p53	P04637	61	46		*
E3 ubiquitin-protein ligase RNF168	Q8IYW5	55	1	Imm	RIDDLE syndrome
CD2-associated protein	Q9Y5K6	50	1	Uri	Focal segmental glomerulosclerosis
Synaptic functional regulator FMR1	Q06787	47	3	Rep	Premature ovarian failure
Low-density lipoprotein receptor-related protein 2	P98164	44	1	Mal	Donnai–Barrow syndrome
Eukaryotic translation initiation factor 4 gamma 1	Q04637	44	1	Ner	Parkinson disease
DNA (cytosine-5)-methyltransferase 1	P26358	41	1	Ner	Hereditary sensory and autonomic neuropathy
Period circadian protein homolog 2	O15055	40	1	Ner	Familial advanced sleep phase syndrome
Latent-transforming growth factor β-binding protein 2	Q14767	40	1	Ner	Primary congenital glaucoma
Low-density lipoprotein receptor-related protein 6	O75581	39	3	Can Car Dig	Breast cancer Coronary artery disease Tooth agenesis
DNA damage-inducible transcript 3 protein	P35638	39	1	Can	Myxoid liposarcoma
KN motif and ankyrin repeat domain-containing protein 1	Q14678	39	1	Ner	Spastic quadriplegic cerebral palsy
Retinoic acid-induced protein 1	Q7Z5J4	36	1	Oco	Smith–Magenis syndrome
Histone-lysine N-methyltransferase 2D	O14686	35	2	Can Mal	Follicular lymphoma Kabuki syndrome
FYN-binding protein 1	O15117	35	1	Car	Thrombocytopenia
Low-density lipoprotein receptor adapter protein 1	Q5SW96	33	1	Dme	Familial autosomal recessive hypercholesterolemia
Catenin β-1	P35222	32	8	Can Can Can Can Can Oth Ski	Thyroid cancer Medulloblastoma Endometrial cancer Colorectal cancer Gastric cancer Hepatocellular carcinoma Autosomal dominant mental retardation Pilomatricoma
Sp110 nuclear body protein	Q9HB58	31	1	Dig	Hepatic veno-occlusive disease with immunodeficiency
Low-density lipoprotein receptor-related protein 5	O75197	30	6	Mal Mal Mal Mus Mus Ner	Osteopetrosis Worth type autosomal dominant osteosclerosis Osteoporosis-pseudoglioma syndrome Hyperostosis corticalis generalisata Osteoporosis Familial exudative vitreoretinopathy
LEM domain-containing protein 2	Q8NC56	30	1	Ner	Cataract
Single-stranded DNA cytosine deaminase	Q9GZX7	30	1	Imm	Hyper IgM syndromes, autosomal recessive type

* The list of diseases involving p53 is found in Supplementary Table S2. Can: Cancers; Car: Cardiovascular diseases; Dme: Congenital disorders of metabolism; Mal: Congenital malformations; Dig: Digestive system diseases; End: Endocrine and metabolic diseases; Imm: Immune system diseases; Mus: Musculoskeletal diseases; Ner: Nervous system diseases; Oco: Other congenital disorders; Rep: Reproductive system diseases; Res: Respiratory diseases; Ski: Skin diseases; Uri: Urinary system diseases; Oth: Other diseases.

In Figure 3 and the following sections, we illustrate how annotations can be found in IDRs of the disease-related proteins.

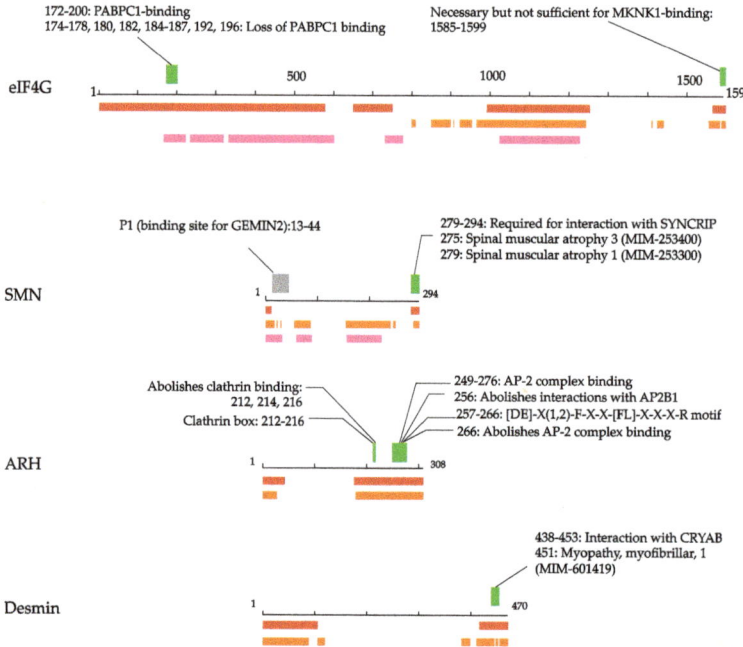

Figure 3. Examples of proteins with pProS. The black line in the middle represents the amino acid chain, and the IDR predictions are presented below. Pink, orange, and red represent the results by MobiDB-lite, DISOPRED3, and DICHOT, respectively. The green bars represent pProSs, and the annotations defining pProS are shown above with the residue numbers of the annotations. The gray bar in the example of survival of motor neuron (SMN) represents the regions of a pseudo-pProS, which was not taken as pProS because the region of the annotation is longer than 30. In the case of low-density lipoprotein receptor adaptor protein 1 (ARH) and desmin, MobiDB-lite does not predict any IDRs. The scale of eIF4G1 (eukaryotic translation initiation factor 4 gamma 1) differs from other three.

3.1. Eukaryotic Translation Initiation Factor 4 Gamma 1

Parkinson's disease is a progressive neurodegenerative movement disorder caused by the death of dopaminergic neurons in the substantia nigra pars compacta (KEGG: H00057). Although deleterious mutations in α-synuclein (OMIM-163890) [47], leucine-rich repeat kinase 2 (OMIM-609007) [48], vesicular protein sorting 35 (OMIM-601501) [49], parkin (OMIM-602544) [50], PTEN induced putative kinase 1 (OMIM-608309) [51], and DJ-1 (OMIM-602533) [52] have been found in multi-incident families with parkinsonism, mutations in the translation initiator, eukaryotic translation initiation factor 4 gamma 1 (eIF4G1, UniProt: Q04637), have also been reported [53]. The eIF4G1 is a component of the protein complex eIF4F, which is involved in the recognition of the mRNA cap, ATP-dependent unwinding of the 5'-terminal secondary structure and recruitment of mRNA to the ribosome. eIF4G1 has long IDRs in its 1599 amino acid residues. In the IDRs, the region from residues 172 to 200 possesses polyadenylate-binding protein 1 (PABPC) binding ability [54], and the region from residues 1585 to 1599 has an annotation of "necessary for binding of MAP kinase-interacting serine/threonine-protein kinase 1 (MKNK1)". Although IDRs in this study were defined by computer predictions, the region of PABPC binding is reported to be unfolded in the isolated state [54]. The eIF4G1 has been found to have five Parkinson's disease-associated mutations: Ala502Val; Gly686Cys; Ser1164Arg; Arg1197Trp;

and Arg1205His. Out of five mutations, Ala502Val and Arg1205His appear to disrupt eIF4E or eIF3E binding and share haplotypes consistent with ancestral founders [53]. These two mutations reside on IDRs, suggesting an association of binding sites on IDRs with Parkinson's disease.

3.2. Survival of Motor Neuron Protein

Spinal muscular atrophy (SMA) is a neuromuscular disease characterized by degeneration of motor neurons, resulting in progressive muscle atrophy and paralysis. The most common form of SMA is caused by mutation of the survival of motor neuron (SMN, UniProt: Q16637) protein (KEGG: H00455). Survival of motor neuron (SMN) protein is in a complex with several proteins, including Gemin2, Gemin3, and Gemin4, and plays important roles in small nuclear ribonucleoprotein (snRNP) biogenesis and pre-mRNA splicing. The SMN protein has two highly homologous genes, SMN1 and SMN2, which lie within the telomeric and centromeric halves of a large inverted repeat on chromosome 5q. The coding sequence of SMN2 differs from that of SMN1 by a single nucleotide in exon 7 (840C-T) [55–57]. Thirty-eight patients with SMA have a homozygous deletion of exon 7 of the SMN1 gene, and the deletion is associated with homozygous deletion of exon 8 in 31 of 34 patients [58]. Exon 7 and 8 cover the region from residues 242 to 294, which is predicted to be an IDR. The region from residues 252 to 281 contains the YG-box for forming helical oligomers (PDB: 4gli) [59]. In the oligomers, the C-terminal region from residues 281 to 297 is disordered [59]. This C-terminal region contains a binding region for heterogeneous nuclear ribonucleoprotein (hnRNP) Q, and the most common SMN mutant found in SMA patients is defective in its interactions with snRNPs [60]. Thus, SMN protein provides an example that a defect of IDR binding ability causes a serious disorder. SMN has another IDR in its N-terminal; this region also contains binding sites for GEMIN2, though the length of the annotation and IDR coverage do not meet the threshold of pProS in this study.

3.3. Low-Density Lipoprotein Receptor Adaptor Protein 1

A known cause of hypercholesterolemia is deficiency of low-density lipoprotein receptors (LDLR) or apolipoprotein B [61]. Recently, mutations in the low-density lipoprotein receptor adapter protein 1 (ARH, UniProt: Q5SW96) were found to cause the autosomal recessive form of hypercholesterolemia [62]. Low-density lipoprotein receptors -mediated endocytosis in the liver is the primary pathway for clearance of circulating LDL, to prevent LDL accumulation. The ARH protein is an adaptor protein required for efficient endocytosis of the LDL receptor. The ARH protein can interact with the internalization sequence in the cytoplasmic tail of LDLR, and the N-terminal region of the clathrin heavy chain, a component of a polyhedral lattice on the transport vesicles in the clathrin-mediated membrane traffic. It also binds upon the beta subunit of adaptor protein complex 2 (AP-2), which is a vesicle coat component involved in cargo selection and vesicle formation. The ARH protein is predicted to have two IDRs in its N- and C-terminus. The IDRs in the C-terminal end have two functional regions: clathrin binding and AP-2 complex binding, which are crucial interactions for LDLR-mediated endocytosis. Although the IDRs are defined only by the computer predictions, the clathrin-binding region of auxilin has been found to be disordered [63], and the tertiary structure of the AP-2 complex binding region of ARH ([DE]-X(1,2)-F-X-X-[FL]-X-X-X-R motif) in the complex with AP-2 β subunit has been solved (PDB: 2g30) [64]. Supplementary Figure S2 shows the structure of this segment binding upon AP-2 β subunit, together with a typical ProS structure of nuclear receptor co-activator 1 (IDEAL: IID50084) binding upon nuclear receptor subfamily 1 group I. Nuclear receptor co-activators or co-repressors have the LXXLL motif in their binding site for nuclear receptors. This motif is one of the annotations frequently found to be a pProS in this study (Supplementary Table S1) and has been shown to be disordered in the isolated state, as mentioned above. The AP-2 binding region shows a similar α-helix structure attached to the globular structure of the partner protein.

3.4. Desmin

Desminopathy belongs to a genetically heterogeneous group of disorders named myofibrillar myopathy, caused by mutations in desmin, αB-crystallin, myotilin, Z-band alternatively spliced PDZ-containing protein, filamin, or Bcl-2-associated athanogene. Desmin (Uniprot: P17661) is the main intermediate filament (IF) protein. It interacts with other proteins to support myofibrils at the level of the Z-disc and forms a continuous cytoskeletal IF network [65]. Desmin has two predicted IDRs in its N- and C-terminus, and the binding region for αB-crystallin (CRYAB) is located in the C-terminal IDR [66]. Several mutations in this region have been reported to cause severe disturbance of filament formation. The desmin mutations Thr442Ile, Arg454Trp, and Ser460Ile reveal a severe disturbance of filament formation competence and filament interactions [66–68], and Thr453Ile exhibits significantly delayed filament assembly kinetics [69,70]. These sites locate on one of the predicted IDRs.

We analyzed the disease-related proteins from subcellular localizations in Figure 4. The location distributions of all disease-related proteins ("all" shown in the right bottom panel) showed that pProS-containing proteins are rich in cytoplasm and nuclear (CN) proteins and nucleus (N) proteins. The distribution of the non-pProS proteins shows a shortage of CN and N proteins. Ota et al. [71] pointed out the IDR richness in the mobile proteins shuttling from cytoplasm to nucleus and vice versa. Cytoplasm and nuclear proteins localize both in the cytoplasm and nucleus, and thus, the results of this study also showed that these CN proteins have functional regions on their IDRs. Although most of the localizations by the disease category showed this trend, some of them show some divergence. "cancers", "cardiovascular diseases", "endocrine and metabolic diseases", "other congenital disorders", "reproductive system diseases", "skin diseases", and "other diseases" showed similarity to that of all disease-related proteins. On the other hand, "congenital disorders of metabolism", "digestive system diseases", "nervous system diseases", and "urinary system diseases" showed another trend. The pProS-containing proteins in these categories do not have many CN proteins and N proteins but have proteins in other locations. It has been indicated that IDRs are found in large numbers in nuclear proteins, such as transcription factors and proteins in the signaling pathways [4,6]. The CN proteins and N proteins are those proteins under such categories because stimulus from outside of the cell is received by receptors and must be transmitted to the nucleus. The system therefore needs to have mobile proteins from cytoplasm to the nucleus. Additionally, in order to regulate such systems, information flow from the nucleus to the cytoplasm is required. Then, the pProS-containing proteins under the first trend can be the typical IDPs previously reported. The other locations contain "endoplasmic reticulum", "cell projection", and "cell junction", etc. The proteins under the second trend suggest that IDPs not belonging to typical IDPs, such as transcription factors, can have functional sites in their IDRs and are involved in human diseases. For example, ARH as shown in Figure 3 has functions in the endocytosis in cytoplasm, and its IDRs have the key regions associated with hypercholesterolemia.

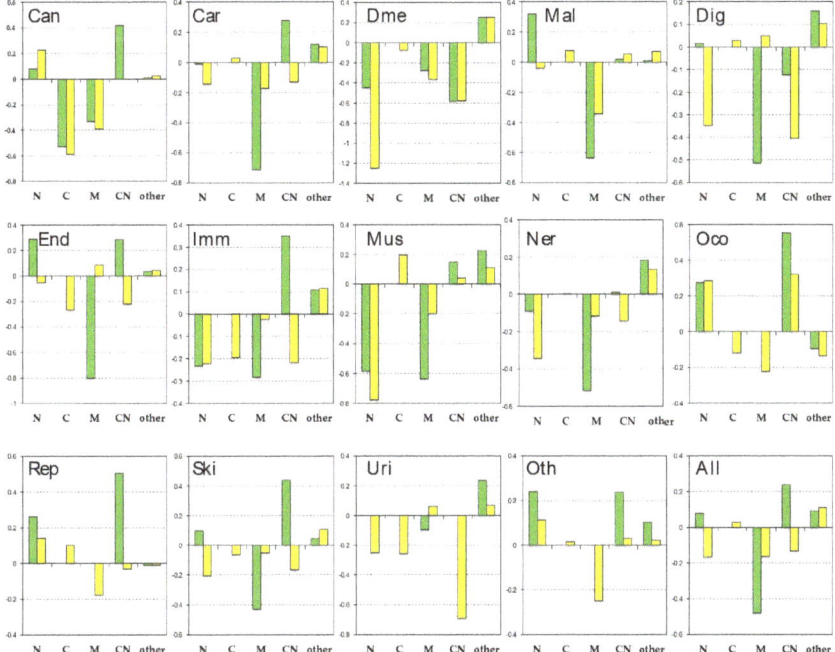

Figure 4. Subcellular localizations by disease category. The bars represent the degree of over-representation in each of the location categories, where green represents pProS-containing proteins, and yellow represents non-pProS proteins (see also Materials and Methods). N: Nuclear; C: Cytoplasm; M: Membrane; CN: Cytoplasm and nuclear; Can: Cancers; Car: Cardiovascular diseases; Dme: Congenital disorders of metabolism; Mal: Congenital malformations; Dig: Digestive system diseases; End: Endocrine and metabolic diseases; Imm: Immune system diseases; Mus: Musculoskeletal diseases; Ner: Nervous system diseases; Oco: Other congenital disorders; Rep: Reproductive system diseases; Ski: Skin diseases; Uri: Urinary system diseases; Oth: Other diseases; All: All disease-related proteins.

4. Discussion

This study is based on IDR predictions and database annotations. We employed consensus methods to define IDRs using three predictors. Because the MobiDB-lite program contains eight different prediction models, we substantially used ten predictors to make consensus IDRs. We found experimental evidence for predicted IDRs in the detailed analysis of some proteins. For example, the annotations frequently found in the IDRs (Supplementary Table S1) were found in the regions experimentally verified as IDRs, and the examples of eIF4G1, SMN protein, and ARH also showed that some parts of the predicted IDRs have been experimentally verified to be IDRs (Figure 3). Due to these examples, we were convinced that the IDRs in this study were promising. Even with the conservative IDR definition, we found more than 1000 pProSs. If the condition to select IDRs was relaxed, more candidates for functional regions in IDRs could be obtained.

Functional segments on IDRs have been collected as the databases such as SLiM/ELM [72]. A proteome-wide analysis combined with high-throughput sequencing data showed that disease-related mutations were enriched in SLiMs on IDRs and occurred more frequently at functionally important residues in SLiMs [73]. Most of these motifs are annotated as "short sequence motif" in UniProt. In this sense, the analysis in this study covers not only these motifs but also potential functional segments annotated as "mutagenesis site" and "region of interest". The ratio of the numbers of "short sequence motif" annotations to those of the other two is one-eighth (Table 1). This result suggests that knowledge of functional segments on IDRs can exist other than the information stored in the motif databases.

We searched potential binding segments in IDRs by referring to the UniProt annotations. The UniProt annotations are human-curated and highly reliable. Some of the information on a protein, however, does not appear in the FT section of the UniProt annotation. For example, the N–terminal IDR of p53 has 11 binding partners, and the C-terminal IDR has 15 partners solved in PDB structures (IDEAL: IID00015). The UniProt annotations in these IDRs are concise, as shown in Figure 2, although the links to the PDB entries are described in the "cross reference" section in UniProt. We picked eIF4G1 as an example in Figure 3. In this example, we found the pProS of the PABPC1-binding region in the UniProt annotation. However, this region also binds upon rotavirus nonstructural protein 3 [74], and this information does not appear in the feature table. In this sense, this study does not cover all of the knowledge of potential functional regions in IDRs. Thus, detailed analysis of each of the proteins would provide more information about functional segments on IDRs in the disease-related proteins.

In fact, we found potential functional sites from another information in UniProt. As shown in Figure 3, some of pProSs coincide with mutation sites associated with human disease. UniProt describes these associations as the link of mutation sites to the OMIM database, which are not directly linked with the feature annotations used in this study. Although we did not use such mutation site information to define pProS, we found considerable numbers of mutation sites in the predicted IDRs. We found 1611 mutation sites in the predicted IDRs of 572 proteins. Among them, UniProt describes links to the OMIM database for 919 mutation sites in 359 proteins. The list of these mutation sites can be found in Supplementary Table S3. Although it is not clear whether these mutation sites are binding sites for other molecules, these sites may possibly be regarded as functional regions in IDRs. Some of the readers may be interested in other model organisms. We briefly surveyed some of the represented model organisms, as shown in Supplementary Table S4. Although the results are preliminary, considerable numbers of annotations were found in the predicted IDRs for the mouse, rat, *Arabidopsis thaliana*, and yeast. These organisms have been long used for model organisms, and knowledge verified by experiments has been accumulated. Thus, for such model organisms, the strategy of the present study can be applied.

When we simply count the numbers of pProSs in the disease categories, the statistics were different from Table 2. The statistics are shown in Supplementary Table S5. The "pProS counts" represent how many times pProSs occur in each of the categories. "Cancers" were top ranked, followed by "congenital malformation" and "nervous system diseases". The large numbers of proteins can account for the large numbers of "pProS counts" of "nervous system diseases" and "congenital malformation". "Cancers", however, does not have as many proteins as these two categories, in spite of many "pProS counts." This is due to the multiple involvement of a protein in different diseases. When a protein having a pProS and is assigned to two diseases, we counted two for the pProS count. Thus, when a protein is assigned to multiple diseases in a disease category, redundant counts in the disease category occur. Supplementary Table S6 lists the top 10 redundant proteins in terms of multiple disease annotations. p53 Has the maximum multiple disease annotations, and most of these diseases are in the category "cancers". The multiple annotations on the other proteins tend to be also redundant in "cancers". The pProS redundancy in Supplementary Table S5, which is the ratio of the numbers of unique pProS to the numbers of pProS counts, shows the trend of this multiple disease association. "cancers" has a remarkably high value of pProS redundancy, suggesting that pProS-containing proteins in "cancers" tend to associate with several kinds of cancers.

p53 is involved in an extremely large number of diseases and has been also known as a hub protein that has great numbers of binding partners in PPI networks. In fact, the BioGRID database [75] lists 1056 interactors for p53, which is ranked 11th in terms of the number of PPIs in the human proteome. Then, we looked at the relation between the number of diseases assigned by KEGG DISEASE and the number of protein interactors. Figure 5 shows the relationship between the two. The correlation coefficients between the mean and median values of the numbers of interactors to the numbers of assigned diseases were 0.86 and 0.87. The distribution of the numbers of assigned diseases likely follows the power law. Therefore, most of the samples are found in the bins of the left side of the chart, and only small numbers of samples are found in the right side of the chart, as suggested by the long boxes. Even within the data of less than 10 assigned diseases, the correlation coefficient of the mean value is 0.73. It can therefore be said that there is generally a correlation between the numbers of interactors and the numbers of diseases involved. It has been pointed out that hub proteins in PPI networks are rich in IDRs [76,77]. If we accept the relationship between the number of protein interactors and the number of diseases involved, these hub proteins, namely IDPs, must be associated with many human diseases.

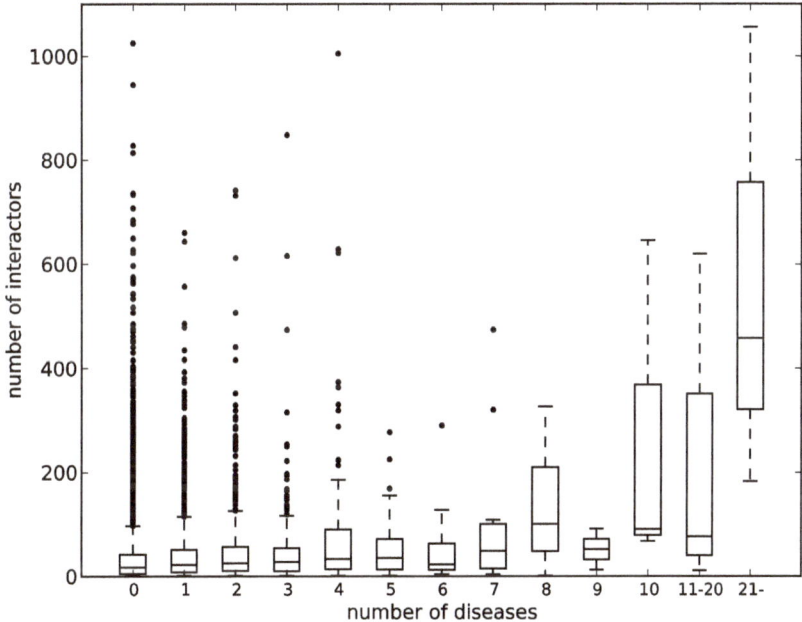

Figure 5. The correlation between the number of protein–protein interactions and the number of diseases involved. The horizontal axis represents the number of diseases, and the vertical one represents the number of interactors. A box and a pair of whiskers represent quartiles, and the line in the middle of the box represents the median. The dots represent outliers.

Post-translational modifications (PTM) are an important modification on proteins to regulate their function. In particular, phosphorylation has been known to occur preferentially on IDRs [78] to regulate signaling pathways and other many biological processes. We surveyed phosphorylation sites of the pProS-containing proteins by using the UniProt annotations and found that 876 phosphorylation sites coincide with pProS regions in 290 proteins. Most of these phosphorylation related pProSs have the annotations relating to protein binding, suggesting that the PPI via these pProSs may be regulated by phosphorylation. We also checked links of these regions to the OMIM database and found that about 30 phosphorylation sites have the links to the OMIM database. Although the number of the direct link to OMIM is short, a lot of phosphorylation sites can regulate PPIs, and the defect of these phosphorylation related pProSs may make an impact on PPI networks.

We analyzed localizations of disease-related proteins to find the richness of the mobile proteins coming and going between the cytoplasm and nucleus in pProS-containing proteins. Recently, proteins and protein-nucleic acid mixtures can undergo liquid–liquid phase separation (LLPS) to form non-membrane organelles or lipid droplets, and have several important biological functions [79–82].

Intrinsically disordered regions have been shown to play important roles in LLPS [83–85]. Some of the non-membrane organelles appeared in the UniProt annotations of subcellular localization. Supplementary Figure S3 shows the distributions of these non-membrane organelles found in disease-related proteins. It is clear that the pProS-containing proteins are over-represented, while the non-pProS proteins are not, with the exception of "lipid droplet" and "P-body". Although the numbers of annotations for these non-membrane organelles are small, these results suggest that IDPs play an important role in forming such organelles and have functional segments on their IDRs.

5. Conclusions

We conducted bioinformatics analyses to survey our knowledge on functional segments in IDRs from the perspective of disease-related proteins. We found more than a thousand annotations in the predicted IDRs, and considerable fractions of the disease-related proteins contained functional segments on IDRs. The detailed analysis on some of the examples showed that the pProSs found in this study were located in the experimentally verified IDRs and could directly associate with the diseases. Hub proteins in the PPI network tend to be involved in many human diseases, and some of the pProS-containing proteins are embedded in non-membrane organelles. We should note that the statistics in this study convey only current research, and more than 100,000 functional segments are expected to exist in IDRs. However, even with limited information, this study showed the power of database search for retrieving knowledge of functional segments in IDRs. The complete lists of pProSs can be found in Supplementary Table S7.

Supplementary Materials: The following are available online at http://www.mdpi.com/2218-273X/9/3/88/s1, Figure S1: The brief outline of the procedure to obtain pProSs; Figure S2: A structural example of a functional fragment found in an experimentally verified IDR; Figure S3: The non-membrane organelles found in the annotations of the disease-related proteins; Table S1: pProSs frequently found in the disease-related proteins; Table S2: The list of disease involving p53; Table S3: The disease associated mutation sites found in the predicted IDRs; Table S4: The numbers of annotations found on IDRs in the other model organisms; Table S5: The redundancy of pProS by the disease categories; Table S6: Proteins involved in multiple diseases; Table S7: The list of pProSs found in this study.

Author Contributions: Investigation, H.A., M.S., A.O. and S.F.; writing—original draft preparation, H.A. and S.F.; supervision, S.F.

Funding: This research received no external funding.

Acknowledgments: We are grateful to the IDEAL development team for their effort to develop and maintain the IDEAL database.

Conflicts of Interest: The authors declare no conflict of interest.

References

1. Dunker, A.K.; Brown, C.J.; Lawson, J.D.; Iakoucheva, L.M.; Obradovic, Z. Intrinsic disorder and protein function. *Biochemistry* **2002**, *41*, 6573–6582. [CrossRef] [PubMed]
2. Dyson, H.J.; Wright, P.E. Intrinsically unstructured proteins and their functions. *Nat. Rev. Mol. Cell Biol.* **2005**, *6*, 197–208. [CrossRef] [PubMed]
3. Tompa, P. The interplay between structure and function in intrinsically unstructured proteins. *FEBS Lett.* **2005**, *579*, 3346–3354. [CrossRef] [PubMed]
4. Fukuchi, S.; Hosoda, K.; Homma, K.; Gojobori, T.; Nishikawa, K. Binary classification of protein molecules into intrinsically disordered and ordered segments. *BMC Struct. Biol.* **2011**, *11*, 29. [CrossRef] [PubMed]
5. Minezaki, Y.; Homma, K.; Kinjo, A.R.; Nishikawa, K. Human transcription factors contain a high fraction of intrinsically disordered regions essential for transcriptional regulation. *J. Mol. Biol.* **2006**, *359*, 1137–1149. [CrossRef] [PubMed]
6. Ward, J.J.; Sodhi, J.S.; McGuffin, L.J.; Buxton, B.F.; Jones, D.T. Prediction and functional analysis of native disorder in proteins from the three kingdoms of life. *J. Mol. Biol.* **2004**, *337*, 635–645. [CrossRef] [PubMed]
7. Iakoucheva, L.M.; Brown, C.J.; Lawson, J.D.; Obradovic, Z.; Dunker, A.K. Intrinsic disorder in cell-signaling and cancer-associated proteins. *J. Mol. Biol.* **2002**, *323*, 573–584. [CrossRef]

8. Babu, M.M.; van der Lee, R.; de Groot, N.S.; Gsponer, J. Intrinsically disordered proteins: Regulation and disease. *Curr. Opin. Struct. Biol.* **2011**, *21*, 432–440. [CrossRef] [PubMed]
9. Uversky, V.N.; Oldfield, C.J.; Dunker, A.K. Intrinsically disordered proteins in human diseases: Introducing the D2 concept. *Ann. Rev. Biophys.* **2008**, *37*, 215–246. [CrossRef] [PubMed]
10. Wu, H.; Fuxreiter, M. The structure and dynamics of higher-order assemblies: Amyloids, signalosomes, and granules. *Cell* **2016**, *165*, 1055–1066. [CrossRef] [PubMed]
11. Toretsky, J.A.; Wright, P.E. Assemblages: Functional units formed by cellular phase separation. *J. Cell Biol.* **2014**, *206*, 579–588. [CrossRef] [PubMed]
12. Calabretta, S.; Richard, S. Emerging roles of disordered sequences in RNA-binding proteins. *Trends Biochem. Sci.* **2015**, *40*, 662–672. [CrossRef] [PubMed]
13. Aguzzi, A.; Altmeyer, M. Phase separation: Linking cellular compartmentalization to disease. *Trends Cell Biol.* **2016**, *26*, 547–558. [CrossRef] [PubMed]
14. Molliex, A.; Temirov, J.; Lee, J.; Coughlin, M.; Kanagaraj, A.P.; Kim, H.J.; Mittag, T.; Taylor, J.P. Phase separation by low complexity domains promotes stress granule assembly and drives pathological fibrillization. *Cell* **2015**, *163*, 123–133. [CrossRef] [PubMed]
15. Knowles, T.P.; Vendruscolo, M.; Dobson, C.M. The amyloid state and its association with protein misfolding diseases. *Nat. Rev. Mol. Cell Biol.* **2014**, *15*, 384–396. [CrossRef] [PubMed]
16. Chiti, F.; Dobson, C.M. Protein misfolding, functional amyloid, and human disease. *Ann. Rev. Biochem.* **2006**, *75*, 333–366. [CrossRef] [PubMed]
17. Mark, W.Y.; Liao, J.C.; Lu, Y.; Ayed, A.; Laister, R.; Szymczyna, B.; Chakrabartty, A.; Arrowsmith, C.H. Characterization of segments from the central region of BRCA1: An intrinsically disordered scaffold for multiple protein–protein and protein–DNA interactions? *J. Mol. Biol.* **2005**, *345*, 275–287. [CrossRef] [PubMed]
18. Chene, P. The role of tetramerization in p53 function. *Oncogene* **2001**, *20*, 2611–2617. [CrossRef] [PubMed]
19. Oliner, J.D.; Pietenpol, J.A.; Thiagalingam, S.; Gyuris, J.; Kinzler, K.W.; Vogelstein, B. Oncoprotein MDM2 conceals the activation domain of tumour suppressor p53. *Nature* **1993**, *362*, 857–860. [CrossRef] [PubMed]
20. Raychaudhuri, S.; Dey, S.; Bhattacharyya, N.P.; Mukhopadhyay, D. The role of intrinsically unstructured proteins in neurodegenerative diseases. *PLoS ONE* **2009**, *4*, e5566. [CrossRef] [PubMed]
21. Qian, J.; Voorbach, M.J.; Huth, J.R.; Coen, M.L.; Zhang, H.; Ng, S.C.; Comess, K.M.; Petros, A.M.; Rosenberg, S.H.; Warrior, U.; et al. Discovery of novel inhibitors of Bcl-xL using multiple high-throughput screening platforms. *Anal. Biochem.* **2004**, *328*, 131–138. [CrossRef] [PubMed]
22. Real, P.J.; Cao, Y.; Wang, R.; Nikolovska-Coleska, Z.; Sanz-Ortiz, J.; Wang, S.; Fernandez-Luna, J.L. Breast cancer cells can evade apoptosis-mediated selective killing by a novel small molecule inhibitor of Bcl-2. *Cancer Res.* **2004**, *64*, 7947–7953. [CrossRef] [PubMed]
23. Vassilev, L.T.; Vu, B.T.; Graves, B.; Carvajal, D.; Podlaski, F.; Filipovic, Z.; Kong, N.; Kammlott, U.; Lukacs, C.; Klein, C.; et al. In vivo activation of the p53 pathway by small-molecule antagonists of MDM2. *Science* **2004**, *303*, 844–848. [CrossRef] [PubMed]
24. Braisted, A.C.; Oslob, J.D.; Delano, W.L.; Hyde, J.; McDowell, R.S.; Waal, N.; Yu, C.; Arkin, M.R.; Raimundo, B.C. Discovery of a potent small molecule IL-2 inhibitor through fragment assembly. *J. Am. Chem. Soc.* **2003**, *125*, 3714–3715. [CrossRef] [PubMed]
25. Emerson, S.D.; Palermo, R.; Liu, C.M.; Tilley, J.W.; Chen, L.; Danho, W.; Madison, V.S.; Greeley, D.N.; Ju, G.; Fry, D.C. NMR characterization of interleukin-2 in complexes with the IL-2Rα receptor component, and with low molecular weight compounds that inhibit the IL-2/IL-Rα interaction. *Protein Sci.* **2003**, *12*, 811–822. [CrossRef] [PubMed]
26. Li, L.; Thomas, R.M.; Suzuki, H.; De Brabander, J.K.; Wang, X.; Harran, P.G. A small molecule Smac mimic potentiates TRAIL- and TNFα-mediated cell death. *Science* **2004**, *305*, 1471–1474. [CrossRef] [PubMed]
27. Oost, T.K.; Sun, C.; Armstrong, R.C.; Al-Assaad, A.S.; Betz, S.F.; Deckwerth, T.L.; Ding, H.; Elmore, S.W.; Meadows, R.P.; Olejniczak, E.T.; et al. Discovery of potent antagonists of the antiapoptotic protein XIAP for the treatment of cancer. *J. Med. Chem.* **2004**, *47*, 4417–4426. [CrossRef] [PubMed]
28. Ko, A.H.; Chiorean, E.G.; Kwak, E.L.; Lenz, H.-J.; Nadler, P.I.; Wood, D.L.; Fujimori, M.; Inada, T.; Kouji, H.; McWilliams, R.R. Final results of a phase Ib dose-escalation study of PRI-724, a CBP/β-catenin modulator, plus gemcitabine (GEM) in patients with advanced pancreatic adenocarcinoma (APC) as second-line therapy after FOLFIRINOX or FOLFOX. *J. Clin. Oncol.* **2016**, *34*, e15721. [CrossRef]

29. Fukuchi, S.; Amemiya, T.; Sakamoto, S.; Nobe, Y.; Hosoda, K.; Kado, Y.; Murakami, S.D.; Koike, R.; Hiroaki, H.; Ota, M. IDEAL in 2014 illustrates interaction networks composed of intrinsically disordered proteins and their binding partners. *Nucleic Acids Res.* **2014**, *42*, D320–D325. [CrossRef] [PubMed]
30. Fukuchi, S.; Sakamoto, S.; Nobe, Y.; Murakami, S.D.; Amemiya, T.; Hosoda, K.; Koike, R.; Hiroaki, H.; Ota, M. IDEAL: Intrinsically disordered proteins with extensive annotations and literature. *Nucleic Acids Res.* **2012**, *40*, D507–D511. [CrossRef] [PubMed]
31. Piovesan, D.; Tabaro, F.; Micetic, I.; Necci, M.; Quaglia, F.; Oldfield, C.J.; Aspromonte, M.C.; Davey, N.E.; Davidovic, R.; Dosztanyi, Z.; et al. DisProt 7.0: A major update of the database of disordered proteins. *Nucleic Acids Res.* **2017**, *45*, D1123–D1124. [CrossRef] [PubMed]
32. Tompa, P.; Davey, N.E.; Gibson, T.J.; Babu, M.M. A million peptide motifs for the molecular biologist. *Mol. Cell* **2014**, *55*, 161–169. [CrossRef] [PubMed]
33. The UniProt Consortium. UniProt: The universal protein knowledgebase. *Nucleic Acids Res.* **2017**, *45*, D158–D169. [CrossRef] [PubMed]
34. Necci, M.; Piovesan, D.; Dosztanyi, Z.; Tosatto, S.C.E. MobiDB-lite: Fast and highly specific consensus prediction of intrinsic disorder in proteins. *Bioinformatics* **2017**, *33*, 1402–1404. [CrossRef] [PubMed]
35. Jones, D.T.; Cozzetto, D. DISOPRED3: Precise disordered region predictions with annotated protein-binding activity. *Bioinformatics* **2015**, *31*, 857–863. [CrossRef] [PubMed]
36. Monastyrskyy, B.; Kryshtafovych, A.; Moult, J.; Tramontano, A.; Fidelis, K. Assessment of protein disorder region predictions in CASP10. *Proteins* **2014**, *82* (Suppl. S2), 127–137. [CrossRef] [PubMed]
37. Kanehisa, M.; Sato, Y.; Furumichi, M.; Morishima, K.; Tanabe, M. New approach for understanding genome variations in KEGG. *Nucleic Acids Res.* **2018**. [CrossRef] [PubMed]
38. The IDEAL database. Available online: http://www.ideal.force.cs.is.nagoya-u.ac.jp/IDEAL/ (accessed on 22 January 2019).
39. Rubin, S.M.; Gall, A.L.; Zheng, N.; Pavletich, N.P. Structure of the Rb C-terminal domain bound to E2F1-DP1: A mechanism for phosphorylation-induced E2F release. *Cell* **2005**, *123*, 1093–1106. [CrossRef] [PubMed]
40. Fontes, M.R.; Teh, T.; Jans, D.; Brinkworth, R.I.; Kobe, B. Structural basis for the specificity of bipartite nuclear localization sequence binding by importin-α. *J. Biol. Chem.* **2003**, *278*, 27981–27987. [CrossRef] [PubMed]
41. Pawson, T.; Nash, P. Assembly of cell regulatory systems through protein interaction domains. *Science* **2003**, *300*, 445–452. [CrossRef] [PubMed]
42. Lee, H.J.; Zheng, J.J. PDZ domains and their binding partners: Structure, specificity, and modification. *Cell Commun. Signal.* **2010**, *8*, 8. [CrossRef] [PubMed]
43. Nomine, Y.; Masson, M.; Charbonnier, S.; Zanier, K.; Ristriani, T.; Deryckere, F.; Sibler, A.P.; Desplancq, D.; Atkinson, R.A.; Weiss, E.; et al. Structural and functional analysis of E6 oncoprotein: Insights in the molecular pathways of human papillomavirus-mediated pathogenesis. *Mol. Cell* **2006**, *21*, 665–678. [CrossRef] [PubMed]
44. Greschik, H.; Althage, M.; Flaig, R.; Sato, Y.; Chavant, V.; Peluso-Iltis, C.; Choulier, L.; Cronet, P.; Rochel, N.; Schule, R.; et al. Communication between the ERRα homodimer interface and the PGC-1α binding surface via the helix 8-9 loop. *J. Biol. Chem.* **2008**, *283*, 20220–20230. [CrossRef] [PubMed]
45. Kallen, J.; Schlaeppi, J.M.; Bitsch, F.; Filipuzzi, I.; Schilb, A.; Riou, V.; Graham, A.; Strauss, A.; Geiser, M.; Fournier, B. Evidence for ligand-independent transcriptional activation of the human estrogen-related receptor alpha (ERRα): Crystal structure of ERRα ligand binding domain in complex with peroxisome proliferator-activated receptor coactivator-1α. *J. Biol. Chem.* **2004**, *279*, 49330–49337. [CrossRef] [PubMed]
46. KEGG DISEASE Database. Available online: https://www.genome.jp/kegg-bin/get_htext?br08402.keg (accessed on 22 January 2019).
47. Giasson, B.I.; Duda, J.E.; Murray, I.V.; Chen, Q.; Souza, J.M.; Hurtig, H.I.; Ischiropoulos, H.; Trojanowski, J.Q.; Lee, V.M. Oxidative damage linked to neurodegeneration by selective α-synuclein nitration in synucleinopathy lesions. *Science* **2000**, *290*, 985–989. [CrossRef] [PubMed]
48. Gandhi, P.N.; Wang, X.; Zhu, X.; Chen, S.G.; Wilson-Delfosse, A.L. The Roc domain of leucine-rich repeat kinase 2 is sufficient for interaction with microtubules. *J. Neurosci. Res.* **2008**, *86*, 1711–1720. [CrossRef] [PubMed]
49. Vilarino-Guell, C.; Wider, C.; Ross, O.A.; Dachsel, J.C.; Kachergus, J.M.; Lincoln, S.J.; Soto-Ortolaza, A.I.; Cobb, S.A.; Wilhoite, G.J.; Bacon, J.A.; et al. VPS35 mutations in Parkinson disease. *Am. J. Hum. Genet.* **2011**, *89*, 162–167. [CrossRef] [PubMed]

50. Yoshii, S.R.; Kishi, C.; Ishihara, N.; Mizushima, N. Parkin mediates proteasome-dependent protein degradation and rupture of the outer mitochondrial membrane. *J. Biol. Chem.* **2011**, *286*, 19630–19640. [CrossRef] [PubMed]
51. Poole, A.C.; Thomas, R.E.; Andrews, L.A.; McBride, H.M.; Whitworth, A.J.; Pallanck, L.J. The PINK1/Parkin pathway regulates mitochondrial morphology. *Proc. Natl. Acad. Sci. USA* **2008**, *105*, 1638–1643. [CrossRef] [PubMed]
52. Ottolini, D.; Cali, T.; Negro, A.; Brini, M. The Parkinson disease-related protein DJ-1 counteracts mitochondrial impairment induced by the tumour suppressor protein p53 by enhancing endoplasmic reticulum-mitochondria tethering. *Hum. Mol. Genet.* **2013**, *22*, 2152–2168. [CrossRef] [PubMed]
53. Chartier-Harlin, M.C.; Dachsel, J.C.; Vilarino-Guell, C.; Lincoln, S.J.; Lepretre, F.; Hulihan, M.M.; Kachergus, J.; Milnerwood, A.J.; Tapia, L.; Song, M.S.; et al. Translation initiator EIF4G1 mutations in familial Parkinson disease. *Am. J. Hum. Genet.* **2011**, *89*, 398–406. [CrossRef] [PubMed]
54. Safaee, N.; Kozlov, G.; Noronha, A.M.; Xie, J.; Wilds, C.J.; Gehring, K. Interdomain allostery promotes assembly of the poly(A) mRNA complex with PABP and eIF4G. *Mol. Cell* **2012**, *48*, 375–386. [CrossRef] [PubMed]
55. Biros, I.; Forrest, S. Spinal muscular atrophy: Untangling the knot? *J. Med. Genet.* **1999**, *36*, 1–8. [PubMed]
56. Wirth, B. An update of the mutation spectrum of the survival motor neuron gene (*SMN1*) in autosomal recessive spinal muscular atrophy (SMA). *Hum. Mutat.* **2000**, *15*, 228–237. [CrossRef]
57. Ogino, S.; Wilson, R.B. Spinal muscular atrophy: Molecular genetics and diagnostics. *Expert Rev. Mol. Diagn.* **2004**, *4*, 15–29. [CrossRef] [PubMed]
58. Matthijs, G.; Schollen, E.; Legius, E.; Devriendt, K.; Goemans, N.; Kayserili, H.; Apak, M.Y.; Cassiman, J.J. Unusual molecular findings in autosomal recessive spinal muscular atrophy. *J. Med. Genet.* **1996**, *33*, 469–474. [CrossRef] [PubMed]
59. Martin, R.; Gupta, K.; Ninan, N.S.; Perry, K.; Van Duyne, G.D. The survival motor neuron protein forms soluble glycine zipper oligomers. *Structure* **2012**, *20*, 1929–1939. [CrossRef] [PubMed]
60. Mourelatos, Z.; Abel, L.; Yong, J.; Kataoka, N.; Dreyfuss, G. SMN interacts with a novel family of hnRNP and spliceosomal proteins. *EMBO J.* **2001**, *20*, 5443–5452. [CrossRef] [PubMed]
61. Zuliani, G.; Arca, M.; Signore, A.; Bader, G.; Fazio, S.; Chianelli, M.; Bellosta, S.; Campagna, F.; Montali, A.; Maioli, M.; et al. Characterization of a new form of inherited hypercholesterolemia: Familial recessive hypercholesterolemia. *Arterioscler. Thromb. Vasc. Biol.* **1999**, *19*, 802–809. [CrossRef] [PubMed]
62. Garcia, C.K.; Wilund, K.; Arca, M.; Zuliani, G.; Fellin, R.; Maioli, M.; Calandra, S.; Bertolini, S.; Cossu, F.; Grishin, N.; et al. Autosomal recessive hypercholesterolemia caused by mutations in a putative LDL receptor adaptor protein. *Science* **2001**, *292*, 1394–1398. [CrossRef] [PubMed]
63. Scheele, U.; Alves, J.; Frank, R.; Duwel, M.; Kalthoff, C.; Ungewickell, E. Molecular and functional characterization of clathrin- and AP-2-binding determinants within a disordered domain of auxilin. *J. Biol. Chem.* **2003**, *278*, 25357–25368. [CrossRef] [PubMed]
64. Edeling, M.A.; Mishra, S.K.; Keyel, P.A.; Steinhauser, A.L.; Collins, B.M.; Roth, R.; Heuser, J.E.; Owen, D.J.; Traub, L.M. Molecular switches involving the AP-2 β2 appendage regulate endocytic cargo selection and clathrin coat assembly. *Dev. Cell* **2006**, *10*, 329–342. [CrossRef] [PubMed]
65. Goldfarb, L.G.; Dalakas, M.C. Tragedy in a heartbeat: Malfunctioning desmin causes skeletal and cardiac muscle disease. *J. Clin. Investig.* **2009**, *119*, 1806–1813. [CrossRef] [PubMed]
66. Sharma, S.; Conover, G.M.; Elliott, J.L.; Der Perng, M.; Herrmann, H.; Quinlan, R.A. αB-crystallin is a sensor for assembly intermediates and for the subunit topology of desmin intermediate filaments. *Cell Stress Chaperones* **2017**, *22*, 613–626. [CrossRef] [PubMed]
67. Bar, H.; Goudeau, B.; Walde, S.; Casteras-Simon, M.; Mucke, N.; Shatunov, A.; Goldberg, Y.P.; Clarke, C.; Holton, J.L.; Eymard, B.; et al. Conspicuous involvement of desmin tail mutations in diverse cardiac and skeletal myopathies. *Hum. Mutat.* **2007**, *28*, 374–386. [CrossRef] [PubMed]
68. Vattemi, G.; Neri, M.; Piffer, S.; Vicart, P.; Gualandi, F.; Marini, M.; Guglielmi, V.; Filosto, M.; Tonin, P.; Ferlini, A.; et al. Clinical, morphological and genetic studies in a cohort of 21 patients with myofibrillar myopathy. *Acta Myol.* **2011**, *30*, 121–126. [PubMed]
69. Arbustini, E.; Pasotti, M.; Pilotto, A.; Pellegrini, C.; Grasso, M.; Previtali, S.; Repetto, A.; Bellini, O.; Azan, G.; Scaffino, M.; et al. Desmin accumulation restrictive cardiomyopathy and atrioventricular block associated with desmin gene defects. *Eur. J. Heart Fail.* **2006**, *8*, 477–483. [CrossRef] [PubMed]

70. Baker, L.K.; Gillis, D.C.; Sharma, S.; Ambrus, A.; Herrmann, H.; Conover, G.M. Nebulin binding impedes mutant desmin filament assembly. *Mol. Biol. Cell* **2013**, *24*, 1918–1932. [CrossRef] [PubMed]
71. Ota, M.; Gonja, H.; Koike, R.; Fukuchi, S. Multiple-localization and Hub proteins. *PLoS ONE* **2016**, *11*, e0156455. [CrossRef] [PubMed]
72. Dinkel, H.; Van Roey, K.; Michael, S.; Kumar, M.; Uyar, B.; Altenberg, B.; Milchevskaya, V.; Schneider, M.; Kuhn, H.; Behrendt, A.; et al. ELM 2016-data update and new functionality of the eukaryotic linear motif resource. *Nucleic Acids Res.* **2016**, *44*, D294–300. [CrossRef] [PubMed]
73. Uyar, B.; Weatheritt, R.J.; Dinkel, H.; Davey, N.E.; Gibson, T.J. Proteome-wide analysis of human disease mutations in short linear motifs: Neglected players in cancer? *Mol. Biosyst.* **2014**, *10*, 2626–2642. [CrossRef] [PubMed]
74. Groft, C.M.; Burley, S.K. Recognition of eIF4G by rotavirus NSP3 reveals a basis for mRNA circularization. *Mol. Cell* **2002**, *9*, 1273–1283. [CrossRef]
75. Chatr-Aryamontri, A.; Oughtred, R.; Boucher, L.; Rust, J.; Chang, C.; Kolas, N.K.; O'Donnell, L.; Oster, S.; Theesfeld, C.; Sellam, A.; et al. The BioGRID interaction database: 2017 Update. *Nucleic Acids Res.* **2017**, *45*, D369–D379. [CrossRef] [PubMed]
76. Haynes, C.; Oldfield, C.J.; Ji, F.; Klitgord, N.; Cusick, M.E.; Radivojac, P.; Uversky, V.N.; Vidal, M.; Iakoucheva, L.M. Intrinsic disorder is a common feature of hub proteins from four eukaryotic interactomes. *PLoS Comput. Biol.* **2006**, *2*, e100. [CrossRef] [PubMed]
77. Patil, A.; Kinoshita, K.; Nakamura, H. Hub promiscuity in protein-protein interaction networks. *Int. J. Mol. Sci.* **2010**, *11*, 1930–1943. [CrossRef] [PubMed]
78. Collins, M.O.; Yu, L.; Campuzano, I.; Grant, S.G.; Choudhary, J.S. Phosphoproteomic analysis of the mouse brain cytosol reveals a predominance of protein phosphorylation in regions of intrinsic sequence disorder. *Mol. Cell. Proteomics* **2008**, *7*, 1331–1348. [CrossRef] [PubMed]
79. Brangwynne, C.P.; Eckmann, C.R.; Courson, D.S.; Rybarska, A.; Hoege, C.; Gharakhani, J.; Julicher, F.; Hyman, A.A. Germline P granules are liquid droplets that localize by controlled dissolution/condensation. *Science* **2009**, *324*, 1729–1732. [CrossRef] [PubMed]
80. Brangwynne, C.P.; Mitchison, T.J.; Hyman, A.A. Active liquid-like behavior of nucleoli determines their size and shape in Xenopus laevis oocytes. *Proc. Natl. Acad. Sci. USA* **2011**, *108*, 4334–4339. [CrossRef] [PubMed]
81. Li, P.; Banjade, S.; Cheng, H.C.; Kim, S.; Chen, B.; Guo, L.; Llaguno, M.; Hollingsworth, J.V.; King, D.S.; Banani, S.F.; et al. Phase transitions in the assembly of multivalent signalling proteins. *Nature* **2012**, *483*, 336–340. [CrossRef] [PubMed]
82. Kato, M.; Han, T.W.; Xie, S.; Shi, K.; Du, X.; Wu, L.C.; Mirzaei, H.; Goldsmith, E.J.; Longgood, J.; Pei, J.; et al. Cell-free formation of RNA granules: Low complexity sequence domains form dynamic fibers within hydrogels. *Cell* **2012**, *149*, 753–767. [CrossRef] [PubMed]
83. Banjade, S.; Wu, Q.; Mittal, A.; Peeples, W.B.; Pappu, R.V.; Rosen, M.K. Conserved interdomain linker promotes phase separation of the multivalent adaptor protein Nck. *Proc. Natl. Acad. Sci. USA* **2015**, *112*, E6426–E6435. [CrossRef] [PubMed]
84. Nott, T.J.; Petsalaki, E.; Farber, P.; Jervis, D.; Fussner, E.; Plochowietz, A.; Craggs, T.D.; Bazett-Jones, D.P.; Pawson, T.; Forman-Kay, J.D.; et al. Phase transition of a disordered nuage protein generates environmentally responsive membraneless organelles. *Mol. Cell* **2015**, *57*, 936–947. [CrossRef] [PubMed]
85. Pak, C.W.; Kosno, M.; Holehouse, A.S.; Padrick, S.B.; Mittal, A.; Ali, R.; Yunus, A.A.; Liu, D.R.; Pappu, R.V.; Rosen, M.K. Sequence Determinants of intracellular phase separation by complex coacervation of a disordered protein. *Mol. Cell* **2016**, *63*, 72–85. [CrossRef] [PubMed]

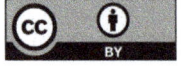 © 2019 by the authors. Licensee MDPI, Basel, Switzerland. This article is an open access article distributed under the terms and conditions of the Creative Commons Attribution (CC BY) license (http://creativecommons.org/licenses/by/4.0/).

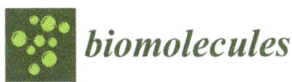

Review

Role of Phosphorylation in the Modulation of the Glucocorticoid Receptor's Intrinsically Disordered Domain

Raj Kumar [1,*] and E. Brad Thompson [2,*]

1 Department of Medical Education, Geisinger Commonwealth School of Medicine, Scranton, PA 18509, USA
2 Department of Biochemistry and Molecular Biology, University of Texas Medical Branch, Galveston, TX 77555, USA
* Correspondence: rkumar@som.geisinger.edu (R.K.); bthompso@utmb.edu (E.B.T.)

Received: 22 December 2018; Accepted: 21 February 2019; Published: 11 March 2019

Abstract: Protein phosphorylation often switches cellular activity from one state to another, and this post-translational modification plays an important role in gene regulation by the nuclear hormone receptor superfamily, including the glucocorticoid receptor (GR). Cell signaling pathways that regulate phosphorylation of the GR are important determinants of GR actions, including lymphoid cell apoptosis, DNA binding, and interaction with coregulatory proteins. All major functionally important phosphorylation sites in the human GR are located in its N-terminal domain (NTD), which possesses a powerful transactivation domain, AF1. The GR NTD exists as an intrinsically disordered protein (IDP) and undergoes disorder-order transition for AF1's efficient interaction with several coregulatory proteins and subsequent AF1-mediated GR activity. It has been reported that GR's NTD/AF1 undergoes such disorder-order transition following site-specific phosphorylation. This review provides currently available information regarding the role of GR phosphorylation in its action and highlights the possible underlying mechanisms of action.

Keywords: glucocorticoid receptor; phosphorylation; intrinsically disordered; transactivation activity; gene regulation; coactivators

---

1. Introduction

The glucocorticoid receptor (GR) is a well-known, ligand-driven transcription factor, essential for many of the functions-physiologic, pathological, and therapeutic of hormonal and synthetic glucocorticoids [1–8]. The GR belongs to the superfamily of the steroid and thyroid hormone-activated intracellular transcription factors, and the larger family of nuclear hormone receptors (NHRs) [9–13]. The GR was the first member of this superfamily to be cloned and characterized [14]. It is a ubiquitously expressed intracellular protein that regulates the expression of glucocorticoid-responsive genes in a cell/tissue- and promoter-specific manner [9,10]. The broad overview of glucocorticoid action (Figure 1) states that the cytosolic GR is part of a large heteromeric complex consisting of several chaperone proteins including HSP90, HSP70, p23, immunophilins of the FK506-binding protein family (FKBP51 and FKBP52) and possibly several others [15–18]. These proteins maintain the receptor in a transcriptionally inactive conformation that favors high affinity ligand binding [15–18].

Glucocorticoid binding to GR's C-terminal ligand binding pocket leads to structural rearrangements, causing the receptor to be released from the complex. At some point, the GR becomes hyper-phosphorylated and active [15–19], enters the nucleus and interacts with site-specific DNA sequences, termed "glucocorticoid response elements" (GREs), and several additional coregulatory proteins. (Figure 1). The GR can also bind at heterodox regulatory elements by "piggybacking" on other transcription factors [10,11,13]. The DNA and protein interactions are highly dynamic in the genomic context, as the receptor rapidly moves from one site to another and interacts with various proteins [9]. One important implication of this model is that the surfaces of the GR must be employed in various ways in order to allow temporary interactions with a variety of other macromolecules, and thus change transcription [9]. In this review, we discuss the structure and functions of the GR, specifically the role of site-specific phosphorylation in the regulation of its intrinsically disordered (ID) NTD.

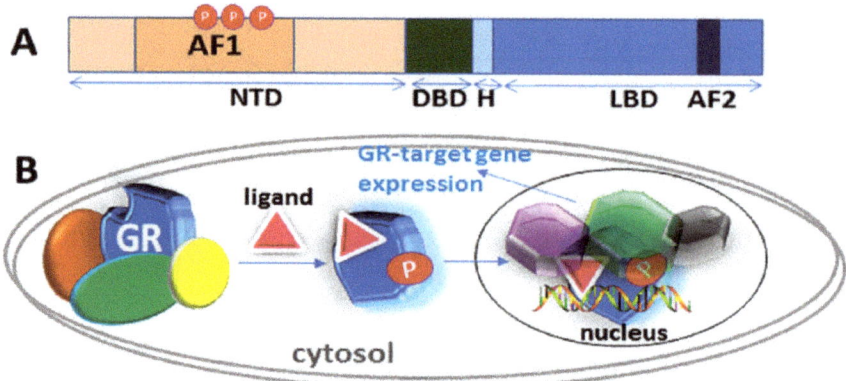

Figure 1. Classical action of the glucocorticoid signaling mediated by the glucocorticoid receptor (GR). (**A**) A topological diagram of human GR protein showing major functional domains and major known AF1 phosphorylation (P) sites (other GR sites not shown) [6]. NTD, N-terminal domain; DBD, DNA binding domain; H, Hinge region, LBD, Ligand binding domain. (**B**) Unliganded receptor is located in the cytosol associated with several heat shock and other chaperone proteins including HSP90, HSP70, CyP-40, P23, and FKBPs (shown by different colors around GR). Ligand binding leads to conformational alterations in the GR, and by doing so GR dissociates from these associated proteins, and ligand bound GR is free to translocate to the nucleus. This process appears to be phosphorylation (P) dependent. Once in the nucleus, GR binds to site-specific DNA binding sequences and interacts with several other coregulatory proteins (shown by different colors and shapes around GR), and subsequently leads to transcriptional regulation. Based on reference [10].

2. The Structure of the Glucocorticoid Receptor and its Gene

The human GR gene consists of 9 exons located on chromosome 5 [20,21]. Like other steroid hormone receptors (SHRs), the GR consists of three well-known major functional domains: N-terminal (NTD), DNA binding (DBD), and ligand-binding (LBD) (Figure 1A). DBD and LBD are separated by a short intrinsically disordered (ID) amino acid sequence known as the "hinge" region [13]. Within the NTD and LBD are two transcription activation function regions, AF1 and AF2, respectively [13]. AF2 is strictly ligand-dependent whereas AF1 is ligand-dependent in the context of the holo-GR but is constitutively active and can regulate GR-target genes in a ligand-independent manner when the LBD is removed [9,13]. In other words, the AF1 can act constitutively in the absence of the LBD and is quite active in stimulating transcription from simple promoters containing cognate GR binding sites [13]. With the discovery of a large cohort of GR forms with unique expression, gene-regulatory, and functional profiles [6], the traditional view that a single GR protein regulates the effects of glucocorticoids has changed in recent years. Alternative exon splicing and translation initiation sites in the human GR mRNA result in a number of receptor sub-types [6].

When interacting with chromosomal DNA, both AF domains of the GR mediate transcriptional activation by recruiting coregulatory multi-subunit complexes that remodel chromatin, target initiation sites, and stabilize the RNA polymerase II machinery for repeated rounds of transcription of target genes [9]. In the conceptual model of receptor:coactivator complexes, the ligand-bound GR recruits one or more cofactors, which subsequently results in the recruitment of additional known cofactors to the assembly of the complex [9,13]. Depending on the GR ligand, these cofactors may lead to increased or reduced transcription of regulated genes. It is likely that additional as yet unknown cofactors are involved, and that different GRs may recruit different components to the complex, thus achieving a level of specificity among GRs and coactivators or corepressors [9].

Though the structures of independently expressed, more stably structured LBD and DBD were solved long ago [22,23], no 3D structure of full-length GR is currently known. From the LBD structural and mutation data, it is clear that ligand binding results in conformational rearrangement of AF2 sub-domain (usually helix 12) such that its surfaces are available for interactions with specific coregulatory proteins through LXXLL motifs [23]. Bound to an agonist ligand, AF2 adopts a conformation that suits for interaction with coactivators, whereas an antagonist binding blocks such interactions and rather opens surfaces for corepressor interactions [23]. However, many ligands originally labeled "antagonists" are actually weak partial agonists that compete for the LBD site. Presumably, when bound with these, the LBD-ligand-coactivator interactions are weaker, so that gene induction is reduced. Furthermore, the GR LBD crystal structure revealed a second charge clamp, which may determine the binding selectivity of a coactivator [23]. The structure of the DBD and how it fits into its GRE has been known for some time [22], though this binding process may be more dynamic than once envisaged [9].

Due to its disordered nature, our understanding about the structure and functions of AF1 has languished until recently. The GR AF1 supplies most of the transcription-controlling power of the GR; and this lack of information about how AF1 interacts with various coregulatory proteins, and the consequences for transcriptional regulation, has hampered understanding of the full spectrum of GR action. The AF1 activation domain was discovered well before AF2 and was initially thought to be the only GR transactivation function. The major obstacle in solving full-length GR structure or that of AF1 alone is the fact that large portion of the GR NTD, including AF1, is IDP [24–30]. A new, quantitative thermodynamic model for allosteric interdomain coupling has been proposed that explains the role of the IDP NTD of the GR in the receptor's function [31]. This model would be applicable to other SHRs and transcription factors generally.

3. The IDP Nature of the GR NTD/AF1 Means that it Can be Thought of as a Large Ensemble of Rapidly Interchanging Conformations

Compared to the LBD and DBD, the GR NTD is most variable in terms of sequence homology and size among various mammals [10]. The AF1 plays an important role in the interaction of the receptor with molecules necessary for the initiation of transcription, such as chromatin modulators and protein from basal transcription factors, including RNA polymerase II, TATA-binding protein (TBP) and a host of TBP-associated proteins [9,28]. The AF1 is also known to interact with many other coregulatory proteins including coactivators and corepressors, which are essential for optimal GR activity in a cell/tissue-specific manner [9,10,12,28]. Several of these coregulatory proteins are also known to interact with the AF2 region [9,10,12,28]. However, unlike the LXXLL binding motif for AF2 interactions, no such motif is known for the AF1 [23], and in fact, IDP regions usually lack a defined interaction motif as in many transcription factors [32–34].

IDPs are subject to combinatorial alternative splicing and post-translational modifications, adding complexity to regulatory networks and providing a mechanism for cell/tissue-specific signaling [35–37]. Thus, the ID ensemble allows molecular recognition by providing protein surfaces capable of binding specific target molecules from the assembly of signaling complexes [35–37]. A variety of computational, biochemical, and biophysical methods have confirmed the IDP nature of the GR AF1 in recent years [24–27,38,39]. It has been proposed that the IDP nature of the GR AF1 allows it rapidly to "sample" its environment until appropriate binding partners are found [38,39]. Then, either by induced-fit or selective binding of a particular AF1 conformer, a high-affinity and more persistent interaction occurs between AF1 and the relevant coregulatory protein(s) [24–27,38,39]. The IDP regions/domains including GR's NTD/AF1 promote molecular recognition primarily through unique combination of high specificity and low binding affinity with their functional binding partners, recognize and bind a number of biological targets, and create propensity to form large interaction surfaces suitable for interactions with their specific binding partners [40–47].

We have reported that several factors can influence AF1 secondary/tertiary structure formation, including binding protein partners, binding of the GR DBD to DNA, post-translational modifications such as site-specific phosphorylation in the NTD and in some circumstances, the type and concentrations of naturally occurring intracellular organic osmolytes [9,25,28,38,39]. We have also reported that such induced conformation in AF1 plays an important role in facilitating AF1's interaction with specific coregulatory proteins and subsequent transcriptional activity [9,24–27,38,39]. The ID domains of many transcription factors have been shown to undergo a disorder-order transition upon interaction with binding partners that act as coregulators [28,35]. We have also shown that interaction of the AF1 with that partner at appropriate concentrations may cause AF1 to adopt higher secondary/tertiary structure that leads to stabilize AF1 structure [24–27,38,39]. For example, the TATA box binding protein (TBP) directly binds to the GR AF1 domain in vitro and in vivo and induces secondary/tertiary structure formation in AF1 such that TBP binding-induced folding in AF1 significantly enhances AF1's interaction with other coactivators and subsequent AF1-mediated, GRE-driven promoter-reporter activity [38,39]. This phenomenon has now been reported for some other SHRs [26].

4. Role of Phosphorylation in the Regulation of Intrinsically Disordered AF1 Structure and Functions

Phosphorylation is an important post translational modification that regulates protein functions, including those of transcription factors in eukaryotic cells [48–52]. For transcription factors, phosphorylation can modulate their DNA binding affinity, interaction with components of the transcription initiation complex, and intracellular translocations [53–55]. Like many other transcription factors, the GR is a phospho-protein; consequently kinases can phosphorylate GR at multiple sites, leading to altered GR transcriptional activity [56–60]. Cell and tissue-specific GR functions are heavily regulated by specific kinases [61]. In the human GR, five serine residues have been identified [59]. All these known phosphorylation sites identified in human GR are found in the IDP NTD [10,59,60]. Three of them (S203, S211, and S226) are located within the AF1 [59].

Phosphorylation of the AF1's core region has been shown to stabilize its structure, i.e. to shift the ensemble of conformers to a higher fraction containing structure [39]. Such phosphorylation is biologically relevant. We have shown that p38 in the MAPK pathways is a potent kinase for in vitro phosphorylation of S211 on the human GR [62,63]. Glucocorticoid treatment of CEM (human leukemic) cells induces the upstream kinase of p38, which phosphorylates and actives p38, which in turn, phosphorylates the GR, establishing a forward-acting functional loop. Because, in vitro and in vivo, p38 phosphorylates the GR at this specific site, we tested the relevance to GR function. The results showed that in transfected cells, the non-phosphorylatable S211A GR mutant was considerably less potent in inducing an AF1-mediated, GRE-driven reporter gene, and in driving GR-mediated apoptosis induced by a synthetic glucocorticoid, dexamethasone [64]. More general relevance to a range of lymphoid malignancies was found when we showed that in several unrelated malignant lymphoid cell lines, a greater proportion of p38 relative to other MAPKs corresponded to relative sensitivity to GR-driven apoptosis [65], Other reports suggest that phosphorylation may affect GR stability and thus alter transcriptional activity of the receptor [66]. We have also shown that site-specific phosphorylation of the ID AF1 leads to disorder-order conformational transition such that AF1's interaction with other critical coregulatory proteins, and subsequent transcriptional activity are significantly enhanced [62,64]. Garabedian and co-workers have also demonstrated that site-specific phosphorylation in GR, particularly S211 and S226, play an important role in gene regulation by the GR, for which AF1 is a main player, as discussed above [36,59,67,68].

Several reports suggest that the state of GR phosphorylation affects its interactions with other proteins. TSG101, a component of the ESCRIT-I complex, has been reported to be preferentially recruited to the nonphosphorylated form of the GR [68]. It has been suggested that TSG101 stabilizes ligand-unbound GR in its unphosphorylated form to protect it from degradation. Thus, TSG101 interaction with GR may be important to keep unliganded GR protected from auto-degradation until the GR becomes hyper-phosphorylated. Interaction with DRIP150 (another GR coregulator and part of mediator complex) also has been reported to be modulated through GR phosphorylation [59]. Thus, it can be concluded that site-specific phosphorylation of the AF1 domain of GR can either enhance or diminish recruitment of coregulators, reflecting the biologic need for the GR to up- or down-regulate gene(s) in a cell- and promoter- specific manner by interactions with specific combinations of cofactors.

5. Discussion

Compared to protein segments with well-define globular structures, protein phosphorylation of Ser residue predominantly occurs within ID regions of signaling molecules [44,69–71]. This is significant because the formation of new hydrogen bonds would be more difficult if the sites of phosphorylation were located within ordered regions [36]. Thus, phosphorylation may regulate protein functions of the GR by affecting the conformational dynamics of the IDP NTD/AF1, leading to altered transcriptional activities [36,37,39,72]. As noted above, the GR exists in several translationally derived forms, successively shortened from the N terminus. The GR-C3 form is several times more active than the full-length, predominant "GRα" form [6,21,31]. It has been shown that this is due to loss of an NTD sub-domain, the R region, which exerts an allosterically repressive effect on GR's AF1 function [31,73]. The structural and functional effects of site-specific phosphorylations of the several GR translational forms will be important to study.

The mechanisms by which GR controls gene expression pose a central problem in molecular biology, and the role of its ID AF1 is of immense importance. Phosphorylation elicits diverse effects on the biological functions of ID proteins by altering the energetics of their conformational landscape and by modulating interactions with other cellular components by stabilizing and/or inducing secondary structural elements [74–77]. There are also reports suggesting that in IDP receptors, poly-electrostatic interactions may also play important role [78]. Thus, signaling cascades that induce phosphorylation of the GR are important factors in determining the physiological actions of its ID NTD/AF1.

6. Summary and Perspectives

Glucocorticoids, working through the GR, regulate a variety of human physiological processes in a cell/tissue-dependent manner at the level of gene regulation. Glucocorticoids have also been frontline therapy for decades in the treatment of several pathological and disease conditions; however, the exact mechanism by which GR passes signals from ligand to regulate specific genes is not fully understood. Knowledge of 3-D structure of the full-length GR will of course be the starting point to provide answers to several questions on the actions of the GR. Post-translational modifications including phosphorylation, ubiquitination, and sumoylation have all been shown to affect functions of NHR family members. There is evidence that that differential phosphorylation stabilizes the structure of the GR's IDP region and thus is a regulator of GR actions; yet it is also quite clear that the role of GR phosphorylation is a remarkably complex phenomenon.

Several outstanding questions remain to be answered: (1) What are the relative levels of phosphorylation of individual sites in specific cell/tissue- types under physiological conditions? (2) How does each phosphorylation site contribute to GR-mediated signaling through conformational rearrangements in the otherwise IDP AF1/NTD? (3) What are the allosteric consequences for the holo-GR? (4) Do the sequence of site-specific phosphorylations and the patterns of multiple-site phosphorylations matter? (5) What is the correlation between cell-based studies and in vivo animal models? (6) What are the effects of phosphorylations on the many GR isoforms?

Based on studies from our laboratory and those of others, we propose that phosphorylation-induced conformational changes in the ID AF1 may be dependent upon the phosphorylation of individual site(s) such that the effects of one phosphorylated GR site may be influenced by the relative phosphorylation of other sites (Figure 2). Cell/tissue-specific effects of GR are tightly regulated through specific kinase(s)/phosphatase(s), and site-specific phosphorylation-induced conformational changes in ID NTD/AF1 and its subsequent effects on transactivation activities may provide critical information on how different surfaces within the ID AF1/NTD may be created and used to manipulate GR target gene expression. How site-specific phosphorylation leads to induced conformations in the ID AF1 and what kind of functional folded conformation it adopts in the full-length receptor are open questions.

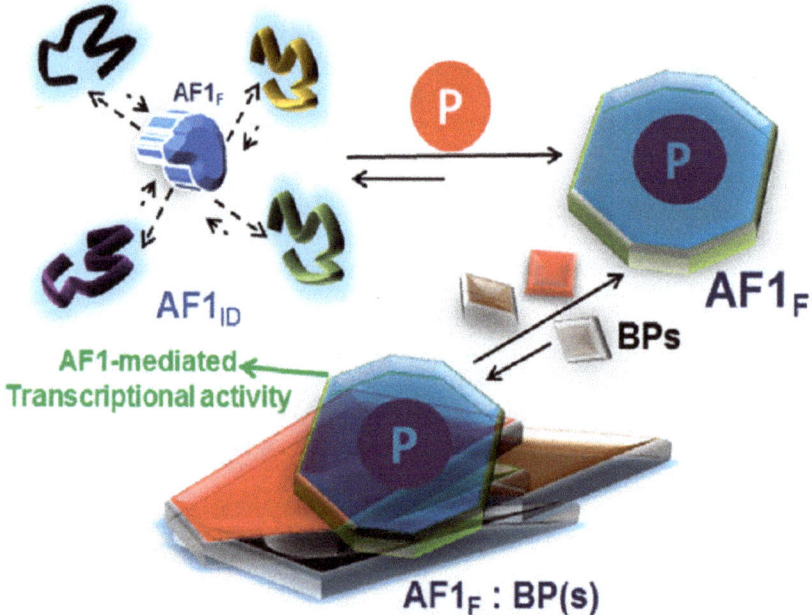

Figure 2. A proposed model of the effect of phosphorylation on the folding of intrinsically disordered (ID) AF1 domain of the glucocorticoid receptor. AF1 exists in equilibrium with mostly unstructured $AF1_{ID}$ and a small fraction of folded ($AF1_F$) conformers. Due to AF1's site-specific phosphorylation (P), the equilibrium is shifted in favor of folded conformers. This structural rearrangement in AF1 creates surfaces well suited for interaction with coregulatory binding partner (BP) proteins (shown by different shapes and colors). The interaction with these BPs results in the regulation of AF1-mediated transcription of GR target gene(s). Based on references [62,72].

Author Contributions: Conceptualization: R.K. and E.B.T.; writing-original draft, R.K.; writing review and editing: R.K. and E.B.T.

Funding: This research received no external funding.

Conflicts of Interest: The authors declare no conflict of interest.

References

1. Caratti, G.; Matthews, L.; Poolman, T.; Kershaw, S.; Baxter, M.; Ray, D. Glucocorticoid receptor function in health and disease. *Clin. Endocrinol.* **2015**, *83*, 441–448. [CrossRef] [PubMed]

2. Sapolsky, R.M.; Romero, L.M.; Munck, A.U. How do glucocorticoids influence stress responses? Integrating permissive, suppressive, stimulatory, and preparative actions. *Endocr. Rev.* **2000**, *21*, 55–89. [CrossRef] [PubMed]
3. Rhen, T.; Cidlowski, J.A. Antiinflammatory action of glucocorticoids–new mechanisms for old drugs. *N. Engl. J. Med.* **2005**, *353*, 1711–1723. [CrossRef] [PubMed]
4. Busillo, J.M.; Cidlowski, J.A. The five Rs of glucocorticoid action during inflammation: Ready, reinforce, repress, resolve, and restore. *Trends Endocrinol. Metab.* **2013**, *24*, 109–119. [CrossRef] [PubMed]
5. Barnes, P.J. Anti-inflammatory actions of glucocorticoids: Molecular mechanisms. *Clin. Sci.* **1998**, *94*, 557–572. [CrossRef] [PubMed]
6. Oakley, R.H.; Cidlowski, J.A. The Biology of the Glucocorticoid Receptor: New Signaling Mechanisms in Health and Disease. *J. Allergy Clin. Immunol.* **2013**, *132*, 1033–1044. [CrossRef] [PubMed]
7. Miner, J.N.; Hong, M.H.; Negro-Vilar, A. New and improved glucocorticoid receptor ligands. *Expert Opin. Investig. Drugs* **2005**, *14*, 1527–1545. [CrossRef] [PubMed]
8. Shah, D.S.; Kumar, R. Steroid resistance in leukemia. *World J. Exp. Med.* **2013**, *3*, 21–25. [CrossRef] [PubMed]
9. Miranda, T.B.; Morris, S.A.; Hager, G.L. Complex genomic interactions in the dynamic regulation of transcription by the glucocorticoid receptor. *Mol. Cell. Endocrinol.* **2013**, *380*, 16–24. [CrossRef] [PubMed]
10. Kumar, R.; Thompson, E.B. Gene regulation by the glucocorticoid receptor: Structure and functions relationship. *J. Steroid Biochem. Mol. Biol.* **2005**, *94*, 383–394. [CrossRef] [PubMed]
11. Kumar, R.; Johnson, B.H.; Thompson, E.B. Overview of the structural basis for transcription regulation by nuclear hormone receptors. *Essay Biochem.* **2004**, *40*, 27–39. [CrossRef]
12. Kumar, R.; Thompson, E.B. Transactivation functions of the N-terminal domains of nuclear receptors: Protein folding and coactivator interactions. *Mol. Endocrinol.* **2003**, *17*, 1–10. [CrossRef] [PubMed]
13. Kumar, R.; Thompson, E.B. The structure of the nuclear hormone receptors. *Steroids* **1999**, *64*, 310–319. [CrossRef]
14. Hollenberg, S.M.; Weinberger, C.; Ong, E.S.; Cerelli, G.; Oro, A.; Lebo, R.; Thompson, E.B.; Rosenfeld, M.G.; Evans, R.M. Primary structure and expression of a functional human glucocorticoid receptor cDNA. *Nature* **1985**, *318*, 635–641. [CrossRef] [PubMed]
15. Pratt, W.B.; Toft, D.O. Steroid receptor interactions with heat shock protein and immunophilin chaperones. *Endocr. Rev.* **1997**, *18*, 306–360. [CrossRef] [PubMed]
16. Pratt, W.B.; Morishima, Y.; Osawa, Y. The Hsp90 chaperone machinery regulates signaling by modulating ligand binding clefts. *J. Biol. Chem.* **2008**, *283*, 22885–22889. [CrossRef] [PubMed]
17. Kaul, S.; Murphy, P.J.; Chen, J.; Brown, L.; Pratt, W.B.; Simons, S.S., Jr. Mutations at positions 547–553 of rat glucocorticoid receptors reveal that hsp90 binding requires the presence, but not defined composition, of a seven-amino acid sequence at the amino terminus of the ligand binding domain. *J. Biol. Chem.* **2002**, *277*, 36223–36232. [CrossRef] [PubMed]
18. Picard, D.; Khursheed, B.; Garabedian, M.J.; Fortin, M.G.; Lindquist, S.; Yamamoto, K.R. Reduced levels of hsp90 compromise steroid receptor action in vivo. *Nature* **1990**, *348*, 166–168. [CrossRef] [PubMed]
19. Freeman, B.C.; Yamamoto, K.R. Disassembly of transcriptional regulatory complexes by molecular chaperones. *Science* **2002**, *296*, 2232–2235. [CrossRef] [PubMed]
20. Yudt, M.R.; Jewell, C.M.; Bienstock, R.J.; Cidlowski, J.A. Molecular origins for the dominant negative function of human glucocorticoid receptor beta. *Mol. Cell. Biol.* **2003**, *23*, 4319–4330. [CrossRef] [PubMed]
21. Lu, N.Z.; Cidlowski, J.A. Translational regulatory mechanisms generate N-terminal glucocorticoid receptor isoforms with unique transcriptional target genes. *Mol. Cell* **2005**, *18*, 331–342. [CrossRef] [PubMed]
22. Luisi, B.F.; Xu, W.X.; Otwinowski, Z.; Freedman, L.P.; Yamamoto, K.R.; Sigler, P.B. Crystallographic Analysis of the Interaction of The Glucocorticoid Receptor with DNA. *Nature* **1991**, *352*, 497–505. [CrossRef] [PubMed]
23. Bledsoe, R.B.; Montana, V.G.; Stanley, T.B.; Delves, C.J.; Apolito, C.J.; Mckee, D.D.; Consler, T.G.; Parks, D.J.; Stewart, E.L.; Willson, T.M.; et al. Crystal Structure of the Glucocorticoid Receptor Ligand Binding Domain Reveals a Novel Mode of Receptor Dimerization and Coactivator Recognition. *Cell* **2002**, *110*, 93–105. [CrossRef]

24. Khan, S.H.; Awasthi, S.; Guo, C.; Goswami, D.; Ling, J.; Griffin, P.R.; Simons, S.S., Jr.; Kumar, R. Binding of the N-terminal region of coactivator TIF2 to the intrinsically disordered AF1 domain of the glucocorticoid receptor is accompanied by conformational reorganizations. *J. Biol. Chem.* **2012**, *287*, 44546–44560. [CrossRef] [PubMed]
25. Kumar, R.; Lee, J.C.; Bolen, D.W.; Thompson, E.B. The conformation of the glucocorticoid receptor af1/tau1 domain induced by osmolyte binds co-regulatory proteins. *J. Biol. Chem.* **2001**, *276*, 18146–18152. [CrossRef] [PubMed]
26. Kumar, R.; Moure, C.M.; Khan, S.H.; Callaway, C.; Grimm, S.L.; Goswami, D.; Griffin, P.R.; Edwards, D.P. Regulation of the structurally dynamic disordered amino-terminal domain of progesterone receptor by protein induced folding. *J. Biol. Chem.* **2013**, *288*, 30285–30299. [CrossRef] [PubMed]
27. Khan, S.H.; Arnott, J.A.; Kumar, R. Naturally occurring osmolyte, trehalose induces functional conformation in an intrinsically disordered region of the glucocorticoid receptor. *PLoS ONE* **2011**, *6*, e19689. [CrossRef] [PubMed]
28. Kumar, R.; McEwan, I.J. Allosteric modulators of steroid hormone receptors: Structural dynamics and gene regulation. *Endocr. Rev.* **2012**, *33*, 271–299. [CrossRef] [PubMed]
29. Dahlman-Wright, K.; Almlöf, T.; McEwan, I.J.; Gustafsson, J.A.; Wright, A.P. Delineation of a small region within the major transactivation domain of the human glucocorticoid receptor that mediates transactivation of gene expression. *Proc. Natl. Acad. Sci. USA* **1994**, *91*, 1619–1623. [CrossRef] [PubMed]
30. Dahlman-Wright, K.; Baumann, H.; McEwan, I.J.; Almlöf, T.; Wright, A.P.; Gustafsson, J.A.; Härd, T. Structural characterization of a minimal functional transactivation domain from the human glucocorticoid receptor. *Proc. Natl. Acad. Sci. USA* **1994**, *92*, 1699–1703. [CrossRef]
31. Li, J.; White, J.T.; Saavedra, H.; Wrabl, J.O.; Motlagh, H.N.; Liu, K.; Sowers, J.; Schroer, T.A.; Thompson, E.B.; Hilser, V.J. Genetically tunable frustration controls allostery in an intrinsically disordered transcription factor. *Elife* **2017**, *12*, 6. [CrossRef] [PubMed]
32. Goswami, D.; Pascal, B.; Kumar, R.; Edwards, D.P.; Griffin, P.R. Influence of Domain Interactions on Conformational Mobility of the Progesterone Receptor Detected by Hydrogen/Deuterium Exchange Mass Spectrometry. *Structure* **2014**, *22*, 961–973. [CrossRef] [PubMed]
33. Simons, S.S.; Edwards, D.P.; Kumar, R. Dynamic Structures of Nuclear Hormone Receptors: New Promises and Challenges. *Mol. Endocrinol.* **2014**, *28*, 173–182. [CrossRef] [PubMed]
34. Kumar, R.; Betney, R.; Li, J.; Thompson, E.B.; McEwan, I.J. Induced alpha-helix structure in AF1 of the androgen receptor upon binding transcription factor TFIIF. *Biochemistry* **2004**, *43*, 3008–3013. [CrossRef] [PubMed]
35. Wright, P.E.; Dyson, H.J. Intrinsically Disordered Proteins in Cellular Signaling and Regulation. *Nat. Rev. Mol. Cell Biol.* **2015**, *16*, 18–29. [CrossRef] [PubMed]
36. Kulkarni, P.; Jolly, M.K.; Jia, D.; Mooney, S.M.; Bhargava, A.; Kagohara, L.T.; Chen, Y.; Hao, P.; He, Y.; Veltri, R.W.; et al. Phosphorylation-induced conformational dynamics in an intrinsically disordered protein and potential role in phenotypic heterogeneity. *Proc. Natl. Acad. Sci. USA* **2017**, *114*, E2644–E2653. [CrossRef] [PubMed]
37. Dunker, A.K.; Uversky, V.N. Signal transduction via unstructured protein conduits. *Nat. Chem. Biol.* **2008**, *4*, 229–230. [CrossRef] [PubMed]
38. Khan, S.H.; Ling, J.; Kumar, R. TBP binding-induced folding of the glucocorticoid receptor AF1 domain facilitates its interaction with steroid receptor coactivator-1. *PLos ONE* **2011**, *6*, e21939. [CrossRef] [PubMed]
39. Kumar, R.; Volk, D.E.; Li, J.; Gorenstein, D.G.; Lee, J.C.; Thompson, E.B. TBP binding induces structure in the recombinant glucocorticoid receptor AF1 domain. *Proc. Natl. Acad. Sci. USA* **2004**, *101*, 16425–16430. [CrossRef] [PubMed]
40. Liu, J.; Perumal, N.B.; Oldfield, C.J.; Su, E.W.; Uversky, V.N.; Dunker, A.K. Intrinsic disorder in transcription factors. *Biochemistry* **2006**, *45*, 6873–6888. [CrossRef] [PubMed]
41. Iakoucheva, L.M.; Brown, C.J.; Lawson, J.D.; Obradovic, Z.; Dunker, A.K. Intrinsic disorder in cell-signaling and cancer-associated proteins. *J. Mol. Biol.* **2002**, *323*, 573–584. [CrossRef]
42. Ward, J.J.; Sodhi, J.S.; McGuffin, L.J.; Buxton, B.F.; Jones, D.T. Prediction and functional analysis of native disorder in proteins from the three kingdoms of life. *J. Mol. Biol.* **2004**, *337*, 635–645. [CrossRef] [PubMed]
43. Tompa, P. Intrinsically unstructured proteins. *Trends Biochem. Sci.* **2002**, *27*, 527–533. [CrossRef]

44. Dyson, H.J.; Wright, P.E. Coupling of folding and binding for unstructured proteins. *Curr. Opin. Struct. Biol.* **2002**, *12*, 54–60. [CrossRef]
45. Namba, K. Roles of partly unfolded conformations in macromolecular self-assembly. *Genes Cells* **2001**, *6*, 1–12. [CrossRef] [PubMed]
46. Crivici, A.; Ikura, M. Molecular and structural basis of target recognition by calmodulin. *Annu. Rev. Biophys. Biomol. Struct.* **1995**, *24*, 85–116. [CrossRef] [PubMed]
47. Romero, P.; Obradovic, Z.; Dunker, A.K. Natively disordered proteins: Functions and predictions. *Appl. Bioinformat.* **2004**, *3*, 105–113. [CrossRef]
48. Ostertag, M.S.; Messias, A.C.; Sattler, M.; Popowicz, G.M. The Structure of the SPOP-Pdx1 Interface Reveals Insights into the Phosphorylation-Dependent Binding Regulation. *Structure* **2019**, *27*, 1–8. [CrossRef] [PubMed]
49. Mattiske, T.; Tan, M.H.; Dearsley, O.; Cloosterman, D.; Hii, C.S.; Gécz, J.; Shoubridge, C. Regulating transcriptional activity by phosphorylation: A new mechanism for the ARX homeodomain transcription factor. *PLoS One* **2018**, *13*, e0206914. [CrossRef] [PubMed]
50. Orea-Soufi, A.; Dávila, D.; Salazar-Roa, M.; de Mar Lorente, M.; Velasco, G. Phosphorylation of FOXO Proteins as a Key Mechanism to Regulate Their Activity. *Methods Mol. Biol.* **2019**, *1890*, 51–59. [CrossRef] [PubMed]
51. Puertollano, R.; Ferguson, S.M.; Brugarolas, J.; Ballabio, A. The complex relationship between TFEB transcription factor phosphorylation and subcellular localization. *EMBO J.* **2018**, *37*, e98804. [CrossRef] [PubMed]
52. Wang, L.G.; Liu, M.X.; Kreis, W.; Budman, D.R. Phosphorylation/dephosphorylation of androgen as a determinant of androgen agonistic or antagonistic activity. *Biochem. Biophys. Res. Commun.* **1999**, *259*, 21–28. [CrossRef] [PubMed]
53. Bai, W.; Weigel, N.L. Phosphorylation and steroid hormone action. *Vit. Horm.* **1995**, *51*, 289–313.
54. Gioeli, D.; Ficarro, S.B.; Kwiek, J.J.; Aaronson, D.; Hancock, M.; Catling, A.D.; White, F.M.; Christian, R.E.; Settlage, R.E.; Shabanowitz, J.; et al. Androgen receptor phosphorylation. *J. Biol. Chem.* **2002**, *32*, 29304–29314. [CrossRef] [PubMed]
55. Rogatsky, I.; Waase, C.L.; Garabedian, M.J. Phosphorylation and inhibition of rat glucocorticoid receptor transcriptional activation by glycogen synthase kinase-3 (GSK-3). Species-specific differences between human and rat glucocorticoid receptor signaling as revealed through GSK-3 phosphorylation. *J. Biol. Chem.* **1998**, *273*, 14315–14321. [CrossRef] [PubMed]
56. Krstic, M.D.; Rogatsky, I.; Yamamoto, K.R.; Garabedian, M.J. Mitogen-activated and cyclin-dependent protein kinases selectively and differentially modulate transcriptional enhancement by the glucocorticoid receptor. *Mol. Cell. Biol.* **1997**, *17*, 3947–3954. [CrossRef] [PubMed]
57. Bodwell, J.E.; Webster, J.C.; Jewell, C.M.; Cidlowski, J.A.; Hu, J.M.; Munck, A. Glucocorticoid receptor phosphorylation: Overview, function and cell cycle-dependence. *J. Steroid Biochem. Mol. Biol.* **1998**, *65*, 91–99. [CrossRef]
58. Bodwell, J.E.; Orti, E.; Coull, J.M.; Pappin, D.J.C.; Smith, L.I.; Swift, F. Identification of phosphorylated sites in the mouse glucocorticoid receptor. *J. Biol. Chem.* **1991**, *266*, 7549–7555. [PubMed]
59. Ismaili, N.; Garabedian, M.J. Modulation of glucocorticoid receptor function via phosphorylation. *Ann. N. Y. Acad. Sci.* **2004**, *1024*, 86–101. [CrossRef] [PubMed]
60. Mason, S.A.; Housley, P.R. Site-directed mutagenesis of the phosphorylation sites in the mouse glucocorticoid receptor. *J. Biol. Chem.* **1993**, *268*, 21501–21504. [PubMed]
61. Duma, D.; Jewell, C.M.; Cidlowski, J.A. Multiple glucocorticoid receptor isoforms and mechanisms of post-translational modification. *J. Steroid Biochem. Mol. Biol.* **2006**, *102*, 11–21. [CrossRef] [PubMed]
62. Garza, A.M.; Khan, S.H.; Kumar, R. Site-specific phosphorylation induces functionally active conformation in the intrinsically disordered N-terminal activation function (AF1) domain of the glucocorticoid receptor. *Mol. Cell. Biol.* **2010**, *30*, 220–230. [CrossRef] [PubMed]
63. Miller, A.L.; Webb, M.S.; Copik, A.J.; Wang, Y.; Johnson, B.H.; Kumar, R.; Thompson, E.B. p38 mitogen-activated protein kinase (MAPK) is a key mediator in glucocorticoid-induced apoptosis of lymphoid cells: Correlation between p38 MAPK activation and site-specific phosphorylation of the human glucocorticoid receptor at serine 211. *Mol. Endocrinol.* **2005**, *19*, 1569–1583. [CrossRef] [PubMed]

64. Khan, S.H.; McLaughlin, W.A.; Kumar, R. Site-specific phosphorylation regulates the structure and function of an intrinsically disordered domain of the glucocorticoid receptor. *Sci. Rep.* **2017**, *7*, 15440. [CrossRef] [PubMed]
65. Garza, A.S.; Miller, A.L.; Johnson, B.H.; Thompson, E.B. Converting cell lines representing hematological malignancies from glucocorticoid-resistant to glucocorticoid-sensitive: Signaling pathway interactions. *Leuk. Res.* **2009**, *33*, 717–727. [CrossRef] [PubMed]
66. Zhou, J.; Cidlowski, J.A. The human glucocorticoid receptor: One gene, multiple proteins and diverse responses. *Steroids* **2005**, *70*, 407–417. [CrossRef] [PubMed]
67. Wang, Z.; Chen, W.; Kono, E.; Dang, T.; Garabedian, M.J. Modulation of glucocorticoid receptor phosphorylation and transcriptional activity by a C-terminal-associated protein phosphatase. *Mol. Endocrinol.* **2007**, *21*, 625–634. [CrossRef] [PubMed]
68. Ismaili, N.; Blind, R.; Garabedian, M.J. Stabilization of the unliganded glucocorticoid receptor by TSG101. *J. Biol. Chem.* **2005**, *280*, 11120–11126. [CrossRef] [PubMed]
69. Iakoucheva, L.M.; Radivojac, P.; Brown, C.J.; O'Connor, T.R.; Sikes, J.G.; Obradovic, Z.; Dunker, A.K. The importance of intrinsic disorder for protein phosphorylation. *Nucleic Acids Res.* **2004**, *32*, 1037–1049. [CrossRef] [PubMed]
70. Bah, A.; Forman-Kay, J.D. Modulation of Intrinsically Disordered Protein Function by Post-translational Modifications. *J. Biol. Chem.* **2016**, *291*, 6696–6705. [CrossRef] [PubMed]
71. Khan, S.H.; Kumar, R. Role of an intrinsically disordered conformation in AMPK-mediated phosphorylation of ULK1 and regulation of autophagy. *Mol. Biosyst.* **2012**, *8*, 91–96. [CrossRef] [PubMed]
72. Kumar, R.; Calhoun, W.J. Differential regulation of the transcriptional activity of the glucocorticoid receptor through site-specific phosphorylation. *Biol. Targets Ther.* **2008**, *2*, 845–854. [CrossRef]
73. Kumar, R.; Thompson, E.B. Influence of flanking sequences on signaling between the activation function AF1 and DNA-binding domain of glucocorticoid receptor. *Arch. Biochem. Biophys.* **2010**, *496*, 140–145. [CrossRef] [PubMed]
74. Dyson, H.J.; Wright, P.E. Intrinsically unstructured proteins and their functions. *Nat. Rev. Mol. Cell Biol.* **2005**, *6*, 197–208. [CrossRef] [PubMed]
75. Baker, J.M.; Hudson, R.P.; Kanelis, V.; Choy, W.Y.; Thibodeau, P.H.; Thomas, P.J.; Forman-Kay, J.D. CFTR regulatory region interacts with NBD1 predominantly via multiple transient helices. *Nat. Struct. Mol. Biol.* **2007**, *14*, 738–745. [CrossRef] [PubMed]
76. He, Y.; Chen, Y.; Mooney, S.M.; Rajagopalan, K.; Bhargava, A.; Sacho, E.; Weninger, K.; Bryan, P.N.; Kulkarni, P.; Orban, J. Phosphorylation-induced conformational ensemble switching in an intrinsically disordered cancer/testis antigen. *J. Biol. Chem.* **2015**, *290*, 25090–25102. [CrossRef] [PubMed]
77. Bah, A.; Vernon, R.M.; Siddiqui, Z.; Krzeminski, M.; Muhandiram, R.; Zhao, C.; Sonenberg, N.; Kay, L.E.; Forman-Kay, J.D. Folding of an intrinsically disordered protein by phosphorylation as a regulatory switch. *Nature* **2015**, *519*, 106–109. [CrossRef] [PubMed]
78. Borg, M.; Mittag, T.; Pawson, T.; Tyres, M.; Forman-Kay, J.D.; Chan, H.S. Polyelectrostatic interactions of disordered ligands suggest a physical basis for ultrasensitivity. *Proc. Natl. Acad. Sci. USA* **2007**, *104*, 9650–9655. [CrossRef] [PubMed]

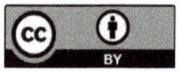

© 2019 by the authors. Licensee MDPI, Basel, Switzerland. This article is an open access article distributed under the terms and conditions of the Creative Commons Attribution (CC BY) license (http://creativecommons.org/licenses/by/4.0/).

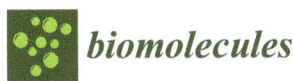

Review

Structure and Functions of Microtubule Associated Proteins Tau and MAP2c: Similarities and Differences

Kateřina Melková [1,2,†], Vojtěch Zapletal [1,2,†], Subhash Narasimhan [1,†], Séverine Jansen [1], Jozef Hritz [1], Rostislav Škrabana [3,4], Markus Zweckstetter [5,6], Malene Ringkjøbing Jensen [7], Martin Blackledge [7] and Lukáš Žídek [1,2,*]

1. Central European Institute of Technology, Masaryk University, Kamenice 5, 625 00 Brno, Czech Republic; katerina.melkova@ceitec.muni.cz (K.M.); vojtech.zapletal@ceitec.muni.cz (V.Z.); subhash.narasimhan@ceitec.muni.cz (S.N.); severine@chemi.muni.cz (S.J.); jozef.hritz@ceitec.muni.cz (J.H.)
2. Faculty of Science, National Centre for Biomolecular Research, Masaryk University, Kamenice 5, 625 00 Brno, Czech Republic
3. Institute of Neuroimmunology, Slovak Academy of Sciences, Dúbravská cesta 9, 845 10 Bratislava, Slovakia; rostislav.skrabana@savba.sk
4. Axon Neuroscience R&D Services SE, Dvořákovo nábrežie 10, 811 02 Bratislava, Slovakia
5. German Center for Neurodegenerative Diseases (DZNE), Von-Siebold-Str. 3a, 37075 Göttingen, Germany; Markus.Zweckstetter@dzne.de
6. Department of NMR-Based Structural Biology, Max Planck Institute for Biophysical Chemistry, Am Fassberg 11, 37077 Göttingen, Germany
7. University Grenoble Alps, CEA, CNRS, 38000 Grenoble, France; malene.ringkjobing-jensen@ibs.fr (M.R.J.); martin.blackledge@ibs.fr (M.B.)
* Correspondence: lzidek@chemi.muni.cz; Tel.: +420-549-498-393
† These authors contributed equally to this work.

Received: 30 January 2019; Accepted: 13 March 2019; Published: 16 March 2019

Abstract: The stability and dynamics of cytoskeleton in brain nerve cells are regulated by microtubule associated proteins (MAPs), tau and MAP2. Both proteins are intrinsically disordered and involved in multiple molecular interactions important for normal physiology and pathology of chronic neurodegenerative diseases. Nuclear magnetic resonance and cryo-electron microscopy recently revealed propensities of MAPs to form transient local structures and long-range contacts in the free state, and conformations adopted in complexes with microtubules and filamentous actin, as well as in pathological aggregates. In this paper, we compare the longest, 441-residue brain isoform of tau (tau40), and a 467-residue isoform of MAP2, known as MAP2c. For both molecules, we present transient structural motifs revealed by conformational analysis of experimental data obtained for free soluble forms of the proteins. We show that many of the short sequence motifs that exhibit transient structural features are linked to functional properties, manifested by specific interactions. The transient structural motifs can be therefore classified as molecular recognition elements of tau40 and MAP2c. Their interactions are further regulated by post-translational modifications, in particular phosphorylation. The structure-function analysis also explains differences between biological activities of tau40 and MAP2c.

Keywords: microtubule associated protein; tau; intrinsically disordered protein; phosphorylation; nuclear magnetic resonance

1. Introduction

The stability and dynamic behavior of the cytoskeleton are regulated by structural microtubule associated proteins (MAPs) [1]. Major structural MAPs in brain nerve cells are the MAP2 and tau protein [2]. Polypeptide chains of MAP2 and tau have a bipolar character; their microtubule binding repeats (MTBRs) and projection domain (PD) lie at C- and N-terminal part of molecule, respectively. Both proteins exist as multiple alternatively spliced isoforms (Figure 1), differing in the presence of the second MTBR (exon 10 of tau and exon 16 of MAP2) and of several exons in PD (including long exon 9 distinguishing high-molecular weight isoforms of MAP2). Expression of individual isoforms is developmentally and regionally regulated. Most notably, adult neurons express high-molecular weight MAP2 isoforms specifically in cell bodies and dendrites [2], whereas the six tau protein isoforms are found predominantly in axons [3]. Low molecular weight MAP2 isoforms are expressed in developing neurons, mostly prenatally, whereas high-molecular weight tau isoforms comprising exons 4a and 6 are expressed only in peripheral tissues [4].

Both high- and low-molecular weight isoforms of the discussed MAPs have been studied extensively. However, detailed and residue-specific description of transient structural features is currently available only for MAP2c and for the tau isoforms presented in Figure 1. Although the structure-function relationship is not described for MAP2a and MAP2b in such details, it is evident that high-molecular weight isoforms of MAP2 play important and specific biological roles. The increased expression of MAP2a (and decreased expression of MAP2c) correlates with the reduction of cytoskeleton dynamics during neuronal maturation [5]. Presence or absence of long PD seems to be one of the factors (together with messenger RNA (mRNA) compartmentalization) controlling cellular localization of MAP2 isoforms [2,5]. Transfection experiments suggested that the presence of long PD prevents MAP2a/b from entering the axons [6]. The size of PD also influences properties of microtubule (MT) bundles induced by MAP2 isoforms, with a potential impact on the kinesin- and dynein-dependent transport along microtubules [2]. It has been suggested that the length of PD of MAP2 and tau isoforms regulates the spacing of MTs inside MT bundles in dendrites and axons [7]. Experiments with tau adsorbed on mica surface (a proxy for the MTs) suggested that the MT distance spacer may be formed by an antiparallel charge-dependent dimerization of PDs from opposing tau molecules [8]. Direct measurement of forces between tau-coated MTs at physiological, sub-stoichiometric tau:tubulin ratio revealed that a structure of the PD layer may depend on both the amount of bound tau and the molecular crowding, where the isoforms with longer PD conferred a much higher resistance to MT bundling under increased osmotic pressure [9]. Interestingly, MAP2 and tau isoforms may bind and crosslink MTs with F-actin by partially overlapping multiple interaction sites in the MTBRs [10,11]. The apparent binding affinity of tau to F-actin is comparable to its affinity to MTs [12]. Mice with either MAP2 or tau gene knockout were apparently normal, but simultaneous disruption of MAP1b gene led to a high prenatal mortality [13–15]. It suggested an important role of MAP2/tau in neurogenesis, which can be (partially) rescued by MAP1b.

Despite the similarity in overall molecular organization and physiological function, along with a high sequence identity of the MTBRs, MAP2 and tau have contrasting significance in pathophysiological processes resulting in chronic diseases. The involvement of MAP2 in pathogenesis (based on detection of high-molecular weight isoforms in adult tissues) is relatively modest. Depletion of MAP2 has been associated with a Lewy body variant of Alzheimer's disease [16], whereas colocalization of MAP2 with α-synuclein in Lewy bodies was shown in Parkinson's disease [17]. Disappearance of dendritic high-molecular weight MAP2 isoforms was recently described in striatum of patients with Huntington's disease [18]. 3β-methoxy-pregnenolone, which binds to MAP2 isoforms in vitro and increases its ability to stimulate tubulin assembly, has antidepressant efficacy in rats [19]. In contrary, tau protein has been long known for its involvement in various neurodegenerative illnesses. Tau was discovered as the constituent of neurofibrillary pathology in Alzheimer's disease and other tauopathies, comprised of more than 20 individual disorders; for review see [3,20]. Tens of exonic and intronic mutations in tau gene with direct implications for neuropathological conditions were described. As the extent of tau pathology correlates with the disease progression, tau has become an appealing target for various therapeutic strategies including small-molecule inhibition of tau aggregation and phosphorylation, anti-sense oligonucleotide therapy, passive and active immunotherapy [21–23]. Pathological forms of tau include high-molecular weight oligomers and polymers, in which the tau molecules associate via their MTBRs, forming tightly ordered amyloid structures [20,24]. The fact that MAP2 was never found polymerized in vivo despite 90% sequence homology of respective MTBRs, aggregation properties of chimeric proteins, and site-directed mutagenesis indicate a key role of individual tau residues for initiation and propagation of polymerization [25,26].

Isoforms of MAP2c and tau are subjects to frequent post-translational modifications [27]. Modifications at specific sites regulate binding to MTs and MT dynamics [28–31]. Importantly, MAP2 and tau isoforms have a highly disordered polypeptide backbone (see below), which can be selectively modulated by protein phosphorylation. Apart from introducing two negative charges per phosphate group (at physiological pH), which can influence the long-range contacts, phosphate oxygens may form specific local interactions with neighbouring main chain polar groups (carbonyl, amine) [32,33], changing the distribution of preferred transient conformations in the conformational ensemble. For instance, using short tau phosphopeptides it has been shown that phosphorylation of proline-rich regions of tau may induce local conformational changes to polyproline II helix [31,34]. Physiological phosphorylation of MAP2 exceeds that of tau (1–2.5 and 0.5–1 phosphates per 100 residues in MAP2 and tau, respectively). However, phosphorylation of tau increases four-fold under pathological conditions and has been associated with tau toxic gain of function [3,28]. In developing brain both proteins exhibit elevated phosphate content, whereas in adulthood the overall phosphorylation decreases. Kinases phosphorylating tau and MAP2 isoforms have been reviewed previously [5,35–37]. Tyrosine kinases include Fyn, Syk, c-Abl, Arg. The list of serine/threonine kinases is long, those discussed as examples in this paper are listed in Table 1.

Table 1. List of Ser/Thr kinases discussed in this review.

Kinase	Abbreviation	Proline-Directed	Activator
cAMP-dependent protein kinase	PKA	no	–
MT-affinity-regulating kinases	MARK1–4	no	–
extracellular signal-regulated kinase 2	ERK2	yes	MEK [a]
glycogen-synthase kinase 3β	GSK3β	yes	–
cyclin dependent kinase 5	CDK5	yes	p35, p39
c-Jun N-terminal kinase 1	JNK1	yes	–
stress-activated protein kinase 4	SAPK4/p38δ	yes	–

[a] MAPK/ERK kinase (also known as itogen-activated protein kinase kinase).

Both tau and MAP2 isoforms are intrinsically disordered in the free state and interact with complex cytoskeletal structures. It makes them challenging targets for structural studies. Nevertheless, improved resolution of nuclear magnetic resonance (NMR) spectroscopy and electron microscopy (EM) made detailed studies of free and interacting MAPs possible. Structural features of highly flexible free tau40 [38,39] and MAP2c [40] isoforms have been described using liquid-state NMR, complemented by quantitative conformational analysis. Recently published atomic and near-atomic resolution data allow us to look for molecular mechanisms of physiological processes altered in chronic diseases. Combination of cryo-electron microscopy (cryo-EM), NMR, and computational analysis provided reliable high-resolution models of tau interacting with microtubules (MTs) [41–43], actin filaments [10], and forming filaments in brains of patients suffering from the Alzheimer's disease [24,44]. Our goal is not to provide here a complete list of physiological and pathological roles of the reviewed proteins or a summary of all experimental structural data. Instead, we discuss (i) how molecular functions and dysfunctions of tau and MAP2 can be traced to sequence motifs forming transient, but well defined local structures with distinct dynamics; and (ii) how differences in such motifs explain functional diversity of tau and MAP2. Specifically, we limit the discussion to the longest, 441-residue brain isoform of human tau (clone htau40, splicing variant 2N4R), and the shortest, 467-residue isoform of rat MAP2 (94% sequence identity with the corresponding human isoform), referred to as tau40 and MAP2c in this paper, respectively. Residue numbering is referred to these two isoforms as well.

Our selection of these MAPs mostly reflects the amount of available experimental data reported in the literature. Also, the similar lengths of the chosen isoforms simplify direct comparison of both proteins.

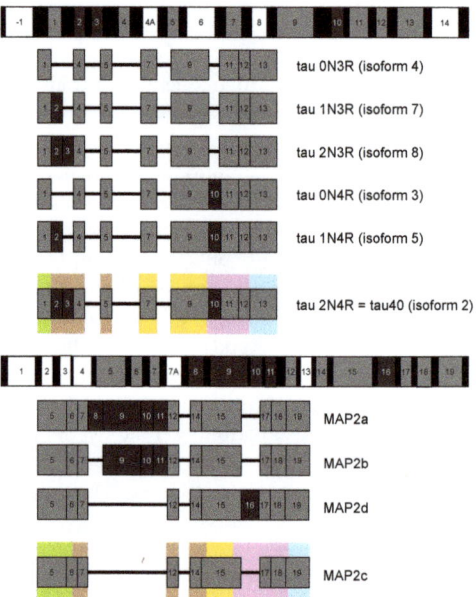

Figure 1. Organization of the DNA sequences of tau (top) and MAP2 (bottom) and splicing isoforms expressed in brain. Exons not expressed in brain isoforms are shown in white, exons expressed in all isoforms are shown in light gray, and exons expressed in some isoforms are shown in dark gray. Regions of isoforms discussed in this review are shown in boxes of different colors. The exons of tau and MAP2 are numbered according to Cailet-Boudin et al. [4] and Sündermann et al. [45], tau isoforms are numbered according to the National Center for Biotechnology Information (NCBI) RefSeq database.

2. Measurement and Presentation of Transient Local Structures

As mentioned above, our goal is to relate the biological functions of tau40 and MAP2c to transient secondary structures observable in a free state. Therefore, we start our discussion by briefly commenting how the structural data were obtained, and how they are presented in this paper.

So-called intrinsically disordered proteins (IDPs), including tau40 and MAP2c, do not adopt a random conformation as many synthetic polymers. Instead, they exist in multiple rapidly inter-converting structures defined by the same interactions as well-ordered proteins. Therefore, transient secondary structure motifs and long-range order are present in IDP samples, and their populations can be estimated by analyzing experimental data.

Formation of transient local structures discussed in this paper was inferred from NMR chemical shifts, measured in several studies [38,40,46–55], and converted to populations of conformers occupying different regions of the Ramachandran diagram by the ASTEROIDS algorithm [39,56,57]. The ASTEROIDS analysis also included results of NMR paramagnetic relaxation enhancements and small-angle X-ray scattering, describing long-range contacts and overall shapes of the studied molecules, respectively. Technically, the result of the analysis was a set of three-dimensional structures selected to match the experimental data. This allowed us to statistically evaluate not only populations of backbone torsion angles of individual amino acids, but also occurrence of their specific combinations, which give rise to secondary structure elements (Figures S1–S4 in Supplementary Materials). Distribution of these parameters are presented in this paper as an experimental measure of the propensity to form such structural motifs.

Although full-length tau40 and MAP2c can be studied by current NMR techniques, analysis of shorter fragments provides useful information about the influence of long-range contacts on local structure. Based on a comparison of $^{13}C^{\alpha}$ chemical shifts, secondary structures of full-length tau40 and of three shorter constructs are very similar [38] and similar results were obtained also for MAP2c and its fragments (Figure S5 in Supplementary Materials). This similarity underlines the fact that secondary structure propensities are highly specific properties of the sequence motifs. However, it should be stressed that although long-range contacts do not change the overall statistics of secondary structures in free tau40 and MAP2c, they define distinct global ("tertiary") structures. External factors such as interactions with binding partners or molecular truncation [58] may result in conformational selection of minor, but functionally important global states. For example, interaction of tau MTBRs with the monoclonal antibody DC8E8 was enhanced up to 25 times after removal of N- and C-termini of the molecule [59].

Visualization of the local structures is not trivial because multiple locally ordered structural motifs cannot be aligned in a single three-dimensional structural model. Therefore, in this paper we discuss conformations of tau40 and MAP2c without showing the three-dimensional structures explicitly. Occurrence of two secondary structure motifs that were present most often in the ensembles of conformers selected by the ASTEROIDS analysis (α-helix and polyproline II) is schematically depicted in Figure 2. To give more quantitative description of the propensity to form secondary structures, populations of continuous stretches of seven residues found in the same conformation in the selected ensembles are plotted for individual tau40 and MAP2c regions in Figures 3–7 [57]. Residues with increased populations of β-turn conformations [60] are also marked in Figures 3–7.

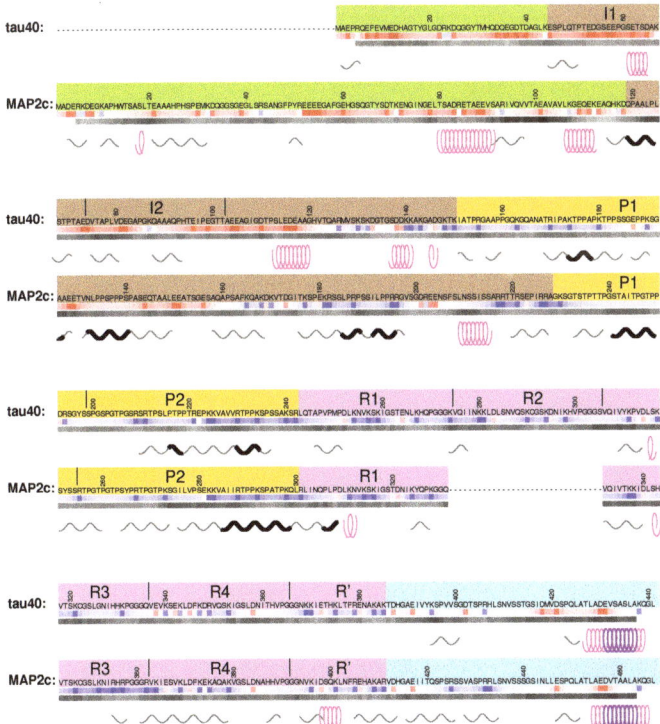

Figure 2. Sequences of human tau40 and rat MAP2c shown with backgrounds distinguishing individual regions. The pale green background indicates the N-terminal region, the brown background indicates

the variable central region preceding the proline-rich domains, the yellow background indicates the proline-rich domains, the violet background indicates MT binding domains, and the cyan background indicates the C-terminal region. Charge distribution, hydropathicity, and preferred secondary structures are shown below the sequences. The charge distribution is represented by the color in the upper rows of squares below the sequences, corresponding to a relative electrostatic potential approximated by $\sum_j CQ_i/(d_0 + d_1|n_i - n_j|)$, where Q_i and n_i are charge and sequential number of the i-th residue, C is a constant including the electric permittivity, and d_k are distance constants. The ratio d_1/d_0 was set to 2.0 and the colors were chosen so that red and blue correspond to the highest negative and positive potential, respectively, which makes the color code independent of C/d_0 [40]. The hydropathicity index according to Kyte and Doolittle [61] is shown as darkness of the lower rows of squares below the sequences (white and black correspond to the values of −4.5 and +4.5, respectively). Formation of transient α-helices is shown as pink and purple symbols (corresponding to more than 5% and 15%, respectively, of structures with continuous stretches of four amino acids in α-helical conformation in the ensembles selected by the ASTEROIDS analysis of NMR chemical shifts [39,57]), formation of transient polyproline II structures is shown as gray and black symbols (corresponding to more than 5% and 15%, respectively, of structures with continuous stretches of four amino acids in polyproline II conformation in the ensembles selected by the ASTEROIDS analysis).

3. N-Terminal Regions

The sequences of tau40 and MAP2c start with PDs, involved in the regulation of microtubule spacing. N-terminal regions of PDs (pale green boxes in Figures 1 and 2) are rich in acidic and hydrophobic amino acids. As the N-terminal regions of tau and MAP2 differ in size, structural properties, and physiological functions, structural characteristics and examples of biological roles associated with these regions are discussed separately for tau40 and MAP2c in this section.

3.1. Structural Properties of N-Terminal Region of tau40

In the free form, the N-terminal region of tau exhibits low content of secondary structure, but makes transient contacts with the positively charged proline-rich regions and strongly helical C-terminus [38,39,62]. These intramolecular electrostatic interactions contribute to formation of bent "paper-clip" tertiary structure of tau (together with contacts between MTBRs and the C-terminal region) [62], and to consequent functional links between distant regions. The intramolecular contacts also compete with intermolecular interactions. In the following paragraphs, we present biological roles that seem to depend on balance between intra- and intermolecular interactions of functionally important sequence at the very N-terminus of tau.

3.2. Phosphatase Activation by Tau N-Terminus and Axonal Transport

The first role of tau discussed in this section is modulation of the axonal transport, closely related to the localization of tau in axons. The motif shown in the pale green box in Figure 3 was described as the phosphatase-activating domain (PAD) because a peptide consisting of amino acids Ala2–Tyr18 activates a signaling cascade involving protein phosphatase 1 (PP1) and GSK3β kinase [63,64]. Phosphatase-activating domain contains an imperfect consensus PP1 binding motif $_5$RQEF$_8$ [65], which explains why Tau specifically interacts with PP1 and targets PP1 to MTs. The PP1 converts GSK3β to its active (dephosphorylated) form, which phosphorylates kinesin light chain. This inhibits fast axonal transport mediated by kinesin moving along MTs since phosphorylation of the kinesin releases the kinesin-bound cargo. It was suggested that a lack of the native intramolecular contacts in aggregates and other pathological forms of tau lead to axonal transport dysfunction accompanying Alzheimer's disease and other neurodegenerative diseases. In the absence of the native contacts, PAD is more exposed, the PP1-GSK3β pathway is hyperactivated, and the axonal transport is inhibited.

The N-terminal region of tau also represents an excellent example of regulation of biologically important interactions by post-translational modifications. The last amino acid of PAD is highly conserved Tyr18 and its neighboring residues match the ideal recognition sequence of the Fyn kinase (GTYG, preceded by an acidic and an aromatic residue) identified by a phage display [66]. Tyr18 is indeed preferentially phosphorylated by several kinases including Fyn [36,67]. It has been shown that the phosphomimetic mutation Y18E prevents the inhibition of axonal transport by PAD. Based on this finding, it was proposed that phosphorylation of Tyr18 regulates the cargo delivery [68].

The N-terminus of tau also binds another protein involved in axonal transport, dynactin. Dynactin is a multi-protein complex essential for axonal transport, playing an important role in mediating the binding of the MT motor dynein to its membranous cargoes [69,70]. The dynactin complex forms an actin-like filament and a lateral arm able to interact with MTs. The major component of the arm is p150. Its N-terminal domain binds MTs, while C-terminal 230 amino acids contribute to a structure, called shoulder, sitting on the filament. It has been reported that tau sequences encoded by exons 1 and 4 interact independently with the C-terminus of p150 and stabilize MT binding to the dynactin complex [71]. Interaction with exon 1 is affected by mutation of Arg5, associated with frontotemporal dementia and parkinsonism linked to chromosome 17 (FTDP-17). Therefore, PAD is most likely involved in the binding and mutations in PAD can cause defects in axonal transport.

3.3. Interactions of Tau with Neuronal Membranes

Another physiological role regulated by phosphorylation of Tyr18 is tau's interaction with neuronal membranes [72]. It has been shown that phosphorylated Tyr18 interacts with the Src-homology 2 (SH2) domain of the tyrosine kinase Fyn, and that Fyn-mediated phosphorylation induces trafficking of tau to detergent-resistant membrane microdomains in mouse primary cortical neurons [73]. These membrane microdomains are involved in intracellular signaling and therefore regulation of the Tyr18 phosphorylation may be an important factor in keeping normal physiological conditions. Furthermore, tau is recruited to the lipid rafts and phosphorylated at Tyr18 when SHSY-5Y cells are treated with the Aβ peptide [74]. It indicates that Tyr18 phosphorylation and interactions of tau with membranes may play a role in the Aβ-induced neurotoxicity.

3.4. Structural Properties of N-Terminal Region of MAP2c

Physiologically important structural features of the N-terminal region of free MAP2c are more complex than those described for tau40. Occurrence of turns (Figure 3) between more extended segments suggests formation of transient hairpin structures. NMR relaxation [57] suggests that aromatic amino acids, frequent among the first 80 residues of MAP2c (most notably Trp14, Phe48, and Tyr50), are parts of a more ordered structure that is not observed in tau40 [38] and that includes also the following segment (Ser81–Glu113), where all hydrophobic residues are aliphatic. Similar to tau40, the N-terminal region of free MAP2c interacts with the proline-rich and MT-binding domains [57]. Unlike in tau40, a very distinct secondary structure motif is present in the N-terminal region of MAP2c. Residues Ser81–Glu113 exhibit a strong propensity to form an α-helix interrupted by a more extended segment. Biological relevance of this motif is discussed in Section 3.6.

3.5. Neurosteroid Binding to the N-Terminal Region of MAP2c

Neural activities are regulated by steroid compounds (neurosteroids) synthesized directly in the brain, independently of the peripheral endocrine glands [75]. Neurosteroids specifically bind to MAP2 isoforms and stimulate MT polymerization and consequently neurite extension [76]. Experiments with truncated MAP2c suggested that the N-terminal region is essential for binding [77,78]. Our unpublished NMR data confirm that neurosteroids bind to the N-terminal region, but presence of C-terminal regions is needed too (Figure S6 in Supplementary Materials). This is consistent with the NMR relaxation data, showing formation of a more ordered structure, and with a homology model predicting residues Met1–Lys71 to form the major portion of a binding pocket [77,78] for neurosteroids.

Therefore, the N-terminal region of MAP2c can be viewed as a transiently structured receptor of steroids controlling neurite extension and thus affecting neuronal plasticity.

3.6. Binding Site for the RII Regulatory Subunit of PKA in the N-Terminal Region of MAP2c

Residues Ser81–Glu113 (encoded by C-terminus of exon 5 and N-terminal half of exon 6, yellow box in Figure 3) represent a very characteristic structural and functional motif of MAP2c, a binding site for the RII regulatory subunit of PKA. The dimeric RI and RII PKA subunits recognize long amphiphilic α-helices (at least five turns) of well-folded A-kinase anchoring proteins (AKAPs, see sequence comparison with MAP2c in Figure 3) [79]. As mentioned above, the terminal parts of the sequence Ser81–Glu113, $_{81}$SADRETAEEVSA$_{92}$ and $_{107}$KGEQEKE$_{113}$, have a high propensity to form α-helix. However, the middle part of the binding site is extended, with increased propensity to form polyproline II conformation. Remarkably, the middle region is most rigid, as revealed by NMR relaxation [57]. The second α-helix of the RII-binding motif also contributes to the proposed steroid binding pocket. The regions interacting with the RII subunit of PKA and with neurosteroids thus form one structural unit, most ordered in the whole molecule, and presumably stabilized by hydrophobic interactions of aromatic residues clustered in the N-terminal region of MAP2c.

3.7. Phosphorylation of MAP2c Tyr67 and SH2 Binding

The N-terminal region of MAP2 isoforms is also a target of post-translational modification. Tyr67 is present in a sequence resembling the Fyn recognition motif [66] (like Tyr18 of tau), and it is the only tyrosine phosphorylated by Fyn in vitro. It is therefore likely that Tyr67 of MAP2 isoforms is an important regulatory point. For example, Tyr67 of human MAP2c is present in the SH2 binding motif pYxN, recognized by the adaptor protein Grb2 [80]. Grb2 links tyrosine kinases with the Ras signaling pathway and it has been postulated that phosphorylation of Tyr67 followed by recruitment of Grb2 are steps of an intracellular signaling cascade in fetal human brains [80]. Furthermore, Grb2 is overexpressed in Alzheimer's disease brains and it was reported to partially revert pathological disassembly of the cytoskeleton [81]. The overlap of the target site of Tyr kinase Fyn and the binding site of a subunit regulating Ser/Thr kinase PKA with the proposed neurosteroid receptor region suggests a possible functional connection of phosphorylation cascades and steroid signaling.

3.8. Summary

Acidic N-terminal regions in both proteins are important for functionally relevant intramolecular tertiary contacts. Moreover, they contain important interaction sites, different in tau40 and MAP2c. The N-terminus of tau interacts with the membranes and inhibits axonal transport. The N-terminal region of MAP2c is ordered to much larger extent than that of tau40, contains a binding motif for the regulatory subunit RII of PKA, and constitutes a large portion of a neurosteroid binding site. The biological activities of the N-terminal regions are regulated by tyrosine phosphorylation.

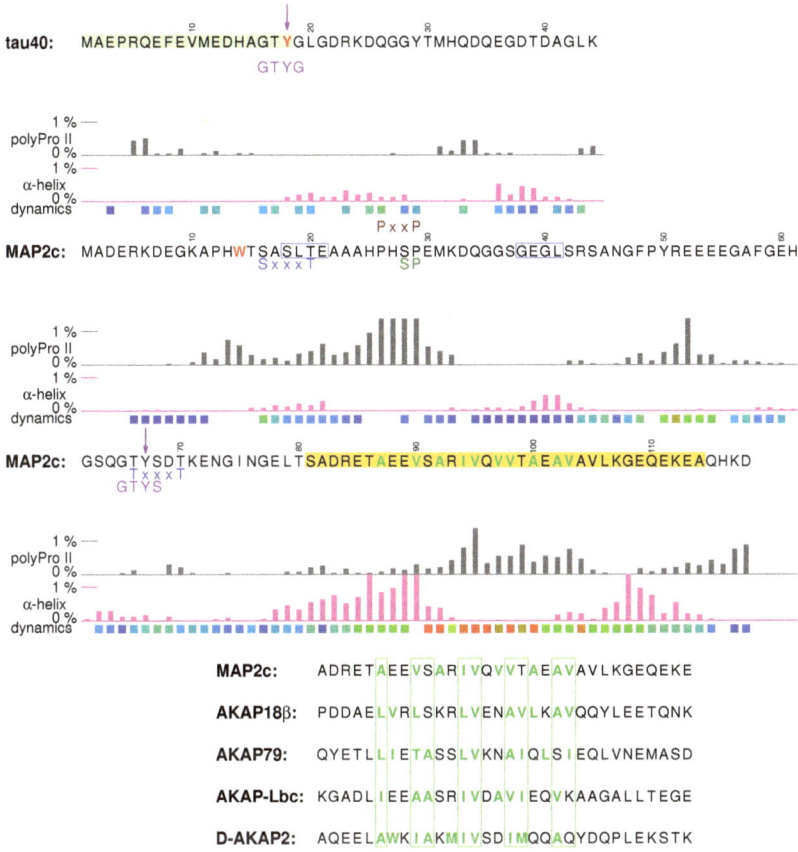

Figure 3. N-terminal sequences of human tau40 and rat MAP2c. The pale green and yellow boxes indicate the region of tau interacting with membranes and the region of MAP2c interacting with the regulatory RII subunit of PKA, respectively. Highly conserved residues are shown in red. Hydrophobic residues in the region interacting with the regulatory RII subunit of PKA are shown in green. Phosphorylated tyrosines are marked with purple arrows. Minimal SH3 interaction motifs (PxxP) are shown in brown above the sequences. Recognition motifs of proline-directed kinases (green) and GSK3β (blue), and Fyn phosphorylation motifs (purple) are shown below the sequences. Populations of continuous stretches of seven amino acids in the α-helical and polyproline II conformations in the ensembles of structures selected by the ASTEROIDS analyses based on measured NMR chemical shifts [31,57] are shown as pink and gray bars placed in the middle of the stretches, respectively. Residues forming β-turns are shown in blue frames. Dynamics of individual amino acids, measured as transverse NMR relaxation rate, is described by colors of the boxes below the secondary structure symbols (blue corresponding to flexible residues with the relaxation rate of $2\,s^{-1}$ or lower, red corresponding to the most ordered residues with the relaxation rate of $10\,s^{-1}$ or higher). The presented values are the relaxation rates measured at 700 MHz and 5 °C for tau40 [38] and values recalculated from relaxation rates measured at 950 MHz and 27 °C for MAP2c [57] in order to account for the magnetic field difference. No temperature correction was applied because relaxation rates of IDPs cannot be easily recalculated for a different temperature. Alignment with the sequences of well-ordered AKAPs is shown under the region interacting with the regulatory RII subunit of PKA (preferred positions of hydrophobic residues in the amphiphilic binding α-helices are shown in green frames).

4. Variable Central Regions Preceding Proline-Rich Domains

Different tau and MAP2 isoforms greatly vary in the length of the sequence between N-terminal and proline-rich domains (brown boxes in Figures 1 and 2), called *variable central region* in this paper. As mentioned above, the resulting variability in the size of PDs seems to allow the nerve cells to regulate spacing of MTs. Features of these parts of MAPs are discussed below separately for tau and MAP2 isoforms.

4.1. Structural Properties of Variable Central Region of tau40

All tau isoforms contain relatively short stretches encoded by exons 4 and 5, but vary in the expression of two 29-amino acid long inserts, encoded by exons 2 and 3, and labeled I1 and I2, respectively (pale green and pale blue boxes in Figure 4, respectively). Both I1 and I2 are present in the longest brain isoform discussed here. I1 and I2 are highly negatively charged and prefer polyproline II conformation, with an exception of a proline-free segment $_{60}$GSETSD$_{65}$ forming transient α-helix. Exon 4 encodes a flexible sequence Glu104–Pro112, connected to a transient α-helix formed by residues Ser113–Val122. In brain variants of tau, the sequence continues by short exon 5, containing a transient helix Ser137–Lys143. In the high-molecular weight isoforms of tau, not expressed in the central nervous system, exon 5 is preceded and followed by long inserts encoded by exons 4a and 6, respectively.

4.2. Regulatory Post-Translational Modifications: Phosphorylation of Tau Insert I1 and Truncation

Little is known about physiological function(s) of the variable central region of tau40. Nevertheless, presence of phosphorylation sites suggests possible regulatory role(s). For example, I1 of human tau contains three recognition sites of proline-directed Ser/Thr kinases (shown in green in Figure 4). Ser46 and Thr50 are phosphorylated by ERK1/2 and GSK-3β kinases in vitro [82–84]. Importantly, Ser46 and Thr50 are, together with Ser202, the only sites phosphorylated solely in the interphase in a Chinese hamster ovary cell line transfected by human tau40 [82]. SAPK4/p38δ is the major kinase phosphorylating Thr50, when cells are exposed to osmotic stress and the phosphomimicking mutation T50E increases the ability of tau to promote tubulin polymerization [85]. Remarkably, the residue corresponding to Thr50 of human tau40 is present in tau of primates, goats and cows, but not in tau of species not forming tau filaments, such as rodents [85]. Phosphorylated Ser46 and Thr50 were identified in Alzheimer's disease and progressive supranuclear palsy brains [86]. It has been proposed that p38δ-mediated phosphorylation of Thr50 helps neurons to respond to the osmotic shock by stabilizing MTs, but a lack of control of the involved kinases and/or phosphatases may result in hyperphosphorylation with consequent pathological effects.

Another post-translational modification affecting biological activity of tau is truncation in the variable central region. Several truncation sites have been found in situ under physiological [87] or pathological [88] conditions. Some truncations affect biological activity of tau. A tau40-derived fragment beginning at Gln124 exhibited enhanced stabilization of MTs in a neuroblastoma cell line [87], whereas truncation at Ile151 efficiently induced tau polymerization in vitro and in transgenic models of tauopathy [89]. Cleavage of tau inside the unstructured PD may thus represent an important mechanism to regulate its function.

4.3. Interactions of the Region Encoded by Tau Exon 4 with the Dynactin Complex

Another reported physiological role of the central region is facilitation of the MT binding to the dynactin complex. Presence of the region encoded by the short exon 4 is sufficient for binding of tau to the C-terminus of dynactin p150 [71]. Since the C-terminal domain of p150 forms an α-helical bundle [70], one can hypothesize that the only secondary structure motif encoded by exon 4, the transient helix Ser113–Val122, is the structural element responsible for interaction of this region of tau with the dynactin complex. As already discussed in Section 3.2, interactions of tau with p150 enhance binding of dynactin to MTs with a possible impact on the axonal transport.

4.4. Structural Properties of Variable Central Region of MAP2c

The N-terminal part of the central region of MAP2c consists of amino acids $_{119}$QPAALPL$_{125}$ (encoded by the C-terminus of exon 6) with a strong polyproline II propensity and of the sequence encoded by short exon 7, including another polyproline II motif, a proline-rich region $_{134}$PPSPPPSP$_{141}$. In the high-molecular weight MAP2 isoforms, the proline-rich region is followed by long inserts (encoded by exons 8–11 in MAP2a and 9–11 in MAP2b, see Figure 1). In MAP2c and MAP2d, the proline-rich region is directly connected to a flexible linker [57], followed by a sequence with a polyproline II propensity, and by a structural and functional motif not present in tau40 (α-helix flanked by polyproline II, shown in the yellow box in Figure 4).

4.5. Neural-Activity-Dependent Phosphorylation of MAP2c Epitope AP-18

The sequence $_{134}$PPSPPPSP$_{141}$ matches a consensus motif PxSPxP (green box in Figure 4) recognized by proline-directed kinases (e.g., GSK3β). When phosphorylated at Ser136, the motif is specifically recognized by the antibody AP-18 [90]. The amino acid composition, resulting in very high propensity to adopt polyproline II conformation, and increased rigidity [57] document that $_{134}$PPSPPPSP$_{141}$ is a well-defined structural motif in free MAP2c. Phosphorylation of Ser136 does not influence interactions of MAP2c with MTs, but relation to other biological functions has been reported. Greatly reduced phosphorylation of Ser136 was observed in the rat olfactory bulb after olfactory restrictions [91] and in rat hippocampus after behavioral training [92], suggesting association with contextual memory. Epinephrine increased phosphorylation of MAP2c in rat pheochromocytoma cells, most likely by activating α_2-adrenoreceptor mediated, ERK/PKC-dependent signaling pathways, and a role in nerve cell differentiation was proposed [93]. However, it should be noted that molecular mechanisms of the mentioned effects are unknown and influence of other factors cannot be excluded. It is also possible that phosphorylation at Ser136, easily observable using the AP-18 antibody, was accompanied by phosphorylation at other sites that were not probed in the aforementioned studies.

4.6. Helical Motif of MAP2c Flanked by PKA Phosphorylation Sites and Involved in Interactions Interfering with MT Binding

The structural motif shown in the yellow box in Figure 4 contains one of the most populated transient helices in MAP2c, surrounded by polyproline II regions with multiple phosphorylation sites. Here we present an example of interactions controlling cytoskeletal dynamics and of their regulation by one particular kinase. The presence of arginines and lysines creates several consensus sites of Ser/Thr kinases recognizing R/KxxS/T and R/KR/KxS/T motifs (shown in red in Figure 4), such as PKA or protein kinase C. Real-time phosphorylation measurement revealed that Ser184 and Thr220 (red in Figure 4) are preferred targets of PKA in this region [40]. Interestingly, the rates of phosphorylations of Ser184 and Thr220 are comparable but Thr220 is dephosphorylated much faster than Ser184 by Ser/Thr phosphatases PP2b, PP2A$_c$, and PP1A$_c$, indicating that signaling may be also controlled by variations of dephosphorylation rate [94]. When Ser184 and Thr220 are phosphorylated, the flanking regions represent motifs recognized by the regulatory proteins 14-3-3 (phosphate group in an extended conformation [95]). Interactions of these motifs with 14-3-3ζ regulate ability of MAP2c to promote tubulin polymerization [40]. Furthermore, the transient α-helix between the PKA sites is one of the regions which show (together with MTBRs) signs of binding to non-canonical SH3 domain of plectin [57,96]. Plectin cross-links MTs with other cytoskeletal proteins and interferes with the MT-stabilizing function of MAPs [96]. The motif of MAP2c discussed in this subsection thus seems to influence MT dynamics in a complex manner, regulated by PKA phosphorylation. As this motif is present only in MAP2 isoforms, it may represent one of structural determinants distinguishing MAP2 from tau.

4.7. Summary

Segments between acidic N-terminal and basic proline-rich domains of tau40 and MAP2c differ substantially in structural propensities and functions. The central part of tau seems to be a region specifically targeted by proline-directed kinases and potentially influencing function of other regions of tau (regulation of MT dynamics). A unique proline-rich motif of MAP2c includes Ser136, phosphorylated in connection with the neural activity. MAP2c, but not tau40, contains a helical motif interacting with protein partners and surrounded by PKA phosphorylation sites regulating the interactions and consequently MT dynamics.

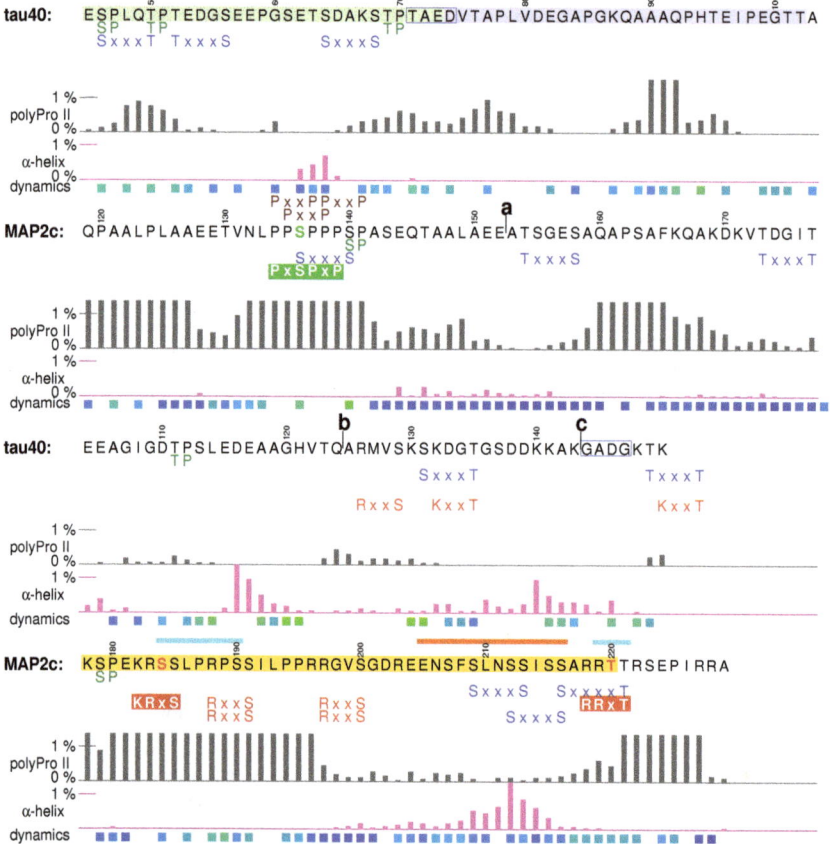

Figure 4. Sequences of variable central regions preceding the proline-rich domains of human tau40 and rat MAP2c. Tau inserts I1 and I2 are shown in pale green and pale blue boxes, respectively. The motif in the yellow box is described in the text. PKA recognition motifs and residues rapidly phosphorylated by PKA in vitro are shown in red. Interactions of MAP2c with plectin and 14-3-3 proteins are shown as orange and cyan bars above the sequence. Letters **a**, **b**, and **c** show position of long exons in the high-molecular weight tau and MAP2 isoforms. Other symbols are used as described for Figure 3.

5. Proline-Rich Domains

The proline-rich regions P1 and P2 (brown boxes in Figures 1 and 2) present in the middle of the tau40 and MAP2c sequences (tau exons 7/9, MAP2c exon 15) exhibit moderate sequence similarity. The proline-rich regions contain multiple SH3-binding (PxxP), phosphorylation (S/TP, R/KxxS/T), and lysine acetylation sites (Figure 5), contribute to the interactions with tubulin and actin [10,42,97], and are involved in intramolecular interactions with the N-terminal regions [38,57]. Structural features and their relation to biological functions are discussed together for proline-rich regions of tau40 and MAP2c in this section.

5.1. Structural Properties of Proline-Rich Domains of Tau and MAP2c

Amino-acid composition of the proline-rich regions determines their general physico-chemical properties: positive charge and tendency to form polyproline II structures. However, the charge distribution and secondary structure propensities are not uniform. The expected polyproline II conformation is most frequent, but the actual population of this structure varies along the sequence (Figures 2 and 5). Segments with the highest populations of polyproline II structures exhibit increased rigidity in NMR relaxation experiments [38,57] (Figure 5), proving that formation of such motifs significantly affects behavior of free tau40 and MAP2c. A slight preference for α-helical conformation was observed only for residues 190–200 and 237–242 in tau40 (Figure 5). Phosphorylation can significantly alter the local conformation. Examples of such phosphorylation effects and their role in regulation of physiological functions of the observed specific structural motifs are discussed below.

5.2. Tubulin-Binding Motif in Tau Region P1

The first discussed structural motif influenced by phosphorylation is the tubulin-binding site in the P1 region of tau40 (Figure 5). Interactions with tubulin were observed for residues Arg170–Ser185, exhibiting the highest polyproline II propensity in the P1 region [41,42]. Phosphorylation of a short synthetic peptide derived from the tau P1 region ($_{174}$KTPPAPKTPP$_{183}$, green frame in Figure 5) further stabilized the polyproline II conformation [34]. It is not known if such phosphorylation-induced structural change plays a role in physiological function of the proline-rich domain, but relation of phosphorylation in the discussed motif to neurodegenerative diseases has been reported: phosphorylation of Thr175 in this region by GSK3β is associated with amyotrophic lateral sclerosis with cognitive impairment [98] and was recently observed also for traumatic brain injury [99]. Furthermore, the phosphomimetic mutation T175D increased GSK3β activity, resulting in phosphorylation of Thr231 [100] in another important structural motif, discussed in Section 5.4.

5.3. Phosphorylation-Controlled Conformational Switch in Tau Epitope AT8

The second motif discussed in this section is the sequence of tau shown in the pale green box in Figure 5. When phosphorylated, the sequence is recognized by the antibody AT8, which is used to determine progression of the Alzheimer's disease *post mortem*. In free, unphosphorylated state, the motif does not prefer any secondary structure. However, phosphorylation at Ser202 and Thr205 induces formation of a helical turn, observable in NMR spectra [101]. Remarkably, this helical structure prevents formation of tau fibers. Phosphorylation of Thr205 mediated by p38γ also leads to disruption of the PSD-95–tau–Fyn complex responsible for Aβ toxicity [102]. Additional phosphorylation at Ser208 disrupts the turn and promotes tau aggregation in vitro [103]. The third phosphorylation seems to favor the polyproline II conformation, as the triply phosphorylated epitope binds to the AT8 antibody in this conformation [104]. This example illustrates how phosphorylation can completely revert local conformational behavior and alter physiological function of the given motif.

From the biological point of view, it is also interesting how is the sequential phosphorylation achieved in the cell. Ser202 and Thr205 can be phosphorylated by activated ERK2 [103], or by the action of CDK5 and GSK3β kinases, known to associate with tau and MTs in the brain [105]. Here we only describe the synergistic phosphorylation by CDK5 and GSK3β, as an example of *substrate priming* in multiple phosphorylation sites. In the normal adult brain, CDK5 activated by protein p35 (or p39) phosphorylates Ser199 and Ser202, and GSK3β is able to phosphorylate only Ser202. If GSK3β is up-regulated, it recognizes the $_{202}$pSPGT$_{205}$ site created e.g., by p35/CDK5, and efficiently phosphorylates Thr205 [105,106]. Additional phosphorylation at Ser208 was achieved in vitro by addition of the rat brain extract [103].

Physiological role of the epitope AT8 is ambiguous. Phosphorylation of Ser202 and Thr205 contributes to the regulation of tau interactions with MTs, but it is not sufficient to inhibit MT binding [107]. Physiological role of the corresponding sequence of MAP2 isoforms is better described. The MAP2c site $_{256}$TPGTPGTPS$_{264}$ closely resembles the AT8 sequence of tau (Figure 5) and seems to be phosphorylated similarly to tau [28]. The c-Jun N-terminal kinase-1 (JNK1) phosphorylates in vitro and in vivo all three threonines of rat MAP2a/b corresponding to tau Ser202, Thr205, and Ser208. In vivo experiments with phosphomimetic mutations of these threonines showed that their phosphorylations increase affinity of high-molecular weight MAP2 isoforms for MTs, stabilize MTs, and induce dendrite growth [108]. Therefore, phosphorylation of the discussed motif in MAP2 isoforms seems to be important for normal neuron morphology.

5.4. Formation of a Salt Bridge in Tau Epitope AT180 Interferes with MT Stabilization

The third example of a functionally important motif in the proline-rich region is the sequence of tau shown in the pale blue box in Figure 5. This site is particularly interesting because NMR line broadening was observed for its amino acids in the presence of tubulin [41,42] and mutagenesis confirmed a direct interaction [42]. However, this region of the tau40-tubulin complex is dynamic [42] and the corresponding electron density was not observed in a recent cryo-EM study of MT-tau interaction [43]. The interactions with MTs are strongly influenced by phosphorylation. Ser235 in the AT180 epitope is the most rapidly phosphorylated residue among the ERK2 sites in vitro [84] and it is also a target of several other kinases including p35/CDK5 or SAPK/p38 [85,105]. Phosphorylation of Thr231 in the same epitope occurs at normal physiological conditions. However, GSK3β phosphorylation of Thr231 is greatly facilitated (primed) by preceding p35/CDK5 phosphorylation of Ser235, in a similar manner as described for the AT8 epitope. The discussed site (pale blue box in Figure 5) phosphorylated at Thr231 and Ser235 is recognized by the antibody AT180 and has a greatly reduced ability to promote MT polymerization. Nuclear magnetic resonance data showed that the structural basis of this effect is formation of a salt bridge between phospho-Thr231 and Arg230, presumably competing with the formation of intermolecular salt bridges to tubulin [31]. Moreover, phosphorylation at Ser235 increases helical propensity of the AT180 epitope, and this trend is further enhanced by phosphorylation of Ser237 and Ser238 [31]. The shift of conformational equilibrium from polyproline II to helical structures does not affect MT binding [31], but may be important for interactions with SH3 domains because the discussed site overlaps with the Class I SH3-recognition motif $_{230}$RTPPKSP$_{236}$ [109] (*vide infra*). The MAP2c site $_{289}$TPPKSPAT$_{296}$ is also similar to the corresponding AT180 site of tau, but the penultimate serine is replaced by alanine (pale blue boxes in Figure 5).

5.5. Specific Phosphorylation of Ser214 by PKA and 14-3-3 Binding in the AT100 Epitope of Tau

The fourth discussed motif, shown in the yellow box in Figure 5, is an example of a site controlled by a very complex regulation network. It contains recognition sites of proline-directed kinases and is also efficiently phosphorylated by PKA. When phosphorylated at Thr212, Ser212, and Thr217, the site is recognized by the antibody AT100 [110]. The mentioned residues are not phosphorylated independently. Phosphorylation of Thr212 by GSK3β is activated by previous phosphorylation of the neighboring AT180 epitope, but inhibited by PKA phosphorylation of Ser214 (shown in red in Figure 5).

Importantly, tau40 is phosphorylated by PKA at Ser214 much more rapidly than at Ser208 in vitro [111]. Furthermore, the PKA-phosphorylated site binds the regulatory proteins 14-3-3, which competes with MT binding [95,112–115]. Finally, the discussed site overlaps with the Class II SH3-recognition motif $_{216}$PTTPTR$_{221}$ [109] (*vide infra*). Please note that the presence of the Class II motif increases population of polyproline II conformation, typical for complexes with both SH3 domains and 14-3-3 proteins.

In contrast to the AT8 and AT180 epitopes, the sequence of the tau epitope AT100 and the corresponding sequence in MAP2c (yellow boxes in Figure 5) differ, resulting in substantially different phosphorylation patterns and intermolecular interactions. The most rapidly phosphorylated target of PKA in the tau molecule, Ser 214 [111], aligns with Gly270 in MAP2c. Therefore, MAP2c is not efficiently phosphorylated by PKA anywhere in P2 [40]. Furthermore, the MAP2c sequence does not exhibit the strong polyproline II propensity of the corresponding tau motif. As a consequence, 14-3-3 protein, primarily recognizing phosphorylation sites with polyproline II conformation [116], binds to P2 of tau [95], but not of MAP2c [40] (Figure 5).

5.6. Binding Sites for the SH3 Domains

In addition to the interactions with MTs, the proline-rich domains specifically interact with SH3 domains of the Fyn kinase and of other proteins. Analysis of the populations of conformations of free tau40 and MAP2c helps to understand the structural basis of these interactions and differences between tau40 and MAP2c. Peptides bound to SH3 domains adopt polyproline II conformation [109]. Tau40 and MAP2c contain 7 and 13 minimal SH3 binding motifs PxxP, respectively, most of them in the P2 region. Among them, one classical Class II motif ($_{216}$PTTPTR$_{221}$) and one classical Class I motif ($_{230}$RTPPKSP$_{236}$) are present in tau and one Class I motif is present in MAP2c ($_{288}$RTPPKSP$_{294}$). Binding assays performed with synthetic biotinylated peptides showed that the Fyn SH3 domain binds preferentially to the Class II site of tau [109] and Class I site of MAP2c [117]. Remarkably, Class I and Class II motifs in free tau40 and MAP2c prefer the polyproline II conformation much more than the minimal SH3-binding motifs PxxP. This suggests that the higher affinity of the Class I and Class II motifs to the SH3 domains are not only due to the presence of the positive charge, but also due to the optimal backbone conformation, highly populated already in the free state.

Binding of SH3 domains to Class I and Class II motifs of tau and MAP2 isoforms is greatly reduced by phosphorylation [109,117]. In addition to introducing a negative charge, phosphorylation can also alter secondary structure propensity. We hypothesize that such conformational changes may distinguish the Class I sites of tau and MAP2c. Sequences of Class I motifs are identical in tau and MAP2c, but the following amino acids differ: slightly helical $_{237}$SSAKS$_{241}$ in tau40 corresponds to $_{295}$ATPKQ$_{299}$ with a strong polyproline II propensity in MAP2c (Figure 5). As mentioned above, the helical propensity around Lys240 in tau40 is greatly enhanced by phosphorylation of two serines missing in MAP2c (Ser237 and Ser 238). Such specific phosphorylation may selectively perturb the Class I SH3 binding site in tau, without affecting it in MAP2c.

5.7. Summary

The proline-rich domains of tau40 and MAP2c represent an important regulatory unit, controlled by multiple kinases and interacting proteins. Several differences in structural features, phosphorylation patterns, and molecular interactions of proline-rich domains of tau40 and MAP2c are likely to represent a basis for functional specificity of these proteins.

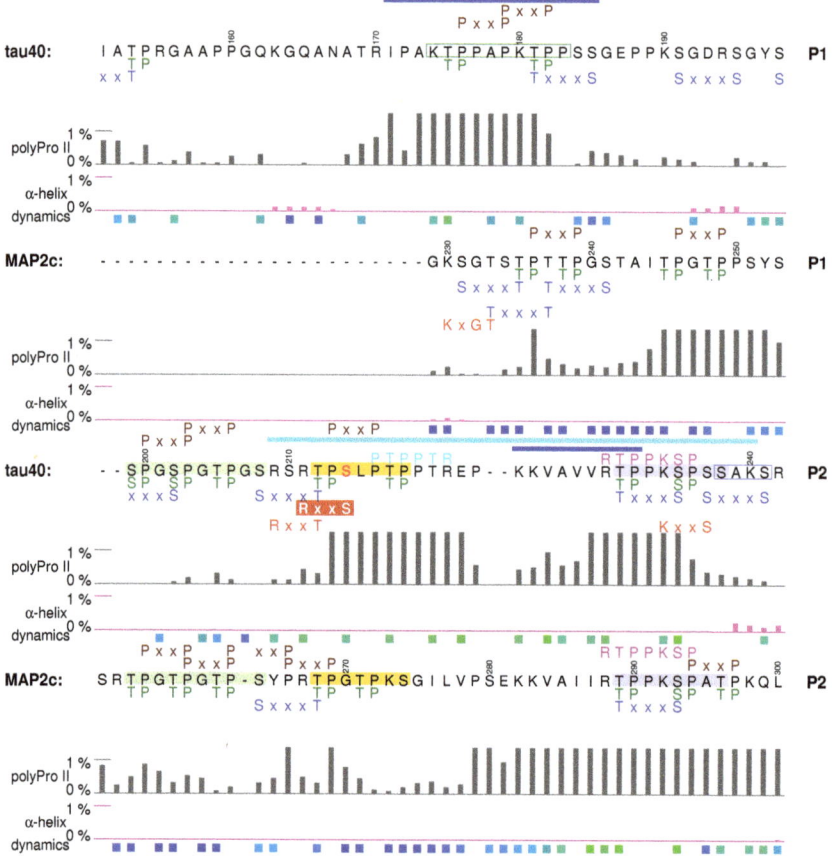

Figure 5. Sequences of proline-rich domains of human tau40 and rat MAP2c. Complex phosphorylation sites shown in the green frame and in pale green, pale blue, and red boxes are described in the text. The classical Class I and Class II SH3 binding sites are presented in magenta and cyan, respectively, above the sequence. Regions of tau interacting with tubulin are indicated by the blue bars above the sequence. Other symbols are used as described for Figures 3 and 4.

6. Microtubule-Binding Domains

Microtubule-binding domain (MTBD, violet boxes in Figures 1 and 2) is the most thoroughly studied region of tau and MAP2 isoforms. It consists of up to four imperfect repeats (R1–R4, R2 is present in MAP2d but missing in MAP2c) of 31 or 32 amino acids (Figure 6). The sequence immediately following MTBR4 (R′) resembles the N-terminus of the aforementioned motif. As sequences, conformation, and dynamics of MTBDs of tau40 and MAP2c are highly similar [38,39,57], they are discussed together in this section.

6.1. Structural Properties of Microtubule-Binding Domains of tau40 and MAP2c

Microtubule-binding repeats in free tau40 and MAP2c contain the same motif, consisting of nine extended and relatively rigid residues, and of a stretch of 22 or 23 more flexible and highly conserved residues, which tends to form turns shown in Figure 6 [38,39,57]. The overall charge of the repeats is positive (Figure 2). The repeats are involved in normal physiological interactions with tubulin [38,41–43], plectin [57,96], actin [10], 14-3-3 [40,95,115,118], and form core structures of pathological tau filaments [24]. To discuss how are the described structural features of tau40 and MAP2c related to their physiological functions, we briefly review what is known about the conformation of tau in complexes with the most important binding partners, tubulin and actin.

6.2. Interactions with Microtubules

Nuclear magnetic resonance [38,41,42,119] and cryo-EM [43] data provided an insight into the specific interactions of tau with MTs. Residues of tau MTBD interacting with MTs and unpolymerized tubulin were identified based on broadening and shifts of peaks in the NMR spectra [38,41,42] (blue bars in Figure 6). Building an atomic-resolution model of the complex with MTs is complicated by presence of multiple potential binding sites on both partners. Due to the favorable time-scale of the interaction, it was possible to gain useful structural details from liquid-state NMR. Transferred nuclear Overhauser effect was recorded for a MT-bound tau fragment consisting of residues Lys268–Asn312, and used to identify hydrogen atoms closer than 0.6 nm in tau conformers bound to MTs [41]. Structural models calculated from the observed contacts converged in two regions folded to hairpin conformations. The hairpins consisted of turns formed by the conserved PGGG motifs and of extended hexapeptides identified previously [120] as the aggregation sites of the second and third MTBR (yellow boxes in Figure 6). Another binding model was derived from cryo-EM data [43]. Local resolution in complexes of MTs with synthetic tau constructs consisting of four identical copies of MTBRs 1 and 2 was sufficient to observe density corresponding to extended chains of tau residues but not to identify individual residues. Using Rosetta [121], the observed density was assigned to stretches of residues including the aforementioned hexapeptides found in extended conformation in the NMR model. The PGGG motifs were not modeled due to the lack of density, but the overall shape of the tau fragment in the cryo-EM model was inconsistent with formation of a hairpin. This discrepancy between cryo-EM and NMR data may reflect different binding modes of tau.

In the cryo-EM study [43], tau was found to bind to the outer surface of MTs along individual protofilaments, in the proximity of tubulin helices 11 and 12 and of the C-terminal tubulin tail. Earlier low-resolution cryo-EM study [122] and sequence homology suggest that MAP2c binds to the MTs in a similar manner. It has been also proposed that tau and MAP2 bind to MTs in a different manner, that MTBRs interact specifically with β-tubulin in the interior of MTs and proline-rich domains bind to the outer surface of MTs [1,123]. This model assumes that the PGGG sequence forms a loop which interacts with the taxol-binding site of β-tubulin, and is thus compatible with the NMR model. Both types of interactions with MTs (binding to the outer and inner surface) are supported by a solid experimental evidence: nanogold particles attached close to the PGGG motif were clearly observed inside [123] and outside [122] MTs. However, high-resolution data are available only for tau bound to the outer surface, despite of efforts to prepare samples with MTBRs interacting with the inner surface [43].

It is obvious that remarkable progress was achieved in characterization of tau-MT complexes, but detailed structures of MT-bound tau or MAP2 isoforms are not available yet. Nevertheless, known structural data already allow us to look for structural features observed in the complexes that are present already in the free state. In all structural models, the first nine amino acids of MTBRs are present in the extended conformation, which is also preferred in free tau40 and MAP2c. A correlation can be also seen between formation of turns in bound and free forms. Turns made by the PGGG motif were identified both in the structural ensembles selected by the ASTEROIDS analysis based on NMR data obtained for free tau40 and MAP2c [39,57], and in the structural models calculated from the contacts observed in NMR spectra observed in complexes of MTs with the tau fragments [41]. This turn was not observed in the Rosetta model based on cryo-EM data, but conformations of other residues are similar to the conformations favored in the ASTEROIDS ensembles. We can therefore conclude that the conformations adopted in the complex with MTs are often most populated in free tau40 and MAP2c.

Interactions with MTs are given not only by conformation of interacting residues, but also by their physical properties that can be regulated by post-translational modifications. For example, MT-stabilizing activity of both tau and MAP2 isoforms is inhibited by MARK phosphorylation [124,125], but phosphorylation by PKA inhibits the stabilizing activity of tau only [126,127]. Subtle differences in phosphorylation patterns and kinetics offer a possible explanation of observed differences. Serines in the middle of MTBRs are present in sequences representing recognition sites of several kinases, most notably the KxGS motif recognized by MARKs [128] (the complex overlapped motifs including the KxGS sites are presented in red boxes under the sequence in Figure 6). In general, PKA recognizes similar motifs. However, in vitro measurements of PKA phosphorylation kinetics revealed an important difference. PKA phosphorylates in vitro Ser324 in the third MTBR of tau40 (R3 in Figure 6) with a medium rate [111], but the in vitro PKA phosphorylation rate is negligible for all serines/threonines in MTBD of MAP2c [40]. Moreover, no serines or threonines are phosphorylated by PKA with a sufficient rate in the proline-rich domain of MAP2c [40], but Ser214 and Ser208 in the proline-rich domain of tau40 are residues of highest in vitro PKA phosphorylation rates [111]. It suggests that specific kinases can selectively control regulation of MT dynamics by tau vs. MAP2 isoforms: the same signal activating PKA can reduce interactions of MTs with tau, but not with MAP2.

6.3. Interactions with Actin and Other Proteins

Microtubule-binding domains of tau and MAP2c do not interact only with MTs, but are also involved in cross-linking and bundling individual actin filaments [11,129]. Liquid state NMR was used to describe interactions of tau40 with filamentous actin in detail [10]. In contrast to the mostly electrostatic interactions of the proline-rich domain [97], MTBD binds to the hydrophobic pocket between actin subdomains 1 and 3 on the surface of the actin filaments. Amino acids involved in the interactions are present in two helical (α or 3_{10}) segments corresponding to residues 260–268 and 277–283. The former region forms a turn in both free and MT-bound tau40. Remarkably, the latter region is extended in a free state and in pathological tau filaments, and overlaps with the aggregation site (*vide infra*). The total number of interacting regions of either type is seven per tau40 molecule. A single helical binding region is sufficient to form a complex with F-actin, but two helical sites have to be present in order to bundle actin filaments. This explains how tau (and other MAPs) can cross-link actin filaments in the nerve cell. Similar to the MT binding, interactions with actin can be affected by post-translational modifications, but the effects may differ as the interactions are of a different nature. It has been reported for MAP2c that phosphorylation of the KxGS motifs favors localization of MAP2c in the actin cytoskeleton, and proposed that such colocalization may directly influence neurite outgrowth [130].

Other proteins described to interact with MTBD are isoforms of regulatory protein 14-3-3 [40,95,115,118]. Although 14-3-3 specifically binds phosphopeptides, it also electrostatically interacts with MTBDs of unphosphorylated tau40 and MAP2c [40,95]. The binding is further stabilized by phosphorylating tau40 and MAP2c in proline-rich and C-terminal regions [40,95,118]. Overlap of the interacting regions for 14-3-3 and for tubulin explains how 14-3-3 regulates interactions of tau40 and MAP2c with MTs. Another example of a protein interfering with MT binding is the cytolinker plectin, whose non-canonical SH3 domain interacts with MTBD and with the helical structure between the PKA sites Ser184 and Thr220 of MAP2c (yellow box in Figure 5), and thus competes with microtubules for MAP2c [57,96].

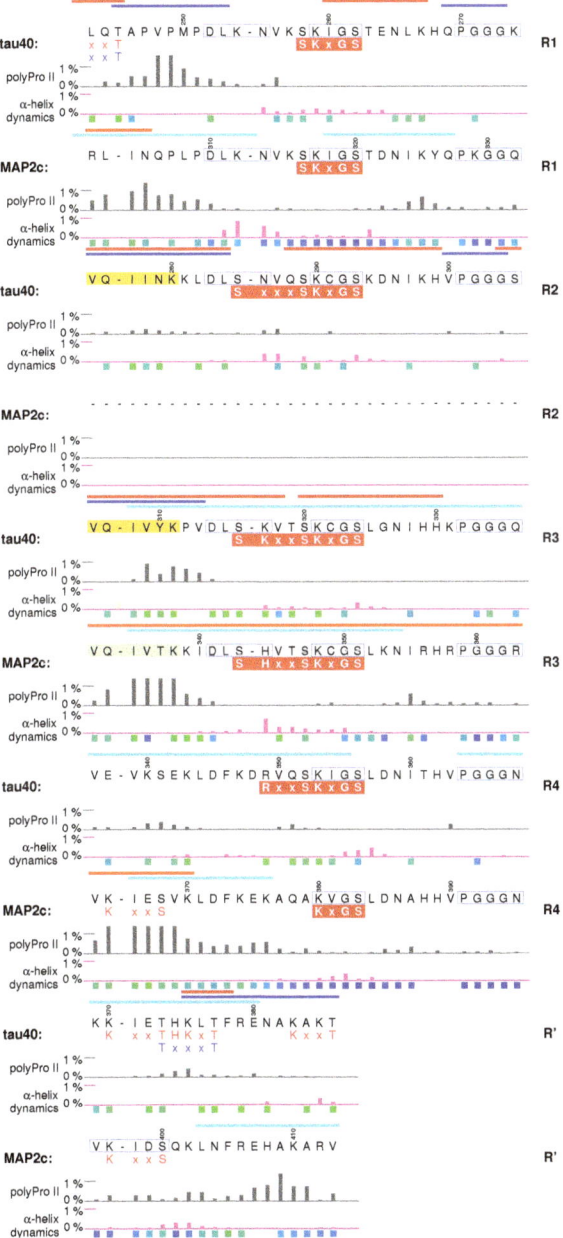

Figure 6. MTBDs of human tau40 and rat MAP2c. MTBRs 1–4 are labeled R1–R4, respectively, the following sequence homologous with the N-terminal sequence of MTBRs is labeled R'. Aggregation sites of tau40 are shown in yellow boxes and the corresponding sequence of MAP2c is shown in a pale green box. Complex phosphorylation sites including the MARK recognition motifs are shown in red boxes. Regions of tau interacting with filamentous actin are indicated by the horizontal red bars above the sequence. Other symbols are used as described for Figures 3 and 4.

6.4. Aggregation of tau40

Despite its central role in normal physiology, MTBD of tau is primarily studied in connection with neuropathological changes involving tau. Stretches of six residues $_{275}$VQIINK$_{280}$ and $_{306}$VQIVYK$_{311}$ (yellow boxes in Figure 6) close to the N-termini of the second and third tau MTBRs, respectively, are able to initiate tau aggregation [120]. Although the actual toxicity of the aggregates and other pathological forms of tau remains to be determined, formation of paired helical filaments in brains is a hallmark of Alzheimer's disease and other neuropathies. A 95-amino-acid fragment of tau40, derived from the PHF core and encompassing the third and fourth MTBR, easily forms filaments in vitro under physiological conditions without the need for other inducers of polymerization [131]. The aggregation also distinguishes tau40 from MAP2c. Although potential role of MAP2 isoforms in neuropathies cannot be excluded, it is clear that MAP2c does not form paired helical filaments or similar aggregates. Comparison of the MTBD sequences immediately suggests two possible causes of the difference: (i) lack of the second MTBR and (ii) difference in three amino acids in the aggregation site of the third MTBR (compare yellow and pale green boxes in Figure 6). Xie et al. investigated these factors systematically, using heparin to induce in vitro aggregation [26,132]. Judging from thioflavin T fluorescence and from amount of sarkosyl-insoluble high-molecular weight products, tau isoform with three MTBRs (0N3R, see Figure 1) aggregated to similar extent as the isoform 0N4R, albeit with a slower kinetics, whereas MAP2c formed very small amount of aggregates. However, replacement of two residues in the tau isoform 0N3R with the corresponding amino acids of MAP2c (double mutation Y310T, P312K, using tau40 numbering) completely abolished the aggregation, while the reciprocal mutation of MAP2c (T337Y, K339P) created a protein aggregating to the similar extent as tau 0N3R, and, furthermore, with much shorter lag-time [26]. Core structures of tau aggregates (paired helical filaments and straight filaments) reconstructed recently from cryo-EM images of samples isolated from brains of Alzheimer's disease patients [24] show that the critical residues pack against Leu376 and His374 of filamentous tau40. NMR data provided additional information about transient interactions with largely disordered "fuzzy coat" regions surrounding the core [44]. These interactions involve P1 region, transient α-helices in C-terminal and central regions, and N-terminal region.

6.5. Summary

Microtubule-binding domain is most intimately related to the physiological roles of MAPs. Populations of conformations of free tau40 and MAP2c resemble the structures observed in the MT-bound state. Distinct conformations were observed in the complexes with actin, where tau was found to form helical structures. The variety of target sites for post-translational modifications is lower in MTBDs than in the proline-rich domains, but the impact of the modifications on the interactions is great. The MT binding is also controlled by interactions (also phosphorylation-dependent) with 14-3-3 proteins.

7. C-Terminal Regions

Regions of potential physiological importance are also located in the sequence between the end of MTBD and the C-terminus of tau40 and MAP2c (cyan boxes in Figures 1 and 2). The overall sequence homology in the C-terminal region of tau40 and MAP2c is high, but the existing small differences have a great impact on the presence of phosphorylation, interaction, and cleavage sites and substantially contribute to the functional differences between tau40 and MAP2c.

7.1. Structural Properties of C-Terminal Regions of tau40 and MAP2c

The first 25 residues of the C-terminal regions of tau40 and MAP2c prefer polyproline II conformation, but the actual propensity differs between tau40 and MAP2c. The middle of the regions is slightly helical, followed by a more extended segment. The sequences of MAP2c and tau40 end by highly conserved segments with a strong α-helical propensity. Conformational analyses (evaluation of populations of structures with continuous stretches of four amino acids in α-helical conformation and estimation of secondary structure propensity from the chemical shift values) revealed more than 20% population of α-helix for both proteins [38,39,55,57]. The C-terminus is also involved in intermolecular interactions with MTBRs and the N-terminal regions [38,57], playing an important role in the "paper-clip" model of tau40 [62].

7.2. Muscarinic Receptor Activation and the PHF-1 Epitope of Tau

The C-terminal region seems to be responsible for activation of cholinergic receptors by extracellular tau. Full-length tau40 and a synthetic peptide $_{391}$EIVYKSPVVSGDTSPRH$_{407}$ (red frame in Figure 7) were reported to interact with cholinergic muscarinic receptors M1 and M3, elevating Ca^{2+} concentration inside neurons. Based on this finding, it has been proposed that neurotoxic effects of tau released from damaged nerve cells are mediated by activating the M1 and M3 muscarinic receptors [133]. The segment of tau activating the M1 and M3 muscarinic receptors and the corresponding segment of MAP2c $_{417}$EIITQSPSRSSVASPRR$_{433}$ (green frame in Figure 7) are less similar in sequence than the rest of the C-terminal domains. Tyr394 of tau, phosphorylated by c-Abl [36], is replaced by threonine in MAP2c, and the whole region is more positively charged in MAP2c (Figure 2). Also, the polyproline II propensity differs between tau and MAP2c. In the M1/M3 muscarinic receptor binding site of tau, it is limited to its N-terminal part [39], but it is observed in the C-terminal region of the motif in MAP2c [57]. These differences suggest that the activation of the M1 and M3 muscarinic receptors and consequent neurotoxic effects are specific features of tau, released to the extracellular space after cell death.

The C-terminal region of tau contains multiple phosphorylation sites, including S/TP motifs (Figure 7). Among them, Ser404 and Ser422 of tau are rapidly phosphorylated by ERK2 [84]. The M1/M3 muscarinic receptor binding site of tau overlaps with an important multiple phosphorylation site (yellow box in Figure 7), recognized by the antibody PHF-1 when Ser404 and Ser396 are phosphorylated. The Ser404, Ser400, and Ser396 residues of tau are phosphorylated subsequently in a similar manner as described for Ser235/Thr231 in P2, and with a similar impact on MT binding and filament formation [134]. Interestingly, tau interacts with the M1 and M3 muscarinic receptors only when the binding site is unphosphorylated [135]. The PHF-1 epitope thus seems to play a dual role in the development of Alzheimer's disease, promoting aggregation in the phosphorylated state but requiring dephosphorylation prior to the muscarinic receptor activation.

7.3. Rapid Phosphorylation at Ser435 and 14-3-3 Binding of MAP2c

As mentioned above, C-terminus of the MAP2c motif shown in the green frame in Figure 7 differs from the corresponding sequence of tau by higher population of polyproline II conformation. Moreover, Ser435 in a close proximity is rapidly phosphorylated in vitro by PKA, while phosphorylation of the corresponding Ser409 in tau is slow. The extended structure and phosphorylation at Ser435 make PKA-phosphorylated MAP2c a better target of 14-3-3 proteins than tau. The differences in PKA phosphorylation and consequently in 14-3-3 binding suggest that PKA represents an important branch point in the signaling pathways. The list of major PKA phosphorylation sites of MAP2c (Ser184 and Thr220 flanking the helical motif preceding the proline-rich region and Ser435, discussed here) and of tau40 (S214 in the proline-rich region and S324 in MTBD) shows that PKA phosphorylates tau inside, but MAP2c outside proline-rich and MT-binding domains. Thus, the same signal (phosphorylation by PKA) has different downstream effects [40].

7.4. Protective Role of the C-Terminal Helix

It is known that C-terminal truncation by apoptotic caspases at Asp421 increases the rate of tau aggregation [136]. The "paper-clip" model of tau explains this observation by transient interactions of the C-terminal α-helix with MTBRs, protecting the aggregation sites. The inherent affinity of the C-terminal α-helix to MTBRs is observed also in filamentous tau, where the helix forms transient contacts with the cross-β core [44]. Interestingly, the last 33 amino acids of tau40 and MAP2c are highly similar, except for the caspase-3 recognition site of tau ($_{418}$DMVD$_{421}$), which aligns with a sequence $_{444}$NLLE$_{447}$ of MAP2c. In fact, MAP2c does not contain any caspase-3 recognition motif DxxD and is not cleaved by this enzyme [137]. The aggregation-promoting caspase-3 cleavage of the C-terminal α-helix of tau40, but not of MAP2c, is another functionally important difference between these MAPs.

7.5. Summary

The C-terminal regions of MAP2c and tau40 consist of less homologous sequences rich in phosphorylation and interaction sites and of the highly homologous α-helical motif at the very terminus. In tau40, but not in MAP2c, the helix is cleaved off by caspase-3, which facilitates aggregation. Similar to the proline-rich regions, the phosphorylation/interaction segment between the C-terminus and MTBD seems to play important regulatory roles specific for MAP2 and tau isoforms.

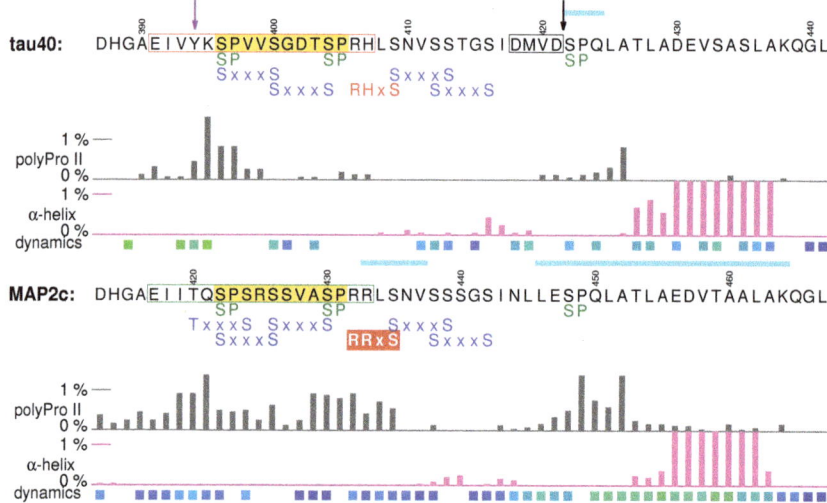

Figure 7. C-terminal sequences of human tau40 and rat MAP2c. The region of tau interacting with cholinergic muscarinic receptors M1 and M3 is shown in the red frame, and the corresponding region of MAP2c is shown in the green frame. The PHF-1 epitope of tau40 is shown in the yellow box and the MAP2c site phosphorylated most rapidly by PKA is shown in the red box. The black frame and the black arrow mark the caspase-3 recognition sequence and cleavage site, respectively. Other symbols are used as described for Figures 3 and 4.

8. Global Structural Features of MAP2c and tau40

Tau40 and MAP2c exhibit distinct structural features also at the level of tertiary structure. The overall shape of the tau40 and MAP2c molecules is mostly given by electrostatic interactions between acidic N-terminal and positively charged C-terminal domains. The structural effect of the intramolecular electrostatic interactions is formation of the bent "paper-clip" conformations [62], discussed above. The "paper-clip" model explains the functional links between distant regions of MAPs, such as effects of the N-terminal regions on MT binding, or phosphorylation of N-terminal tyrosines by the Fyn kinase interacting with the proline-rich domain of tau40 and MAP2c. Moreover, close contacts observed in the N-terminal region of MAP2c, comprising the proposed steroid-binding pocket and the interaction site for the regulatory RII subunit of PKA, indicate formation of a hydrophobic core missing in tau [57]. In addition to electrostatic and hydrophobic interactions, disulfide bonds can be formed between cysteines in the second and third MTBRs of tau and MAP2 isoforms containing all four MTBRs. On one hand, such intramolecular oxidation seems to prevent aggregation of tau40, on the other hand, intermolecular disulfide bridges promote fibrilization of tau isoforms containing three MTBRs [131,138,139].

At higher concentration, formation of antiparallel dimers is expected based on the charge distribution. Both types of structures have been observed in early studies of tau [140,141] and MAP2c [142]. In the cellular environment, the intramolecular contacts contribute to the delicate equilibrium of interactions related to MT dynamics [143], aggregation of tau [38], and interactions with other partners. The biological relevance of the formation of antiparallel dimers is less clear. Quantitative data [80,93,144–147] show that prenatal cytosolic concentrations of tau and MAP2c in adult neurons (5 µM–10 µM) [147] are low compared to the conditions when dimerization was significant in vitro. However, formation of dimers can be expected in regions with locally increased tau and MAP2c concentrations [130]. Electrostatic dimerization of tau and MAP2 isoforms was proposed as a molecular mechanism of MT bundling [8]. The ability to form the dimers is altered by phosphorylation. Proline-directed cdc2-like kinase, phosphorylating P2 and MTBD of tau, promotes tau dimerization [141], whereas PKA, phosphorylating outside P2 and MTBD of MAP2c, reduces intermolecular MAP2c interactions [57]. In the case of tau, anti-parallel dimerization due to the electrostatic interactions competes with formation of paired helical filaments stabilized mostly by hydrophobic interactions and able to form inter-strand disulfide bridges [138]. This additional complexity provides a more complete picture of the balance between normal and pathological physiology of tau, but also complicates interpretation of experimental data.

9. Conclusions

A wealth of structural features revealed on tau40 and MAP2c proteins by state-of-the-art protein NMR, cryo-EM, and computations, summarized above, provided a detailed insight into molecular pathophysiology of an important class of MAPs. Tau40 and MAP2c are complex molecules and their physiological roles are yet not fully understood. The structure-function analysis is further complicated by the transient nature of the structural motifs of free forms of these MAPs. Nevertheless, the available data, discussed in detail in the preceding sections, already show a clear relation of numerous structural motifs of tau40 and MAP2c to various biological functions. The biological role is often manifested by specific interactions of short sequence motifs exhibiting transient, but clearly observable structural features. Such motifs can be therefore classified as molecular recognition elements of tau40 and MAP2c. Figure 8 summarizes structure-function relations discussed above and documents that most of the motifs with well-defined transient secondary structure can be associated with a particular function. Specific functions were also identified for more complex structural elements consisting of combination of several motifs (e.g., of extended and turn structures in MTBRs). Comparison of the transient local structures observed in free tau40 and MAP2c with the conformations in complexes with the binding partners (or in homologous complexes with other proteins sharing the same binding motif) often revealed conformational selection of structural motifs highly populated in the free state. However, conformational changes induced upon binding were also noticed (e.g., interactions of tau40 with actin and possibly of MAP2c with the RII subunit of PKA). Moreover, slower dynamics and presence of intramolecular contacts showed that biological functions also involve formation of compacted three-dimensional ("tertiary") structures (e.g., N-terminal region of MAP2c or "paper-clip" structure of tau40). The physiologically important interactions of tau40 and MAP2c are further regulated by post-translational modifications, the specific phosphorylations and truncations discussed above represent illustrative examples.

The structure-function analysis also helps to understand molecular basis for the distinct biological activities of tau40 and MAP2c. Some of the differences are associated with structurally diverse N-terminal domains, not interacting directly with MTs. Other differences are more subtle, associated with local variation of amino-acid sequences of otherwise homologous C-terminal domains. The emerging picture of sensitive regulations of different tau and MAP2 functions by minor sequence changes, or slightly different phosphorylation kinetics, emphasizes intrinsic ability of disordered proteins to be specialized in interactions [148]. Structural principles observed site by site on related but functionally different tau40 and MAP2c may contribute new clues to decipher their physiological destiny as well as pathological role in chronic neurodegenerative diseases.

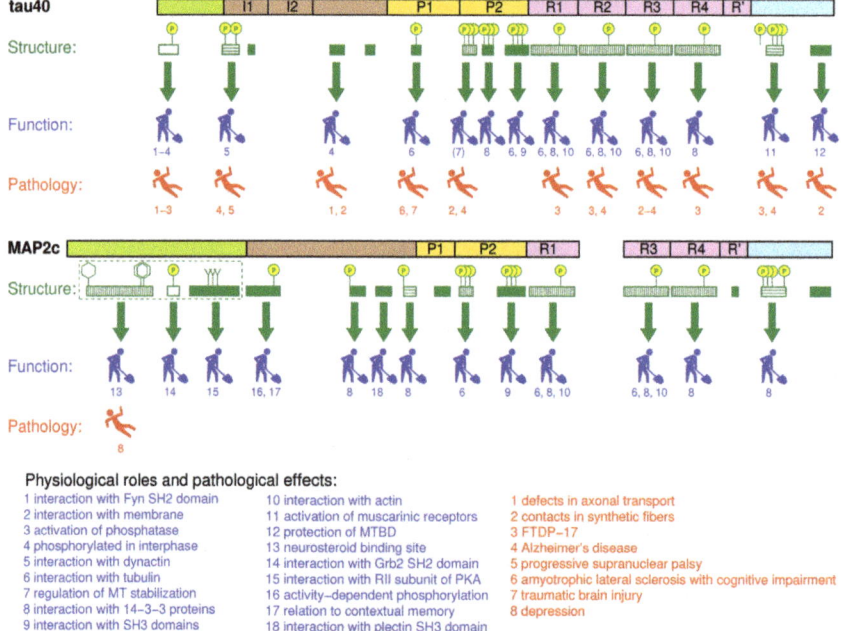

Figure 8. Association of biological functions with the transient structures of tau40 and MAP2c. Schematic representations of structural features (green symbols), normal physiological functions (blue symbols), and pathological effects (red symbols) are placed below horizontal bars showing regions of tau40 and MAP2c, colored as in Figure 2. The filled green rectangles represent all structural motifs with high population of transient secondary structures (continuous stretches of four residues found in polyproline II or α-helical conformation in more than 15% or 5%, respectively, structures in the ensemble selected by the ASTEROIDS analysis based on the experimental data), horizontal hatched green rectangles represent motifs associated with biological functions but with less populated secondary structures, vertical hatched green rectangles represent more complex motifs containing transient turn structures, and open green rectangles represent motifs not exhibiting significant secondary structure propensities but involved in long-range intramolecular interactions. The hexagons, Y-shapes, and circles with "P" above the rectangles indicate functionally important aromatic residues, hydrophobic aliphatic residues, and phosphorylation sites. The transient N-terminal compact structure of MAP2c is marked by the dashed frame. The thick green arrows show which structural motifs are associated with biological functions discussed in this paper, labeled by numbers explained under the diagrams.

Supplementary Materials: The following are available at http://www.mdpi.com/2218-273X/9/3/105/s1, Figure S1: Analysis of transient secondary structures of tau40, Figure S2: Analysis of transient turn structures of tau40, Figure S3: Analysis of transient secondary structures of MAP2c, Figure S4: Analysis of transient β-turn structures of MAP2c, Figure S5: Comparison of secondary chemical shifts of full-length MAP2c and of its fragments, Figure S6: NMR titration of dehydroepiandrosterone by MAP2c and its fragments.

Funding: This research was funded by the Ministry of Education, Youth, and Sport of the Czech Republic, grant number LTC17078 (Inter-Excellence Inter-Cost).

Conflicts of Interest: The authors declare no conflict of interest. The funders had no role in the design of the study; in the collection, analyses, or interpretation of data; in the writing of the manuscript, or in the decision to publish the results.

References

1. Amos, L.A.; Schlieper, D. Microtubules and MAPs. *Adv. Protein Chem.* **2005**, *71*, 257–298. [PubMed]
2. Dehmelt, L.; Halpain, S. The MAP2/Tau family of microtubule-associated proteins. *Genome Biol.* **2004**, *6*, 204. [CrossRef]
3. Arendt, T.; Stieler, J.T.; Holzer, M. Tau and tauopathies. *Brain Res. Bull.* **2016**, *126*, 238–292. [CrossRef] [PubMed]
4. Caillet-Boudin, M.L.; Buée, L.; Sergeant, N.; Lefebvre, B. Regulation of human MAPT gene expression. *Mol. Neurodegener.* **2015**, *10*, 28. [CrossRef] [PubMed]
5. Sánchez, C.; Díaz-Nido, J.; Avila, J. Phosphorylation of microtubule-associated protein 2 (MAP2) and its relevance for the regulation of the neuronal cytoskeleton function. *Prog. Neurobiol.* **2000**, *61*, 133–168. [CrossRef]
6. Kanai, Y.; Hirokawa, N. Sorting mechanisms of Tau and MAP2 in neurons: Suppressed axonal transit of MAP2 and locally regulated microtubule binding. *Neuron* **1995**, *14*, 421–432. [CrossRef]
7. Chen, J.; Kanai, Y.; Cowan, N.J.; Hirokawa, N. Projection domains of MAP2 and tau determine spacings between microtubules in dendrites and axons. *Nature* **1992**, *360*, 674–677. [CrossRef]
8. Rosenberg, K.J.; Ross, J.L.; Feinstein, H.E.; Feinstein, S.C.; Israelachvili, J. Complementary dimerization of microtubule-associated tau protein: Implications for microtubule bundling and tau-mediated pathogenesis. *Proc. Natl. Acad. Sci. USA* **2008**, *105*, 7445–7450. [CrossRef]
9. Chung, P.J.; Choi, M.C.; Miller, H.P.; Feinstein, H.E.; Raviv, U.; Li, Y.; Wilson, L.; Feinstein, S.C.; Safinya, C.R. Direct force measurements reveal that protein Tau confers short-range attractions and isoform-dependent steric stabilization to microtubules. *Proc. Natl. Acad. Sci. USA* **2015**, *112*, E6416–E6425. [CrossRef]
10. Cabrales Fontela, Y.; Kadavath, H.; Biernat, J.; Riedel, D.; Mandelkow, E.; Zweckstetter, M. Multivalent cross-linking of actin filaments and microtubules through the microtubule-associated protein Tau. *Nat. Commun.* **2017**, *8*, 1981. [CrossRef]
11. Elie, A.; Prezel, E.; Guérin, C.; Denarier, E.; Ramirez-Rios, S.; Serre, L.; Andrieux, A.; Fourest-Lieuvin, A.; Blanchoin, L.; Arnal, I. Tau co-organizes dynamic microtubule and actin networks. *Sci. Rep.* **2015**, *5*, 9964. [CrossRef] [PubMed]
12. Goode, B.L.; Chau, M.; Denis, P.E.; Feinstein, S.C. Structural and functional differences between 3-repeat and 4-repeat tau isoforms: Implications for normal tau function and the onset of neurodegenerative disease. *J. Biol. Chem.* **2000**, *275*, 38182–38189. [CrossRef] [PubMed]
13. Harada, A.; Oguchi, K.; Okabe, S.; Kuno, J.; Terada, S.; Ohshima, T.; Sato-Yoshitake, R.; Takei, Y.; Noda, T.; Hirokawa, N. Altered microtubule organization in small-calibre axons of mice lacking tau protein. *Nature* **1994**, *369*, 488–491. [CrossRef]
14. Teng, J.; Takei, Y.; Harada, A.; Nakata, T.; Chen, J.; Hirokawa, N. Synergistic effects of MAP2 and MAP1B knockout in neuronal migration, dendritic outgrowth, and microtubule organization. *J. Cell Biol.* **2001**, *155*, 65–76. [CrossRef]
15. Takei, Y.; Teng, J.; Harada, A.; Hirokawa, N. Defects in Axonal Elongation and Neuronal Migration in Mice with Disrupted *tau* and *map1b* Genes. *J. Cell Biol.* **2000**, *150*, 989–1000. [CrossRef]
16. Mukaetova-Ladinska, E.B.; Xuereb, J.H.; Garcia-Sierra, F.; Hurt, J.; Gertz, H.J.; Hills, R.; Brayne, C.; Huppert, F.A.; Paykel, E.S.; McGee, M.A.; et al. Lewy body variant of Alzheimer's disease: Selective neocortical loss of t-SNARE proteins and loss of MAP2 and α-Synuclein in medial temporal lobe. *Sci. World J.* **2009**, *9*, 1463–1475. [CrossRef] [PubMed]
17. D'Andrea, M.R.; Ilyin, S.; Plata-Salaman, C.R. Abnormal patterns of microtubule-associated protein-2 (MAP-2) immunolabeling in neuronal nuclei and Lewy bodies in Parkinson's disease substantia nigra brain tissues. *Neurosci. Lett.* **2001**, *306*, 137–140. [CrossRef]
18. Cabrera, J.R.; Lucas, J.J. MAP2 Splicing is Altered in Huntington's Disease. *Brain Pathol.* **2016**, *27*, 181–189. [CrossRef] [PubMed]
19. Bianchi, M.; Baulieu, E.E. 3β-Methoxy-pregnenolone (MAP4343) as an innovative therapeutic approach for depressive disorders. *Proc. Natl. Acad. Sci. USA* **2012**, *109*, 1713–1718. [CrossRef]
20. Goedert, M. Tau filaments in neurodegenerative diseases. *FEBS Lett.* **2018**, *592*, 2383–2391. [CrossRef] [PubMed]

21. Congdon, E.E.; Sigurdsson, E.M. Tau-targeting therapies for Alzheimer disease. *Nat. Rev. Neurol.* **2018**, *14*, 399–415. [CrossRef]
22. Novak, P.; Cehlar, O.; Skrabana, R.; Novak, M. Tau Conformation as a Target for Disease-Modifying Therapy: The Role of Truncation. *J. Alzheimers Dis.* **2018**, *64*, S535–S546. [CrossRef]
23. Jadhav, S.; Avila, J.; Schöll, M.; Kovacs, G.G.; Kövari, E.; Skrabana, R.; Evans, L.D.; Kontsekova, E.; Malawska, B.; de Silva, R.; et al. A walk through tau therapeutic strategies. *Acta Neuropathol. Commun.* **2019**, *7*, 22. [CrossRef] [PubMed]
24. Fitzpatrick, A.W.P.; Falcon, B.; He, S.; Murzin, A.G.; Murshudov, G.; Garringer, H.J.; Crowther, R.A.; Ghetti, B.; Goedert, M.; Scheres, S.H.W. Cryo-EM structures of tau filaments from Alzheimer's disease. *Nature* **2017**, *547*, 185–190. [CrossRef] [PubMed]
25. DeTure, M.A.; Di Noto, L.; Purich, D.L. In vitro assembly of Alzheimer-like filaments: How a small cluster of charged residues in Tau and MAP2 controls filament morphology. *J. Biol. Chem.* **2002**, *277*, 34755–34759. [CrossRef] [PubMed]
26. Xie, C.; Soeda, Y.; Shinzaki, Y.; In, Y.; Tomoo, K.; Ihara, Y.; Miyasaka, T. Identification of key amino acids responsible for the distinct aggregation properties of microtubule-associated protein 2 and tau. *J. Neurochem.* **2015**, *135*, 19–26. [CrossRef] [PubMed]
27. Wang, Y.; Mandelkow, E. Tau in physiology and pathology. *Nat. Rev. Nerocsi.* **2016**, *17*, 5–21. [CrossRef]
28. Sánchez, C.; Pérez, M.; Avila, J. GSK3β-mediated phosphorylation of the microtubule-associated protein 2C (MAP2C) prevents microtubule bundling. *Eur. J. Cell Biol.* **2000**, *79*, 252–260. [CrossRef]
29. Fischer, D.; Mukrasch, M.D.; Biernat, J.; Bibow, S.; Blackledge, M.; Griesinger, C.; Mandelkow, E.; Zweckstetter, M. Conformational Changes Specific for Pseudophosphorylation at Serine 262 Selectively Impair Binding of Tau to Microtubules. *Biochemistry* **2009**, *48*, 10047–10055. [CrossRef] [PubMed]
30. Schwalbe, M.; Biernat, J.; Bibow, S.; Ozenne, V.; Jensen, M.R.; Kadavath, H.; Blackledge, M.; Mandelkow, E.; Zweckstetter, M. Phosphorylation of human tau protein by microtubule affinity-regulating kinase 2. *Biochemistry* **2013**, *52*, 9068–9079. [CrossRef] [PubMed]
31. Schwalbe, M.; Kadavath, H.; Biernat, J.; Ozenne, V.; Blackledge, M.; Mandelkow, E.; Zweckstetter, M. Structural Impact of Tau Phosphorylation at Threonine 231. *Structure* **2015**, *23*, 1448–1458. [CrossRef] [PubMed]
32. Tholey, A.; Lindemann, A.; Kinzel, V.; Reed, J. Direct effects of phosphorylation on the preferred backbone conformation of peptides: A nuclear magnetic resonance study. *Biophys. J.* **1999**, *76*, 76–87. [CrossRef]
33. Newberry, R.W.; Raines, R.T. The n→ π* Interaction. *Acc. Chem. Res.* **2017**, *50*, 1838–1846. [CrossRef] [PubMed]
34. Bielska, A.A.; Zondlo, N.J. Hyperphosphorylation of Tau Induces Local Polyproline II Helix. *Biochemistry* **2006**, *45*, 5527–5537. [CrossRef] [PubMed]
35. Martin, L.; Latypova, X.; Wilson, C.M.; Magnaudeix, A.; Perrin, M.L.; Yardin, C.; Terro, F. Tau protein kinases: Involvement in Alzheimer's disease. *Ageing Res. Rev.* **2013**, *12*, 289–309. [CrossRef] [PubMed]
36. Lebouvier, T.; Scales, T.M.E.; Williamson, R.; Noble, W.; Duyckaerts, C.; Hanger, D.P.; Reynolds, C.H.; Anderton, B.H.; Derkinderen, P. The Microtubule-Associated Protein Tau is Also Phosphorylated on Tyrosine. *J. Alzheimers Dis.* **2009**, *18*, 1–9. [CrossRef] [PubMed]
37. Tremblay, M.A.; Acker, C.M.; Davies, P. Tau phosphorylated at tyrosine 394 is found in Alzheimer's disease tangles and can be a product of the abl-related kinase, Arg. *J. Alzheimers Dis.* **2010**, *19*, 721–733. [CrossRef] [PubMed]
38. Mukrasch, M.D.; Bibow, S.; Korukottu, J.; Jeganathan, S.; Biernat, J.; Griesinger, C.; Mandelkow, E.; Zweckstetter, M. Structural polymorphism of 441-residue tau at single residue resolution. *PLoS Biol.* **2009**, *7*, e34. [CrossRef] [PubMed]
39. Schwalbe, M.; Ozenne, V.; Bibow, S.; Jaremko, M.; Jaremko, L.; Gajda, M.; Jensen, M.R.; Biernat, J.; Becker, S.; Mandelkow, E.; et al. Predictive Atomic Resolution Descriptions of Intrinsically Disordered hTau40 and α-Synuclein in Solution from NMR and Small Angle Scattering. *Structure* **2014**, *22*, 238–249. [CrossRef] [PubMed]
40. Jansen, S.; Melková, K.; Trošanová, Z.; Hanáková, K.; Zachrdla, M.; Nováček, J.; Župa, E.; Zdráhal, Z.; Hritz, J.; Žídek, L. Quantitative mapping of microtubule-associated protein 2c (MAP2c) phosphorylation and regulatory protein 14-3-3ζ-binding sites reveals key differences between MAP2c and its homolog Tau. *J. Biol. Chem.* **2017**, *292*, 6715–6727. [CrossRef] [PubMed]

41. Kadavath, H.; Jaremko, M.; Jaremko, Ł.; Biernat, J.; Mandelkow, E.; Zweckstetter, M. Folding of the Tau Protein on Microtubules. *Angew. Chem. Int. Ed.* **2015**, *54*, 10347–10351. [CrossRef] [PubMed]
42. Kadavath, H.; Hofele, R.V.; Biernat, J.; Kumar, S.; Tepper, K.; Urlaub, H.; Mandelkow, E.; Zweckstetter, M. Tau stabilizes microtubules by binding at the interface between tubulin heterodimers. *Proc. Natl. Acad. Sci. USA* **2015**, *112*, 7501–7506. [CrossRef]
43. Kellogg, E.H.; Hejab, N.M.A.; Poepsel, S.; Downing, K.H.; DiMaio, F.; Nogales, E. Near-atomic model of microtubule-tau interactions. *Science* **2018**, *360*, 1242–1246. [CrossRef] [PubMed]
44. Bibow, S.; Mukrasch, M.D.; Chinnathambi, S.; Biernat, J.; Griesinger, C.; Mandelkow, E.; Zweckstetter, M. The dynamic structure of filamentous Tau. *Angew. Chem. Int. Ed.* **2011**, *50*, 11520–11524. [CrossRef] [PubMed]
45. Sündermann, F.; Fernandez, M.P.; Morgan, R.O. An evolutionary roadmap to the microtubule-associated protein MAP Tau. *BMC Genom.* **2016**, *17*, 264. [CrossRef] [PubMed]
46. Smet, C.; Leroy, A.; Sillen, A.; Wieruszeski, J.M.; Landrieu, I.; Lippens, G. Accepting its Random Coil Nature Allows a Partial NMR Assignment of the Neuronal Tau Protein. *ChemBioChem* **2004**, *5*, 1639–1646. [CrossRef]
47. Lippens, G.; Wieruszeski, J.M.; Leroy, A.; Smet, C.; Sillen, A.; Buée, L.; Landrieu, I. Proline-Directed Random-Coil Chemical Shift Values as a Tool for the NMR Assignment of the Tau Phosphorylation Sites. *ChemBioChem* **2004**, *5*, 73–78. [CrossRef] [PubMed]
48. Mukrasch, M.D.; Biernat, J.; von Bergen, M.; Griesinger, C.; Mandelkow, E.; Zweckstetter, M. Sites of tau important for aggregation populate β-structure and bind to microtubules and polyanions. *J. Biol. Chem.* **2005**, *280*, 24978–24986. [CrossRef]
49. Mukrasch, M.D.; von Bergen, M.; Biernat, J.; Fischer, D.; Griesinger, C.; Mandelkow, E.; Zweckstetter, M. The "jaws" of the tau-microtubule interaction. *J. Biol. Chem.* **2007**, *282*, 12230–12239. [CrossRef]
50. Verdegem, D.; Dijkstra, K.; Hanoulle, X.; Lippens, G. Graphical interpretation of Boolean operators for protein NMR assignments. *J. Biomol. NMR* **2008**, *42*, 11–21. [CrossRef]
51. Sibille, N.; Hanoulle, X.; Fanny, B.; Dries, V.; Isabelle, L.; Jean-Michel, W.; Guy, L. Selective backbone labelling of ILV methyl labelled proteins. *J. Biomol. NMR* **2009**, *43*, 219–227. [CrossRef]
52. Lopez, J.; Ahuja, P.; Gerard, M.; Wieruszeski, J.M.; Lippens, G. A new strategy for sequential assignment of intrinsically unstructured proteins based on 15N single isotope labelling. *J. Magn. Reson.* **2013**, *236*, 1–6. [CrossRef] [PubMed]
53. Narayanan, R.L.; Dürr, U.H.N.; Bibow, S.; Biernat, J.; Mandelkow, E.; Zweckstetter, M. Automatic Assignment of the Intrinsically Disordered Protein Tau with 441-Residues. *J. Am. Chem. Soc.* **2010**, *132*, 11906–11907. [CrossRef] [PubMed]
54. Harbison, N.W.; Bhattacharya, S.; Eliezer, D. Assigning Backbone NMR Resonances for Full Length Tau Isoforms: Efficient Compromise between Manual Assignments and Reduced Dimensionality. *PLoS ONE* **2012**, *7*, e34679. [CrossRef] [PubMed]
55. Nováček, J.; Janda, L.; Dopitová, R.; Žídek, L.; Sklenář, V. Efficient protocol for backbone and side-chain assignments of large, intrinsically disordered proteins: Transient secondary structure analysis of 49.2 kDa microtubule associated protein 2c. *J. Biomol. NMR* **2013**, *56*, 291–301. [CrossRef] [PubMed]
56. Nodet, G.; Salmon, L.; Ozenne, V.; Meier, S.; Jensen, M.R.; Blackledge, M. Quantitative description of backbone conformational sampling of unfolded proteins at amino acid resolution from NMR residual dipolar couplings. *J. Am. Chem. Soc.* **2009**, *131*, 17908–17918. [CrossRef]
57. Melková, K.; Zapletal, V.; Jansen, S.; Nomilner, E.; Zachrdla, M.; Hritz, J.; Nováček, J.; Zweckstetter, M.; Jensen, M.R.; Blackledge, M.; et al. Functionally specific binding regions of microtubule-associated protein 2c exhibit distinct conformations and dynamics. *J. Biol. Chem.* **2018**, *293*, 13297–13309. [CrossRef] [PubMed]
58. Kovacech, B.; Skrabana, R.; Novak, M. Transition of Tau Protein from Disordered to Misordered in Alzheimer's Disease. *Neurodegener. Dis.* **2010**, *7*, 24–27. [CrossRef] [PubMed]
59. Kontsekova, E.; Zilka, N.; Kovacech, B.; Skrabana, R.; Novak, M. Identification of structural determinants on tau protein essential for its pathological function: Novel therapeutic target for tau immunotherapy in Alzheimer's disease. *Alzheimers Res. Ther.* **2014**, *6*, 45. [CrossRef] [PubMed]
60. de Brevern, A.G. Extension of the classical classification of β-turns. *Sci. Rep.* **2016**, *6*, 33191. [CrossRef]
61. Kyte, J.; Doolittle, R. A simple method for displaying the hydropathic character of a protein. *J. Mol. Biol.* **1982**, *157*, 105–132. [CrossRef]

62. Jeganathan, S.; von Bergen, M.; Brutlach, H.; Steinhoff, H.J.; Mandelkow, E. Global hairpin folding of tau in solution. *Biochemistry* **2006**, *45*, 2283–2293. [CrossRef] [PubMed]
63. LaPointe, N.E.; Morfini, G.; Pigino, G.; Gaisina, I.N.; Kozikowski, A.P.; Binder, L.I.; Brady, S.T. The amino terminus of tau inhibits kinesin-dependent axonal transport: Implications for filament toxicity. *J. Neurosci. Res.* **2009**, *87*, 440–451. [CrossRef] [PubMed]
64. Kanaan, N.M.; Morfini, G.A.; LaPointe, N.E.; Pigino, G.F.; Patterson, K.R.; Song, Y.; Andreadis, A.; Fu, Y.; Brady, S.T.; Binder, L.I. Pathogenic Forms of Tau Inhibit Kinesin-Dependent Axonal Transport through a Mechanism Involving Activation of Axonal Phosphotransferases. *J. Neurosci.* **2011**, *31*, 9858–9868. [CrossRef]
65. Liao, H.; Li, Y.; Brautigan, D.L.; Gundersen, G.G. Protein phosphatase 1 is targeted to microtubules by the microtubule- associated protein tau. *J. Biol. Chem.* **1998**, *273*, 21901–21908. [CrossRef]
66. Dente, L.; Vetriani, C.; Zucconi, A.; Pelicci, G.; Lanfrancone, L.; Pelicci, P.; Cesareni, G. Modified phage peptide libraries as a tool to study specificity of phosphorylation and recognition of tyrosine containing peptides. *J. Mol. Biol.* **1997**, *269*, 694–703. [CrossRef]
67. Lee, G.; Thangavel, R.; Sharma, V.M.; Litersky, J.M.; Bhaskar, K.; Fang, S.M.; Do, L.H.; Andreadis, A.; Van Hoesen, G.; Ksiezak-Reding, H. Phosphorylation of Tau by Fyn: Implications for Alzheimers Disease. *J. Neurosci.* **2004**, *24*, 2304–2312. [CrossRef]
68. Stern, J.L.; Lessard, D.V.; Hoeprich, G.J.; Morfini, G.A.; Berger, C.L.; Drubin, D.G. Phosphoregulation of Tau modulates inhibition of kinesin-1 motility. *Mol. Biol. Cell* **2017**, *28*, 1079–1087. [CrossRef] [PubMed]
69. Schroer, T.A. Dynactin. *Annu. Rev. Cell Dev. Biol.* **2004**, *20*, 759–779. [CrossRef]
70. Carter, A.P.; Diamant, A.G.; Urnavicius, L. How dynein and dynactin transport cargos: A structural perspective. *Curr. Opin. Struct. Biol.* **2016**, *37*, 62–70. [CrossRef] [PubMed]
71. Magnani, E.; Fan, J.; Gasparini, L.; Golding, M.; Williams, M.; Schiavo, G.; Goedert, M.; Amos, L.A.; Spillantini, M.G. Interaction of tau protein with the dynactin complex. *EMBO J.* **2007**, *26*, 4546–4554. [CrossRef]
72. Brandt, R.; Léger, J.; Lee, G. Interaction of tau with the neural plasma membrane mediated by taus amino-terminal projection domain. *J. Cell Biol.* **1995**, *131*, 1327–1340. [CrossRef]
73. Usardi, A.; Pooler, A.M.; Seereeram, A.; Reynolds, C.H.; Derkinderen, P.; Anderton, B.; Hanger, D.P.; Noble, W.; Williamson, R. Tyrosine phosphorylation of tau regulates its interactions with Fyn SH2 domains, but not SH3 domains, altering the cellular localization of tau. *FEBS J.* **2011**, *278*, 2927–2937. [CrossRef] [PubMed]
74. Hernandez, P.; Lee, G.; Sjoberg, M.; MacCioni, R.B. Tau phosphorylation by cdk5 and Fyn in response to amyloid peptide Aβ25-35: Involvement of lipid rafts. *J. Alzheimers Dis.* **2009**, *16*, 149–156. [CrossRef] [PubMed]
75. Baulieu, E.E. Neurosteroids: Of the Nervous System, By the Nervous System, For the Nervous System. *Recent Progr. Horm. Res.* **1997**, *52*, 1–32. [PubMed]
76. Fontaine-Lenoir, V.; Chambraud, B.; Fellous, A.; David, S.; Duchossoy, Y.; Baulieu, E.E.; Robel, P. Microtubule-associated protein 2 (MAP2) is a neurosteroid receptor. *Proc. Natl. Acad. Sci. USA* **2006**, *103*, 4711–4716. [CrossRef] [PubMed]
77. Laurine, E.; Lafitte, D.; Grégoire, C.; Sérée, E.; Loret, E.; Douillard, S.; Michel, B.; Briand, C.; Verdier, J.M. Specific binding of dehydroepiandrosterone to the N terminus of the microtubule-associated protein MAP2. *J. Biol. Chem.* **2003**, *278*, 29979–29986. [CrossRef] [PubMed]
78. Mizota, K.; Ueda, H. N-terminus of MAP2C as a neurosteroid-binding site. *NeuroReport* **2008**, *19*, 1529–1533. [CrossRef] [PubMed]
79. Götz, F.; Roske, Y.; Schulz, M.S.; Autenrieth, K.; Bertinetti, D.; Faelber, K.; Zühlke, K.; Kreuchwig, A.; Kennedy, E.J.; Krause, G.; et al. AKAP18:PKA-RIIα structure reveals crucial anchor points for recognition of regulatory subunits of PKA. *Biochem. J.* **2016**, *473*, 1881–1894. [CrossRef] [PubMed]
80. Zamora-Leon, S.P.; Bresnick, A.; Backer, J.M.; Shafit-Zagardo, B. Fyn phosphorylates human MAP-2c on tyrosine 67. *J. Biol. Chem.* **2005**, *280*, 1962–1970. [CrossRef] [PubMed]
81. Majumder, P.; Roy, K.; Singh, B.K.; Jana, N.R.; Mukhopadhyay, D. Cellular levels of Grb2 and cytoskeleton stability are correlated in a neurodegenerative scenario. *Dis. Models Mech.* **2017**, *10*, 655–669. [CrossRef]

82. Illenberger, S.; Zheng-Fischhöfer, Q.; Preuss, U.; Stamer, K.; Baumann, K.; Trinczek, B.; Biernat, J.; Godemann, R.; Mandelkow, E.M.; Mandelkow, E. The endogenous and cell cycle-dependent phosphorylation of tau protein in living cells: Implications for Alzheimer's disease. *Mol. Biol. Cell* **1998**, *9*, 1495–1512. [CrossRef] [PubMed]
83. Hanger, D.P.; Byers, H.L.; Wray, S.; Leung, K.Y.; Saxton, M.J.; Seereeram, A.; Reynolds, C.H.; Ward, M.A.; Anderton, B.H. Novel phosphorylation sites in Tau from Alzheimer brain support a role for casein kinase 1 in disease pathogenesis. *J. Biol. Chem.* **2007**, *282*, 23645–23654. [CrossRef] [PubMed]
84. Qi, H.; Prabakaran, S.; Cantrelle, F.X.; Chambraud, B.; Gunawardena, J.; Lippens, X.G.; Landrieu, I. Characterization of neuronal tau protein as a target of extracellular signal-regulated kinase. *J. Biol. Chem.* **2016**, *291*, 7742–7753. [CrossRef] [PubMed]
85. Feijoo, C.; Campbell, D.G.; Jakes, R.; Goedert, M.; Cuenda, A. Evidence that phosphorylation of the microtubule-associated protein Tau by SAPK4/p38δ at Thr50 promotes microtubule assembly. *J. Cell Sci.* **2005**, *118*, 397–408. [CrossRef] [PubMed]
86. Wray, S.; Saxton, M.; Anderton, B.; Hanger, D. Direct analysis of tau from PSP brain identifies new phosphorylation sites and a major fragment of N-terminally cleaved tau containing four microtubule-binding repeats. *J. Neurochem.* **2008**, *105*, 2343–2352. [CrossRef]
87. Derisbourg, M.; Leghay, C.; Chiappetta, G.; Fernandez-Gomez, F.J.; Laurent, C.; Demeyer, D.; Carrier, S.; Buée-Scherrer, V.; Blum, D.; Vinh, J.; et al. Role of the Tau N-terminal region in microtubule stabilization revealed by new endogenous truncated forms. *Sci. Rep.* **2015**, *5*, 9659. [CrossRef] [PubMed]
88. Zilka, N.; Kovacech, B.; Barath, P.; Kontsekova, E.; Novák, M. The self-perpetuating tau truncation circle. *Biochem. Soc. Trans.* **2012**, *40*, 681–686. [CrossRef]
89. Skrabana, R.; Kovacech, B.; Filipcik, P.; Zilka, N.; Jadhav, S.; Smolek, T.; Kontsekova, E.; Novak, M.; Deli, M. Neuronal Expression of Truncated Tau Efficiently Promotes Neurodegeneration in Animal Models: Pitfalls of Toxic Oligomer Analysis. *J. Alzheimers Dis.* **2017**, *58*, 1017–1025. [CrossRef]
90. Berling, B.; Wille, H.; Roll, B.; Mandelkow, E.M.; Garner, C.; Mandelkow, E. Phosphorylation of microtubule-associated proteins MAP2a,b and MAP2c at Ser136 by proline-directed kinases in vivo and in vitro. *Eur. J. Cell Biol.* **1994**, *64*, 120–130.
91. Philpot, B.D.; Lim, J.H.; Halpain, S.; Brunjes, P.C. Experience-Dependent Modifications in MAP2 Phosphorylation in Rat Olfactory Bulb. *J. Neurosci.* **1997**, *17*, 9596–9604. [CrossRef] [PubMed]
92. Woolf, N.; Zinnerman, M.; Johnson, G. Hippocampal microtubule-associated protein-2 alterations with contextual memory. *Brain Res.* **1999**, *821*, 241–249. [CrossRef]
93. Tie, L.; Zhang, J.Z.; Lin, Y.H.; Su, T.H.; Li, Y.H.; Wu, H.L.; Zhang, Y.Y.; Yu, H.M.; Li, X.J. Epinephrine increases phosphorylation of MAP-2c in rat pheochromocytoma cells (PC12 Cells) via a protein kinase C- and mitogen activated protein kinase-dependent mechanism. *J. Proteome. Res.* **2008**, *7*, 1704–1711. [CrossRef]
94. Alexa, A.; Schmidt, G.; Tompa, P.; Ogueta, S.; Vázquez, J.; Kulcsár, P.; Kovács, J.; Dombrádi, V.; Friedrich, P. The phosphorylation state of threonine-220, a uniquely phosphatase-sensitive protein kinase A site in microtubule-associated protein MAP2c, regulates microtubule binding and stability. *Biochemistry* **1992**, *41*, 12427–12435. [CrossRef]
95. Joo, Y.; Schumacher, B.; Landrieu, I.; Bartel, M.; Smet-Nocca, C.; Jang, A.; Choi, H.S.; Jeon, N.L.; Chang, K.A.; Kim, H.S.; et al. Involvement of 14-3-3 in tubulin instability and impaired axon development is mediated by Tau. *FASEB J.* **2015**, *29*, 4133–4144. [CrossRef] [PubMed]
96. Valencia, R.; Walko, G.; Janda, L.; Novaček, J.; Mihailovska, E.; Reipert, S.; Andrä-Marobela, K.; Wiche, G. Intermediate filament-associated cytolinker plectin 1c destabilizes microtubules in keratinocytes. *Mol. Biol. Cell* **2013**, *24*, 768–784. [CrossRef] [PubMed]
97. He, H.J.; Wang, X.S.; Pan, R.; Wang, D.L.; Liu, M.N.; He, R.Q. The proline-rich domain of tau plays a role in interactions with actin. *BMC Cell Biol.* **2009**, *10*, 81. [CrossRef]
98. Gohar, M.; Yang, W.; Strong, W.; Volkening, K.; Leystra-Lantz, C.; Strong, M.J. Tau phosphorylation at threonine-175 leads to fibril formation and enhanced cell death: Implications for amyotrophic lateral sclerosis with cognitive impairment. *J. Neurochem.* **2009**, *108*, 634–643. [CrossRef]
99. Moszczynski, A.J.; Strong, W.; Xu, K.; McKee, A.; Brown, A.; Strong, M.J. Pathologic Thr^{175} tau phosphorylation in CTE and CTE with ALS. *Neurology* **2018**, *90*, e380–e387. [CrossRef]

100. Moszczynski, A.J.; Gohar, M.; Volkening, K.; Leystra-Lantz, C.; Strong, W.; Strong, M.J. Thr^{175}-phosphorylated tau induces pathologic fibril formation via GSK3β-mediated phosphorylation of Thr^{231} in vitro. *Neurobiol. Aging* **2015**, *36*, 1590–1599. [CrossRef]
101. Gandhi, N.S.; Landrieu, I.; Byrne, C.; Kucic, P.; Cantrelle, F.X.; Wieruszeski, J.M.; L, M.R.; Jacquot, Y.; Lippens, G. A Phosphorylation-Induced Turn Defines the Alzheimer's Disease AT8 Antibody Epitope on the Tau Protein. *Angew. Chem. Int. Ed.* **2015**, *54*, 6819–6823. [CrossRef] [PubMed]
102. Ittner, A.; Chua, S.W.; Bertz, J.; Volkerling, A.; van der Hoven, J.; Gladbach, A.; Przybyla, M.; Bi, M.; van Hummel, A.; Stevens, C.H.; et al. Site-specific phosphorylation of tau inhibits amyloid-β toxicity in Alzheimer's mice. *Science* **2016**, *354*, 904–908. [CrossRef]
103. Despres, C.; Byrne, C.; Qi, H.; Cantrelle, F.X.; Huvent, I.; Chambraud, B.; Baulieu, E.E.; Jacquot, Y.; Landrieu, I.; Lippens, G.; et al. Identification of the Tau phosphorylation pattern that drives its aggregation. *Proc. Natl. Acad. Sci. USA* **2017**, *114*, 9080–9085. [CrossRef] [PubMed]
104. Malia, T.J.; Teplyakov, A.; Ernst, R.; Wu, S.J.; Lacy, E.R.; Liu, X.; Vandermeeren, M.; Mercken, M.; Luo, J.; Sweet, R.W.; et al. Epitope mapping and structural basis for the recognition of phosphorylated tau by the anti-tau antibody AT8. *Proteins Struct. Funct. Bioinf.* **2016**, *84*, 427–434. [CrossRef] [PubMed]
105. Hashiguchi, M.; Hashiguchi, T. Chapter Four—Kinase-Kinase Interaction and Modulation of Tau Phosphorylation. In *International Review of Cell and Molecular Biology*; Jeon, K.W., Ed.; Academic Press: Cambridge, MA, USA, 2013; Volume 300, pp. 121–160.
106. Yang, P.H.; Zhu, J.X.; Huang, Y.D.; Zhang, X.Y.; Lei, P.; Bush, A.; Xiang, Q.; Su, Z.; Zhang, Q.H. Human Basic Fibroblast Growth Factor Inhibits Tau Phosphorylation via the PI3K/Akt-GSK3β Signaling Pathway in a 6-Hydroxydopamine-Induced Model of Parkinson's Disease. *Neurodegener. Dis.* **2016**, *16*, 357–369. [CrossRef]
107. Amniai, L.; Barbier, P.; Sillen, A.; Wieruszeski, J.M.; Peyrot, V.; Lippens, G.; Landrieu, I. Alzheimer disease specific phosphoepitopes of Tau interfere with assembly of tubulin but not binding to microtubules. *FASEB J.* **2009**, *23*, 1146–1152. [CrossRef] [PubMed]
108. Komulainen, E.; Zdrojewska, J.; Freemantle, E.; Mohammad, H.; Kulesskaya, N.; Deshpande, P.; Marchisella, F.; Mysore, R.; Hollos, P.; Michelsen, K.A.; et al. JNK1 controls dendritic field size in L2/3 and L5 of the motor cortex, constrains soma size, and influences fine motor coordination. *Front. Cell. Neurosci.* **2014**, *8*, 272. [CrossRef]
109. Reynolds, C.H.; Garwood, C.J.; Wray, S.; Price, C.; Kellie, S.; Perera, T.; Zvelebil, M.; Yang, A.; Sheppard, P.W.; Varndell, I.M.; et al. Phosphorylation regulates tau interactions with Src homology 3 domains of phosphatidylinositol 3-kinase, phospholipase Cγ1, Grb2, and Src family kinases. *J. Biol. Chem.* **2008**, *283*, 18177–18186. [CrossRef]
110. Yoshida, H.; Goedert, M. Sequential phosphorylation of tau protein by cAMP-dependent protein kinase and SAPK4/p38delta or JNK2 in the presence of heparin generates the AT100 epitope. *J. Neurochem.* **2006**, *99*, 154–164. [CrossRef] [PubMed]
111. Landrieu, I.; Lacosse, L.; Leroy, A.; Wieruszeski, J.M.; Trivelli, X.; Sillen, A.; Sibille, N.; Schwalbe, H.; Saxena, K.; Langer, T.; et al. NMR analysis of a Tau phosphorylation pattern. *J. Am. Chem. Soc.* **2006**, *128*, 3575–3583. [CrossRef]
112. Sadik, G.; Tanaka, T.; Kato, K.; Yamamori, H.; Nessa, B.N.; Morihara, T.; Takeda, M. Phosphorylation of tau at Ser214 mediates its interaction with 14-3-3 protein: Implications for the mechanism of tau aggregation. *J. Neurochem.* **2009**, *108*, 33–43. [CrossRef] [PubMed]
113. Sluchanko, N.N.; Seit-Nebi, A.S.; Gusev, N.B. Effect of phosphorylation on interaction of human tau protein with 14-3-3zeta. *Biochem. Biophys. Res. Commun.* **2009**, *379*, 990–994. [CrossRef] [PubMed]
114. Sluchanko, N.N.; Seit-Nebi, A.S.; Gusev, N.B. Phosphorylation of more than one site is required for tight interaction of human tau protein with 14-3-3zeta. *FEBS Lett.* **2009**, *583*, 2739–4272. [CrossRef] [PubMed]
115. Sluchanko, N.N.; Gusev, N.B. 14-3-3 proteins and regulation of cytoskeleton. *Biochemistry* **2010**, *75*, 1528–1546. [CrossRef]
116. Johnson, C.; Crowther, S.; Stafford, M.; Campbell, D.; Toth, R.; MacKintosh, C. Bioinformatic and experimental survey of 14-3-3-binding sites. *Biochem. J.* **2010**, *427*, 69–78. [CrossRef] [PubMed]
117. Zamora-Leon, S.P.; Lee, G.; Davies, P.; Shafit-Zagardo, B. Binding of Fyn to MAP-2c through an SH3 binding domain. *J. Biol. Chem.* **2001**, *276*, 39950–39958. [CrossRef]

118. Andrei, S.A.; Meijer, F.A.; Neves, J.F.; Brunsveld, L.; Landrieu, I.; Ottmann, C.; Milroy, L.G. Inhibition of 14-3-3/Tau by Hybrid Small-Molecule Peptides Operating via Two Different Binding Modes. *ACS Chem. Neurocsi.* **2018**, *9*, 2639–2654. [CrossRef]
119. Gigant, B.; Landrieu, I.; Fauquan, C.; Barbie, P.; Huvent, I.; Wieruszeski, J.M.; Knossow, M.; Lippens, G. Mechanism of Tau-Promoted Microtubule Assembly As Probed by NMR Spectroscopy. *J. Am. Chem. Soc.* **2014**, *136*, 12615–12623. [CrossRef] [PubMed]
120. von Bergen, M.; Friedhoff, P.; Biernat, J.; Heberle, J.; Mandelkow, E.M.; Mandelkow, E. Assembly of tau protein into Alzheimer paired helical filaments depends on a local sequence motif ((306)VQIVYK(311)) forming beta structure. *Proc. Natl. Acad. Sci. USA* **2000**, *97*, 5129–5134. [CrossRef] [PubMed]
121. Wang, R.Y.R.; Song, Y.; Barad, B.A.; Cheng, Y.; Fraser, J.S.; DiMaio, F. Automated structure refinement of macromolecular assemblies from cryo-EM maps using Rosetta. *eLife* **2016**, *5*, e17219. [CrossRef]
122. Al-Bassam, J.; Ozer, R.S.; Safer, D.; Halpain, S.; Milligan, R.A. MAP2 and tau bind longitudinally along the outer ridges of microtubule protofilaments. *J. Cell Biol.* **2002**, *157*, 1187–1196. [CrossRef]
123. Kar, S.; Fan, J.; Smith, M.J.; Goedert, M.; Amos, L.A. Repeat motifs of tau bind to the insides of microtubules in the absence of taxol. *EMBO J.* **2003**, *22*, 70–77. [CrossRef]
124. Drewes, G.; Trinczek, B.; Illenberger, S.; Biernat, J.; Schmitt-Ulms, G.; Meyer, H.E.; Mandelkow, E.M.; Mandelkow, E. Microtubule-associated Protein/Microtubule Affinity-regulating Kinase (p110mark): A novel protein kinase that regulates tau-microtubule interactions and dynamic instability by phosphorylation at the Alzheimer-specific site serine 262. *J. Biol. Chem.* **1995**, *270*, 7679–7688. [CrossRef] [PubMed]
125. Illenberger, S.; Drewes, G.; Trinczek, B.; Biernat, J.; Meyer, H.E.; Olmsted, J.B.; Mandelkow, E.M.; Mandelkow, E. Phosphorylation of microtubule-associated proteins MAP2 and MAP4 by the protein kinase p110^{mark}. Phosphorylation sites and regulation of microtubule dynamics. *J. Biol. Chem.* **1996**, *271*, 10834–10843. [CrossRef]
126. Brandt, R.; Lee, G.; Teplow, D.B.; Shalloway, D.; Abdel-Ghany, M. Differential Effect of Phosphorylation and Substrate Modulation on Tau's Ability to Promote Microtubule Growth and Nucleation. *J. Biol. Chem.* **1994**, *269*, 11776–11782.
127. Itoh, T.J.; Hisanaga, S.; Hosoi, T.; Kishimoto, T.; Hotani, H. Phosphorylation states of microtubule-associated protein 2 (MAP2) determine the regulatory role of MAP2 in microtubule dynamics. *Biochemistry* **1997**, *36*, 12574–12582. [CrossRef] [PubMed]
128. Schneider, A.; Biernat, J.; von Bergen, M.; Mandelkow, E.; Mandelkow, E.M. Phosphorylation that Detaches Tau Protein from Microtubules (Ser262, Ser214) Also Protects It against Aggregation into Alzheimer Paired Helical Filaments. *Biochemistry* **1999**, *38*, 3549–3558. [CrossRef] [PubMed]
129. Sattilaro, R.F. Interaction of microtubule-associated protein 2 with actin filaments. *Biochemistry* **1986**, *25*, 2003–2009. [CrossRef] [PubMed]
130. Ozer, R.S.; Halpain, S. Phosphorylation-dependent localization of microtubule-associated protein MAP2c to the actin cytoskeleton. *Mol. Biol. Cell* **2000**, *11*, 3573–3587. [CrossRef]
131. Al-Hilaly, Y.K.; Pollack, S.J.; Vadukul, D.M.; Citossi, F.; Rickard, J.E.; Simpson, M.; Storey, J.M.; Harrington, C.R.; Wischik, C.M.; Serpell, L.C. Alzheimer's Disease-like Paired Helical Filament Assembly from Truncated Tau Protein Is Independent of Disulfide Crosslinking. *J. Mol. Biol.* **2017**, *429*, 3650–3665. [CrossRef]
132. Xie, C.; Miyasaka, T.; Yoshimura, S.; Hatsuta, H.; Yoshina, S.; Kage-Nakadai, E.; Mitani, S.; Murayama, S.; Ihara, Y. The homologous carboxyl-terminal domains of microtubule-associated protein 2 and TAU induce neuronal dysfunction and have differential fates in the evolution of neurofibrillary tangles. *PLoS ONE* **2014**, *9*, e89796. [CrossRef] [PubMed]
133. Gómez-Ramos, A.; Díaz-Hernández, M.; Rubio, A.; Miras-Portugal, M.T.; Avila, J. Extracellular tau promotes intracellular calcium increase through M1 and M3 muscarinic receptors in neuronal cells. *Mol. Cell. Neurosci.* **2008**, *37*, 673–681. [CrossRef] [PubMed]
134. Li, T.; Paudel, H.K. Glycogen Synthase Kinase 3β Phosphorylates Alzheimer's Disease-Specific Ser396 of Microtubule-Associated Protein Tau by a Sequential Mechanism. *Biochemistry* **2006**, *45*, 3125–3133. [CrossRef] [PubMed]
135. Díaz-Hernández, M.; Gómez-Ramos, A.; Rubio, A.; Gómez-Villafuertes, R.; Naranjo, J.R.; Teresa Miras-Portugal, M.; Avila, J. Tissue-nonspecific alkaline phosphatase promotes the neurotoxicity effect of extracellular tau. *J. Biol. Chem.* **2010**, *285*, 32539–35248. [CrossRef] [PubMed]

136. Berry, R.W.; Abraha, A.; Lagalwar, S.; LaPointe, N.; Gamblin, T.C.; Cryns, V.L.; Binder, L.I. Inhibition of Tau Polymerization by Its Carboxy-Terminal Caspase Cleavage Fragment. *Biochemistry* **2003**, *42*, 8325–8331. [CrossRef] [PubMed]
137. Fifre, A.; Sponne, I.; Koziel, V.; Kriem, B.; Potin, F.T.Y.; Bihain, B.E.; Olivier, J.L.; Oster, T.; Pillot, T. Microtubule-associated Protein MAP1A, MAP1B, and MAP2 Proteolysis during Soluble Amyloid β-Peptide-induced Neuronal Apoptosis: Synergistic Involvement of Calpain and Caspase-3. *J. Biol. Chem.* **2006**, *281*, 229–240. [CrossRef]
138. Walker, S.; Ullman, O.; Stultz, C.M. Using intramolecular disulfide bonds in tau protein to deduce structural features of aggregation-resistant conformations. *J. Biol. Chem.* **2012**, *287*, 9591–9600. [CrossRef]
139. Crowe, A.; James, M.J.; Virginia, M.Y.; Smith, A.B.; Trojanowski, J.Q.; Ballatore, C.; Brunden, K.R. Aminothienopyridazines and methylene blue affect Tau fibrillization via cysteine oxidation. *J. Biol. Chem.* **2013**, *288*, 11024–11037. [CrossRef]
140. De Ancos, J.G.; Correas, I.; Avila, J. Differences in microtubule binding and self-association abilities of bovine brain tau isoforms. *J. Biol. Chem.* **1993**, *268*, 7976–7982.
141. Paudel, H.K. Phosphorylation by neuronal cdc2-like protein kinase promotes dimerization of tau protein in vitro. *J. Biol. Chem.* **1997**, *272*, 28328–28334. [CrossRef] [PubMed]
142. Wille, H.; Mandelkow, E.M.; Mandelkow, E. The Juvenile Microtubule-associated Protein MAP2c Is a Rod-like Molecule That Forms Antiparallel Dimer. *J. Biol. Chem.* **1992**, *267*, 10737–10742.
143. Goode, B.L.; Denis, P.E.; Panda, D.; Radeke, M.J.; Miller, H.P.; Wilson, L.; Feinstein, S.C. Functional interactions between the proline-rich and repeat regions of tau enhance microtubule binding and assembly. *Mol. Biol. Cell* **1997**, *8*, 353–365. [CrossRef] [PubMed]
144. Guo, Y.; Gong, H.S.; Zhang, J.; Xie, W.L.; Tian, C.; Chen, C.; Shi, Q.; Wang, S.B.; Xu, Y.; Zhang, B.Y.; et al. Remarkable reduction of MAP2 in the brains of scrapie-infected rodents and human prion disease possibly correlated with the increase of calpain. *PLoS ONE* **2012**, *7*, e30163. [CrossRef] [PubMed]
145. Ackmann, M.; Wiech, H.; Mandelkow, E. Nonsaturable binding indicates clustering of tau on the microtubule surface in a paired helical filament-like conformation. *J. Biol. Chem.* **2000**, *275*, 30335–30343. [CrossRef] [PubMed]
146. Meixner, A.; Haverkamp, S.; Wässle, H.; Führer, S.; Thalhammer, J.; Kropf, N.; Bittner, R.E.; Lassmann, H.; Wiche, G.; Propst, F. MAP1B is required for axon guidance and Is involved in the development of the central and peripheral nervous system. *J. Cell Biol.* **2000**, *151*, 1169–1178. [CrossRef] [PubMed]
147. Liu, F.; Iqbal, K.; Grundke-Iqbal, I.; Rossie, S.; Gong, C.X. Dephosphorylation of tau by protein phosphatase 5: Impairment in Alzheimer's disease. *J. Biol. Chem.* **2005**, *280*, 1790–1796. [CrossRef]
148. Tompa, P.; Schad, E.; Tantos, A.; Kalmar, L. Intrinsically disordered proteins: Emerging interaction specialists. *Curr. Opin. Struct. Biol.* **2015**, *35*, 49–59. [CrossRef] [PubMed]

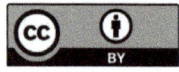

© 2019 by the authors. Licensee MDPI, Basel, Switzerland. This article is an open access article distributed under the terms and conditions of the Creative Commons Attribution (CC BY) license (http://creativecommons.org/licenses/by/4.0/).

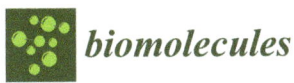

Review

Spontaneous Switching among Conformational Ensembles in Intrinsically Disordered Proteins

Ucheor B. Choi [1], Hugo Sanabria [2], Tatyana Smirnova [3], Mark E. Bowen [4,*] and Keith R. Weninger [5,*]

1. Department of Molecular and Cellular Physiology, Department of Neurology and Neurological Sciences, Department of Structural Biology, Department of Photon Science, Howard Hughes Medical Institute, Stanford University, Stanford, CA 94305, USA; ucheor@stanford.edu
2. Department of Physics and Astronomy, Clemson University, Clemson, SC 29634, USA; hsanabr@clemson.edu
3. Department of Chemistry, North Carolina State University, Raleigh, NC 27695, USA; tismirno@ncsu.edu
4. Department of Physiology and Biophysics, Stony Brook University, Stony Brook, NY 11794, USA
5. Department of Physics, North Carolina State University, Raleigh, NC 27695, USA
* Correspondence: mark.bowen@stonybrook.edu (M.E.B.); krwening@ncsu.edu (K.R.W.); Tel.: +1-919-513-3696 (M.E.B.); +1-631-444-2536 (K.R.W.)

Received: 17 January 2019; Accepted: 15 March 2019; Published: 22 March 2019

Abstract: The common conception of intrinsically disordered proteins (IDPs) is that they stochastically sample all possible configurations driven by thermal fluctuations. This is certainly true for many IDPs, which behave as swollen random coils that can be described using polymer models developed for homopolymers. However, the variability in interaction energy between different amino acid sequences provides the possibility that some configurations may be strongly preferred while others are forbidden. In compact globular IDPs, core hydration and packing density can vary between segments of the polypeptide chain leading to complex conformational dynamics. Here, we describe a growing number of proteins that appear intrinsically disordered by biochemical and bioinformatic characterization but switch between restricted regions of conformational space. In some cases, spontaneous switching between conformational ensembles was directly observed, but few methods can identify when an IDP is acting as a restricted chain. Such switching between disparate corners of conformational space could bias ligand binding and regulate the volume of IDPs acting as structural or entropic elements. Thus, mapping the accessible energy landscape and capturing dynamics across a wide range of timescales are essential to recognize when an IDP is acting as such a switch.

Keywords: dynamic configuration; free energy landscape; intrinsically disordered protein; IDP

---

1. Introduction

In general, proteins do not fold into static structures. Rather, most proteins fluctuate within a pseudocontinuum of accessible configurations about their lowest energy folded state. Often, these fluctuations are coupled to the protein's functional cycle such as catalytic activity or molecular recognition. However, many proteins lack a predominant low-energy state, and instead sample a broad and disparate ensemble of configurations. Such intrinsically disordered proteins (IDPs) lack the stable folded state, which is a central element in the classical structure–function paradigm. Nonetheless, IDPs, and proteins containing intrinsically disordered regions (IDRs), are now understood to play essential roles in cell signaling pathways and regulatory networks [1–6].

Models for how function arises from an ensemble of rapidly interconverting IDP conformers generally fall into two categories: those directly involved in molecular recognition and those acting as linker or structural elements. Unlike molecular recognition by folded domains, wherein the interaction residues are spread across the polypeptide chain, IDP interactions tend to involve short linear motifs (SLiMs), which are contiguous within the chain. Disordered SLiMs adopt an ensemble of conformations and these different conformations of the same sequence may be recognized by distinct binding partners [7]. The timescale of IDP conformational dynamics is an important determinant of the binding mode for IDPs. Rapid conformational dynamics supports the classic induced fit model, where the IDP can reconfigure the binding site before the initial encounter complex dissociates. Many IDPs couple the energy from order transitions to the recognition event, which provides a powerful mechanism for allostery. In other cases, the disorder persists even in the bound state [8,9]. If the timescale for IDP dynamics slows, then the binding mode is limited to conformational selection wherein the interaction is only possible during those windows when the binding competent configuration is present. In this way, the timescale of IDP conformational dynamics plays a key role in differentiating modes of molecular recognition by IDPs.

The dynamic nature of IDPs and IDRs makes them well suited to function as linkers between functional elements such as binding sites or folded domains. For example, the fly-casting model revealed how conformational exchange allows IDPs to explore a large volume in the search for binding partners [10–12]. The entropic clock model showed how the degree of extension of the IDP linker between a pore and its blocking domain controlled the open time of an ion channel [13]. The entropic bristle model suggested that IDPs can fill large volumes of three-dimensional (3D) space during their conformational searching, which can regulate protein interactions [14]. Thus, the timescale and the range of conformational sampling within the ensemble governs the structural properties of IDPs acting as linkers or bristles.

These functional roles for IDPs rely on their dynamic properties to control the energetics of binding reactions as well as for regulating hydrodynamic volume and spacing. Understanding protein structure is the key to describing its function. With IDPs this necessitates extending our understanding beyond minimum energy states to further characterize the ensemble both in terms of the accessible landscape as well as the timescales of conformational dynamics.

The rise of polymer science led to a great foundation of Nobel prize-winning theory to describe the behavior of homopolymers composed of many repeated subunits [15]. Based on different starting assumptions about the polymer, a continuum ensemble of end-to-end distances can be estimated by well-established approximations such as a Gaussian chain, a self-avoiding random coil, or a worm-like chain model [16,17]. While fully appropriate for polymers, in application to IDPs, such models lack molecular detail and rely on assumptions about polymer behavior that are not strictly applicable to polypeptides. Nonetheless, such polymer models still retain great predictive power, particularly for proteins in near ideal solvent conditions. As such, polymer models have shown great utility in describing the ensemble properties of chemically denatured proteins and coil-like IDPs.

Due to the intrinsic flexibility of IDPs, models from polymer physics have proven useful to describe their ensemble properties in many specific cases. A common extrapolation from polymer models is the assumption that the conformational landscape is generally featureless and that the entire landscape is accessible. For proteins selected through evolution to fold, neither of these assumptions is true. The extent to which these assumptions hold true for IDPs depends on their class. Simple swollen coils often follow polymer scaling, but now it is recognized that many IDPs, even polar polypeptides like Huntingtin [18], undergo collapse to form more compact, disordered globules [19,20]. At these higher packing densities, self-interaction becomes more prevalent and conformational dynamics become more complex. In addition, while specific long-range intramolecular interactions are generally absent in IDPs, molecular dynamics simulations have shown that charge patterning does govern IDP conformation through intramolecular electrostatic effects [19,21,22]. Thus, sequence evolution can select for IDPs with limited or biased conformational ensembles such that a continuum of conformations is not possible.

Conformational switching is well accepted in folded proteins, and IDPs may also be able to switch between discrete conformational ensembles while remaining disordered in both states. Here, we will focus on ensemble switching behavior identified in an increasing number of IDPs (Figure 1).

In these cases, IDPs were observed to stochastically switch between distinct states within the entirety of conformational space or showed evidence of dynamics on slow timescales (Figure 1B). Both phenomena are suggestive of large energy barriers between states or the existence of metastable intermediates. A combination of methods from ensemble to single molecule is required to elucidate this individual molecular behavior. Regulating the access to distinct regions of IDP conformational space provides mechanisms to govern IDP activity. Understanding the origins of switch-like transitions will provide new insights into the mechanisms by which IDP conformational dynamics can modulate cell signaling.

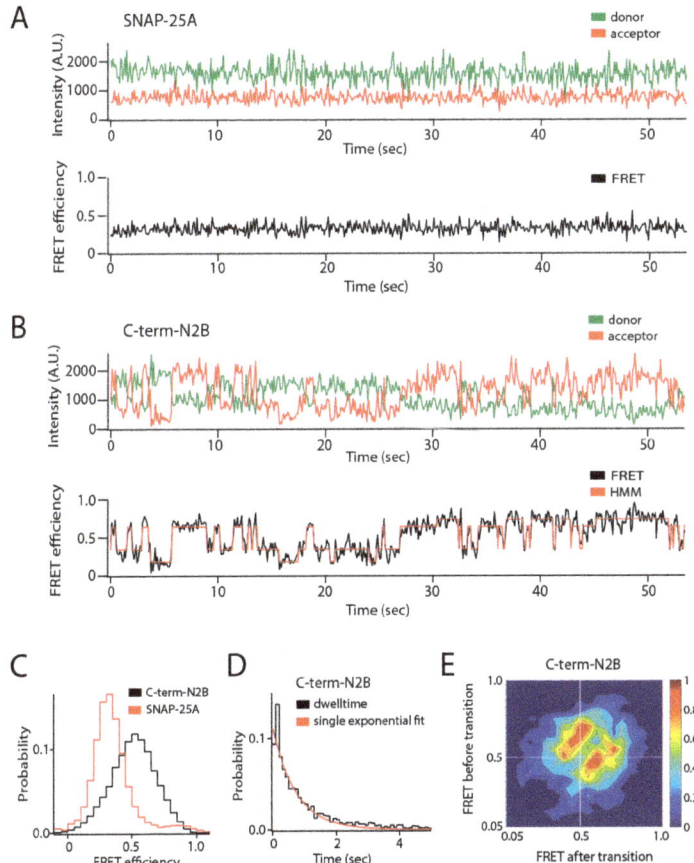

Figure 1. Single molecule observation of state switching in an intrinsically disordered protein (IDP) with single molecule Förster resonance energy transfer (smFRET). The soluble N-ethylmaleimide-sensitive factor activating protein receptor (SNARE) protein synaptosomal nerve-associated protein 25A (SNAP-25A) and the C-terminal tail of the GluN2B subunit of the N-methyl-D-aspartate (NMDA) receptor (NMDAR) (C-term-N2B) are intrinsically disordered in their native states. Residues 20 and 197 of SNAP-25A and residues 1273 and 1394 of C-term-N2B were randomly labeled with donor and acceptor fluorophores for smFRET measurements [23]. Labeled single molecules were encapsulated in liposomes (100 nm in diameter) that were then surface-tethered through biotin–streptavidin linkage on a surface passivated with biotinylated bovine serum albumin (BSA). Fluorescence emission was recorded using an emCCD (electron multiplying charge coupled device) camera at a frame rate of 10 Hz. At this time resolution, rapid conformational dynamics are time-averaged, but surface attachment

allows extended observations of the same molecule for seconds to minutes. (**A**) Representative single molecule fluorescence intensity time trace of SNAP-25A (top panel) does not show spontaneous switching. The fluorescence intensities were converted to Förster resonance energy transfer (FRET) efficiency (bottom panel, black line). SNAP-25A molecules showed a stable FRET efficiency with no switching between different FRET values. (**B**) Representative single molecule fluorescence intensity time trace of C-term-N2B (top panel) and FRET efficiency (bottom panel, black line) fit by hidden Markov modeling (HMM) to obtain the dwell times in each state (bottom panel, red line). Donor and acceptor signals for C-term-N2B molecules show step-wise, anticorrelated changes in intensity, yielding steady FRET for seconds before spontaneously switching to different FRET values, which would correspond to distinct disordered states with a different average size. (**C**) FRET efficiency histogram for C-term-N2B molecules show a broad distribution across the entire range of FRET values (black line) in contrast to SNAP-25A molecules (red lines). (**D**) Histogram of state dwell times for C-term-N2B obtained from HMM. The mean state dwell time is on the order of seconds and showed no correlation with FRET efficiency. (**E**) Transition density plot for C-term-N2B shows the FRET efficiency before a transition (*y*-axis) plotted against the FRET efficiency after that transition (*x*-axis) for all observed transitions. These transitions proved too variable to resolve or assign to specific conformations. A.U.: Arbitrary units.

2. Evidence of Configuration Switching in IDP Studies

One of the best examples of state switching in polypeptides is protein folding. There are two states: the unfolded state, which is characterized by a broad ensemble of disparate, interconverting conformations, and the folded state, which is characterized by local fluctuation within a narrow range of conformational space. In most cases, such folding transitions are unidirectional under physiological conditions. However, some proteins, such as the ankyrin repeat (AR) domain from the IκB transcription inhibitor, undergo reversible order to disorder transitions at room temperature [24]. Only single molecule fluorescence resonance energy transfer (smFRET) of surface attached molecules could detect the "nanospring dynamics" that occurred on the seconds timescale as individual akyrin repeats came "unglued" [25]. Ensemble nuclear magnetic resonance (NMR) measurements on the same protein showed well-resolved NMR cross-peaks and high-order parameters but no signs of dynamic behavior [24]. Such a slow timescale for state switching suggests a large energy barrier separating these regions of conformational space.

A similar conformational state switching has been reported in α-synuclein, an IDP linked to Parkinson's disease that undergoes a disorder-to-order transition upon interaction with amphiphilic small molecules or membranes. However, in this case, the transition is not spontaneous but regulated by functional interactions [26–28]. Other IDPs are known to change their form of disorder in response to physiological signals such as ion influx or posttranslational modifications like phosphorylation [29,30]. A key aspect of state switching in these IDPs is that the entire conformational landscape is not always accessible or there are sharp energy barriers, which separate discrete subregions of conformational space. The conformation is not "continuously tunable" [26].

Given the broad ensemble of conformations an IDP may adopt, it is not always possible to know how much of the conformational landscape is being explored and when such switching is occurring. One hallmark of deeper energy basins within the conformational landscape is the presence of slow timescale dynamics. However, most structural methods are not well suited for detecting slow timescale conformational dynamics.

A comparison of synaptic IDPs and IDRs revealed stochastic conformational switching in two out of five proteins in a test set despite the fact that all proteins appeared similarly intrinsically disordered by other measures [23]. The cytoplasmic domains from both neuroligin and the GluN2B subunit of the *N*-methyl-D-aspartate (NMDA) receptor (NMDAR) showed continuous hop-like conformational diffusion with Förster resonance energy transfer (FRET) shifts equivalent to nanometer scale motions in a single 100 millisecond time bin (Figure 1B). The sensitivity to stoichiometry provided by single molecule detection allows IDP clustering or aggregation to be distinguished from single molecule conformational switching. These IDRs adopted a compact globular form of disorder, yet another IDP (synaptobrevin) with a similar form of disorder failed to show transitions [23].

The transitions in GluN2B were detected with seven different FRET labeling combinations representing dye separations from 83 to 172 residues [31]. Only the shortest separation of 15 residues failed to show any transitions, which is expected because a short polypeptide segment should not be capable of large conformational changes. This important control confirms that photophysical effects on dye environment and orientation are not the origin of the transitioning phenomena. Because of their complexity, the transitions observed in synaptic IDRs proved uninterpretable in terms of structural intermediates [23].

Similar stochastic transitions between FRET efficiency levels were observed in the smFRET traces for protein 4.1, a cytoskeletal adaptor protein that stabilizes spectrin–actin crosslinks [32]. The protein appeared to switch between an unresolved number of discrete conformational states. Interestingly, while binding of protein 4.1 to the nuclear mitotic apparatus (NuMA) protein changed the pattern of transitions, it did not eliminate the transitions, indicating that the complex retains switch-like dynamics. Similarly, binding partner interactions with the synaptic scaffold protein postsynaptic density protein 95 (PSD-95) also showed no effect on conformational switching in the IDR from neuroligin [23]. Conformational switching may play a functional role even after these IDPs interact with downstream factors.

State switching in IDPs is also possible on faster timescales. The yeast prion protein Sup35 is a translation termination factor that forms amyloid fibrils. At low concentrations, smFRET showed that the protein formed a compact disordered globule [33]. However, fluorescence correlation spectroscopy (FCS) analysis of fluorescence quenching revealed at least two well separated components to the dynamics, including a slower component that originated from long-range contacts.

3. Theoretical Framework for Understanding IDP Conformational Switching

Swollen random coils can fully sample a "flat" energy landscape. Fast sampling is possible because little energy is needed to overcome small barriers between different configurations. Such IDPs have been described using equilibrium statistical mechanics as freely joint Gaussian chains, self-avoiding coils, and worm-like chains [17,23,34]. The conformational switching, described above in Section 2, challenges such approaches because these IDPs are sequestered off from the entirety of the conformational space. Thus, in the absence of the simplifying assumption that all states are present and equally probable, one cannot construct a statistical ensemble that represents all the possible states.

Intrinsically disordered protein conformational switching has been likened to the Lorenz attractor in nonlinear chaotic systems [35]. Like the Lorenz attractor, this switching behavior in IDPs has been shown to be sensitive to initial conditions and is also restricted to be near the attractor points in conformational space. Chaos, in dynamical mechanical systems, is dependent on underlying nonlinear relationships in the governing interactions. Intrinsically disordered proteins certainly have interactions within their peptide chain, with other components in solution, and with the host fluid that are likely to involve nonlinearities.

All conformational transitions are noise-assisted reactions of the type described by Kramers' transition state theory [36–38]. The energy for excursions between basins must come from fluctuations where the polypeptide gains enough energy from the thermal milieu. Therefore, the continuum of timescales relates to the continuum of barriers between different regions of conformational space. Polypeptides are not uniform chemical polymers. Within the core of a compact, globular IDP there exists a nonlinear potential as alternate long-range interactions (favorable and unfavorable) are transiently sampled as distinct regions of the polypeptide chain are brought into close proximity. Given such a fluctuating force, thermally activated transitions could occur across a range of timescales. Even rare transitions are possible within some finite time.

Within Kramers' theory, the time to escape a basin is related to the damping factor associated with internal friction. Studies of IDPs have pointed to the important role of internal friction in modulating conformational dynamics and folding [39,40]. Friction within expanded IDPs depends on the quality of solvent interactions. However, in collapsed, globular IDPs, shielding of residues in the interior removes solvent interactions and can create a complex network of coupled and decoupled chain segments [34,41]. Thus, nonlinear dynamics arising from feedback among these different couplings should not be surprising. Large transitions (e.g., folding–unfolding) involve a complex set of possible pathways within the energy landscape [42].

Conformational switching occurs over a wide range of timescales, ranging from very slow processes lasting for seconds down to microsecond timescales [43]. To explain this, a scale-free approach is needed. The energy landscape we have postulated for these IDPs, containing multiple minima with high energy barriers, is also characteristic of glasses (Figure 2). Mean-field theories of disordered glasses can describe the existence of stable and metastable states [44–46]. At low density or low packing fraction (ϕ), glasses remain liquid and can sample all states (Figure 2C). As the packing fraction increases, the individual particles are subject to jamming and undergo a glass transition where they become trapped within individual basins (Figure 2D). In this jammed state, excitations can extend over a wide range of timescales [47].

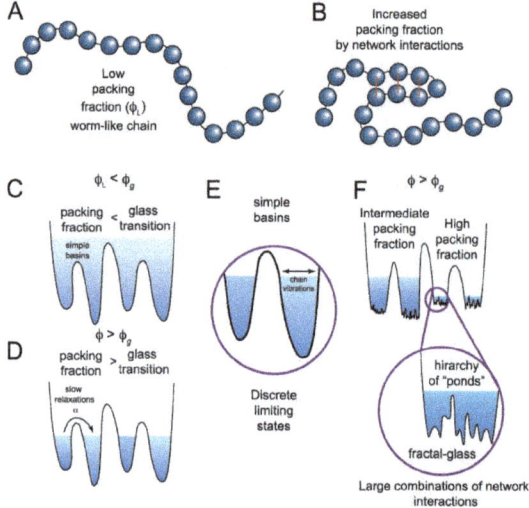

Figure 2. Switching in IDPs shows similarity to structural glasses. (**A**) IDPs can be modeled as worm-like chains when the packing fraction (ϕ) of the constituent particles is low (ϕ_L). Glasses can flow when the packing fraction is low but undergo a phase transition at high packing fractions when particles are caged by interactions with their neighbors. Applying this analogy of glasses to describe IDPs, the amino acids are the constituent particles. (**B**) If amino acids interact, the packing fraction increases, giving rise to a more complex energy landscape with states at different energy levels. (**C**) These states (simple basins) represent the minima of the energy landscape. When the packing fraction is lower than the glass transition (ϕ_g), or collapsed state, the polypeptide can sample a continuum of states following polymer models. Transitions between states would be described by Kramers' transition state theory. (**D**) When there are many network interactions, the packing fraction increases and not all conformations are accessible. The limiting states are separated by deep wells and discrete states can be identified. Such conformational switching could result from a number of different mechanisms including internal friction, long rage potentials, ion mediated interactions, or other forces that modulate the network interactions. (**E**) Discrete limiting states produce conformational switching, yet there is still a subensemble of conformations inside each basin. (**F**) At high packing fractions, the subensemble of states can also become discontinuous, generating potential transitions across widely separated temporal domains. (Figure adapted from reference [47]).

Deep within the glass phase, each individual basin becomes a metabasin composed of a fractal hierarchy of sub-basins (Figure 2F) [48]. This fractal free-energy landscape was recently proposed to explain the roughness transition in structural glasses [47]. A similar fractal hierarchy or scale free-energy landscape could arise from packing of chain segments within an IDP. The packing particles are collapsed chain segments within the polymer along with coordinated ions and bound solvent (Figure 2B). A high packing fraction could lead to jamming and produce metastable configurations, which might switch to other equally stable configurations as intrachain interaction forces evolve with the conformational search. In this model, such local phase transitions would extend to other packed chain segments, leading to the observed IDP conformational switching across a wide temporal regime.

4. Possible Mechanisms to Sequester Regions of Conformational Space in IDPs

The origin of continuous slow timescale dynamics or state switching is not clear. Proline isomerization is one of the conformational changes in polypeptides known to operate on this timescale and can result in state switching. Conformational exchange rates linked to proline isomerization were detected in the IDR of the transcriptional regulator E2 from human papillomavirus (HPV) by collecting NMR nuclear overhauser spectroscopy (NOESY) spectra at different mixing times [20]. This discrete conformational transition in E2 is the rate-limiting step for antibody recognition of this viral antigen. Interestingly, proline depletion of GluN2B reduced the number of molecules that showed any stochastic FRET transitions, but proline-depleted constructs showed similar transition rates to the wild type [49]. Thus, for GluN2B, proline appeared to facilitate switching but not govern the timescale.

Aside from proline isomerization, the major determinant of IDP conformation are self-interactions (i.e., between amino acids in the chain) and solvent interactions. Most intrachain interactions in IDPs are local, yet chain segments can partition into both packed and extended forms of disorder. These chain segments are continuously exposed to one another during the conformational search, with favorable interactions restricting chain motions and unfavorable interactions limiting access to some conformations. Within the disordered globule, the quality and quantity of the solvent is evolving as water and ions interact with local chain segments and are drawn into the "core" of the IDP. For example, ions from solution could neutralize local charge densities stabilizing distinct configuration space from those visited in the absence of the ions. Compacted chain segments of IDPs can temporarily exclude water [34,41,50], which would result in stable local minima that would limit the conformational search. As noted above, the complexity of conformational space within these fractal basins would mean that available thermal energy could be dissipated by small, local rearrangements rather than long-range motions.

Chain reconfiguration could also transiently trap unfavorable interactions within the globular interior. This unfavorable interaction would destabilize any metastable local conformations and drive the system to a new region of conformational space. Reintroduction of water to a temporarily dehydrated chain segment would upset the balance of the chain interactions. Chain reconfiguration will inevitably bring charged amino acids within the globular interior with a finite probability of unfavorable interactions being trapped by approach jamming. These sorts of trapped interactions represent high energy metastable intermediates that could suddenly be released when a random fluctuation exposes a pathway that permits access to alternate regions of conformational space. Such an event would manifest as sudden stochastic changes in the sampled conformational space, or what we have termed IDP conformational switching.

It remains to be established that effects as subtle as sequestering an additional ion or water molecule could generate the spontaneous IDP ensemble switching that is the focus of this discussion. There are some relevant examples where such small perturbations can affect molecular properties. Deoxyribonucleic acid (DNA) certainly can transiently recruit or bind ions from solution changing its polymeric properties [51], bearing in mind that DNA can easily be modeled as a worm-like chain [52,53]. Certainly, changes in proteins at the level of a single amino acid can impact disordered states [54–63]. Changes of the amino acid sequence in IDPs and IDRs have been linked to human diseases. Aggregation of α-synuclein has been linked to sequence composition in familial forms of Parkinson's disease. Familial mutations that enhanced aggregation slowed conformational dynamics, while mutations that sped up intramolecular diffusion inhibited aggregation [64]. De novo missense mutations in the cytoplasmic IDR of the NMDAR, discussed above, are linked familial forms of epilepsy [65,66]. That changes at the level of individual amino acids can reshape the energy landscape of IDPs suggests that transient interactions with ions or water could generate the observed ensemble switching phenomenon.

5. State Switching Can Occur Close to the Boundary of a Folding Transition

Most protein folding studies to date have focused on single domain proteins displaying simple two state behavior. The folding of large multidomain proteins can be more complex with metastable intermediate states in their energy landscapes. At low denaturant concentrations (0.65 M GdmCl), the three-domain, 214 amino acid protein adenylate kinase (AK) began to show stochastic FRET transitions between six states [42]. The transitions were too variable to resolve nor could they all be assigned to specific denatured intermediates. Furthermore, the "situation [became] even more complex at higher concentrations of denaturant." [42]. This shows that a folded protein slightly destabilized by denaturants shows similarly complex transitioning to that observed in switching IDPs.

Thus, transitioning molecules arise when the impetus for a polypeptide to fold is lowered slightly and becomes more complex as more of the conformational landscape becomes available. Ultimately, transitions become faster until they are unresolved and become continuous dynamics of the type described by polymer models. Thus, a similar transition should be possible if an expanded coil is brought close to a folded state. Interestingly, smFRET measured in the presynaptic fusion protein SNAP-25 did show scaling that fit to polymer models [23]. However, stochastic FRET switching was induced in SNAP-25 upon binding the SNARE protein syntaxin, which is a binary intermediate in the formation of the tripartite SNARE complex [67]. This confirms that an expanded coil-like IDP can be converted to state switching as protein interactions restrict access to portions of the conformational landscape.

6. Functional Relevance of IDP Ensemble Switching through Phosphorylation

Aside from transitions involving an ordered state, few biological functions have been directly connected to the modulation of IDP conformational ensembles. Post-translational modifications can change the interaction potential of existing amino acids [29,30,68–71]. Phosphorylation is among the best-documented mechanism for dynamically affecting biological function of proteins. In particular, phosphorylation has been connected with modulating disorder in IDPs [29,68–75].

For example, the ribonucleic acid (RNA) binding protein fused in sarcoma (FUS) forms aggregated protein deposits in neurodegenerative disorders, which are modulated by phosphorylation. Nuclear magnetic resonance studies found that phosphorylation of FUS, or phosphomimetic mutations, did not "alter the disordered structure of FUS" [50]. However, phosphorylation of FUS did decrease transient polypeptide collapse and increase the radius of gyration. These changes in the IDP ensemble were associated with reduced intermolecular interaction and aggregation such that a phosphomimetic variant reduced the toxicity of FUS to live cells [50].

Phosphorylation of an IDR was also linked to biological function of the NMDAR, which uses the energy of neurotransmitter binding to open its ion channel. Allosteric inhibition of channel gating by extracellular zinc can be alleviated by Src kinase phosphorylation of the C-terminal IDR of the GluN2B subunit (C-term-N2B) [76], which switches conformation as noted above (Figure 3A) [23]. The effect of Src phosphorylation is mediated by expansion of this globular IDR without affecting conformational transitions (Figure 3B,C) [31]. Deleting prolines near the phosphorylation sites had the opposite effect and compacted the IDR while reducing the probability of transitions. Both of these modifications, which change the size of the disordered states in opposite directions, eliminated the ability of zinc to allosterically regulate channel gating without disrupting the underlying gating mechanisms [49].

Thus, this IDR appears to have an optimal packing density that supports allosteric coupling between domains of the receptor.

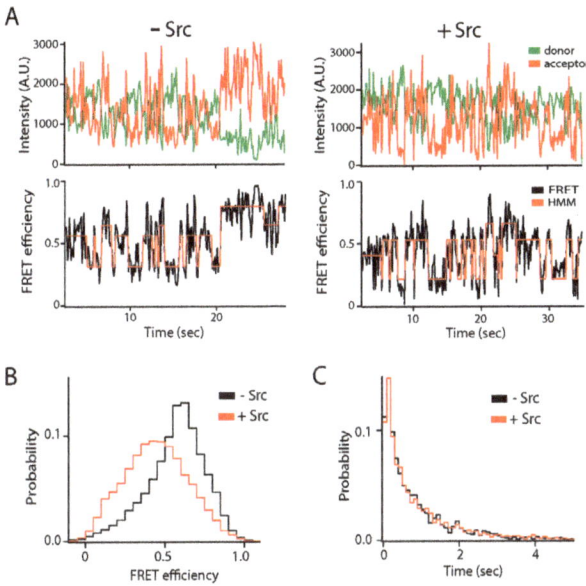

Figure 3. Effect of Src kinase phosphorylation on the conformational ensemble of the NMDA receptor. The C-terminal intrinsically disordered region (IDR) of the GluN2B subunit of the NMDA receptor (C-term-N2B) was randomly labeled with donor and acceptor fluorophores at residues 1323 and 1453 [31]. Src kinase phosphorylates C-term-N2B on tyrosine residues 1336 and 1472. (**A**) Representative single molecule fluorescence intensity (top panels) and fluorescence resonance energy transfer (FRET) efficiency fit by hidden Markov modeling (HMM) (bottom panels) for unphosphorylated (left) and phosphorylated (right) C-term-N2B. Phosphorylation did not induce structure in C-term-N2B as the dynamic transitions continued. (**B**) FRET efficiency histogram of C-term-N2B before (black line) and after (red line) Src phosphorylation. Phosphorylation led to shift towards lower FRET indicating a general expansion of the polypeptide, which was confirmed with hydrodynamic measurements. (**C**) Dwell time histograms for transitions in C-term-N2B, obtained from HMM, before (black line) and after (red line) Src phosphorylation. Although phosphorylation shifted the ensemble FRET efficiency, stochastic transitions were unaffected. A.U.: Arbitrary units.

Phosphorylation-induced modulation of an IDP ensemble was also connected to regulation of cellular signaling processes in prostate cancer. Prostate-associated gene 4 (PAGE4) is an IDP that is expressed exclusively in adult males who have prostate cancer. Interactions between PAGE4 and transcription factors have been suggested to control androgen sensitivity [77–83]. Both homeodomain-interacting protein kinase 1 (HIPK1) and CDC-Like Kinase 2 (CLK2) phosphorylate PAGE4, with CLK2 modifying many more sites. Experiments combining NMR, paramagnetic relaxation enhancement (PRE), small angle X-ray scattering (SAXS) and smFRET have determined that HIPK1 phosphorylation compacts the ensemble, while CLK2 phosphorylation leads to expansion. Molecular dynamics (MD) simulations linked changes in PAGE4 ensembles to distinct phosphorylation patterns [84]. These different phosphorylation patterns influenced transcription factor binding. HIPK1-treated PAGE4 binds to AP-1, whereas CLK2 treatment of PAGE4 decreases its affinity for AP-1. Phosphorylation by HIPK1 effectively disrupts the PAGE4 interaction with c-Jun and consequently stimulated c-Jun dependent transcription in prostate cancer cell models [85,86]. In contrast, CLK2 phosphorylation of PAGE4 inhibited c-Jun dependent transcription. Importantly, HIPK1 is expressed in both androgen-dependent and androgen-independent prostate cancer cells, whereas CLK2 and PAGE4 are expressed only in androgen-dependent cells. A model for the PAGE4–Jun-Fos (AP-1)–AR regulatory circuit suggests phosphorylation patterns in prostate cancer cells can oscillate. Thus, it was proposed that androgen dependence may vary in time [78] with switching between androgen-dependent and androgen-independent phenotypes being a result of details of PAGE4 phosphorylation [77,79,80,84]. This differential phosphorylation is associated with opposing shifts in the conformational ensemble of PAGE4.

7. Conclusions and Prospects for Understanding IDP Switching

Intrinsically disordered proteins are essential components of cellular signaling pathways because of their adaptability to the local environment. Cell signaling events can lead to changes in ionic composition or pH that affect solvent quality while posttranslational modifications affect net charge and hydropathy. Intrinsically disordered proteins can respond instantly to such signals by shifting to alternate conformational ensembles. Their unique capabilities can allow a single IDP to interact with multiple binding partners. Intrinsically disordered proteins also play structural roles as linkers or entropic elements. Additionally, IDPs are linked to the formation of membraneless organelles (i.e., liquid phase separation) [87,88]. These important functions allow for more nuanced coordination of signal transduction.

Here, we have highlighted a recently identified conformational switching phenomenon observed in a small but growing number of IDPs. Intrinsically disordered proteins in this class appear disordered by standard measures of secondary structure or hydrodynamic mobility but also appear to fluctuate between well-separated regions of conformational space. If the conformational ensembles are functionally distinct, then mechanisms that biases conformational sampling will govern protein activity. We suggest such control over IDP switching may be an important regulator of cellular signaling networks.

Few experimental methods are sensitive to conformational switching in IDPs [89]. Integrative structural biology approaches where several methods are applied to a single protein may help inform our understanding of the molecular mechanisms controlling intrinsic disorder in proteins. Several methods including smFRET, NMR, electron paramagnetic resonance double electron–electron resonance (EPR-DEER), paramagnetic relaxation enhancement (PRE), and small-angle neutron scattering (SANS)/small-angle X-ray scattering (SAXS) have all been applied to IDP studies. These different methods are able to provide complementary information about local chain contacts and global disordered structure. Comparing and cross-validating such results with multiple methods may help reveal specific interactions that are critical for determining details of the disordered state. To date, switching has only been observed in vitro, so it remains to be determined if such switching transitions are present within live cells [3], where smFRET may enable direct observation [90–92]. Similarly, switching has been primarily studied under dilute conditions so it remains unknown whether the phenomenon persists in the condensed phase [93,94].

In addition to experimental approaches, MD simulation is a critical tool to understand the mechanisms that govern access to the full conformational ensemble. Molecular dynamics simulations of IDPs are particularly challenging. Details of the force fields are critically important and are a topic of continued development [95,96]. The long timescales required to observe ensemble switching are difficult to achieve for standard MD simulation and require more sophisticated ensemble sampling approaches. Despite these difficulties progress applying MD simulation to IDPs is an area of active work [84,97–103]. Critically, experimental studies and simulations provide essential feedback to each other [103–107]. The molecular mechanisms controlling rapid dynamics in IDPs are becoming clearer through MD simulation [83,101]. However, spontaneous ensemble switching of an IDP has yet to be reported so molecular details remain unknown.

If IDP ensemble switching does regulate signaling, then these mechanisms could be used for therapeutic intervention in those pathways. Efforts are already underway to identify small molecules that can specifically bind IDPs [2,108,109]. An exciting functional connection has been found for the transcription factor TFIID where a drug-like molecule affected the DNA interaction to prevent transcription initiation by RNA polymerase [2,109]. Additional strategies for intervening in signaling pathways within the diseased state will likely emerge as our understanding grows as to how IDP conformational dynamic leads to function within cellular networks.

Author Contributions: Conceptualization, M.E.B., H.S., T.S. and K.R.W.; writing—review and editing, U.B.C., M.E.B., H.S., T.S. and K.R.W.

Funding: This research has thus far been unable to secure any external funding.

Conflicts of Interest: The authors declare no conflict of interest.

References

1. Uversky, V.N.; Dunker, A.K. Understanding protein non-folding. *Biochim. Biophys. Acta Proteins Proteomics* **2010**, *1804*, 1231–1264. [CrossRef] [PubMed]
2. Shammas, S.L. Mechanistic roles of protein disorder within transcription. *Curr. Opin. Struct. Biol.* **2017**, *42*, 155–161. [CrossRef]
3. Wright, P.E.; Dyson, H.J. Intrinsically disordered proteins in cellular signalling and regulation. *Nat. Rev. Mol. Cell Biol.* **2015**, *16*, 18–29. [CrossRef] [PubMed]
4. Oldfield, C.J.; Dunker, A.K. Intrinsically Disordered Proteins and Intrinsically Disordered Protein Regions. *Annu. Rev. Biochem.* **2014**, *83*, 553–584. [CrossRef] [PubMed]
5. Fung, H.Y.J.; Birol, M.; Rhoades, E. IDPs in macromolecular complexes: The roles of multivalent interactions in diverse assemblies. *Curr. Opin. Struct. Biol.* **2018**, *49*, 36–43. [CrossRef]
6. Berlow, R.B.; Dyson, H.J.; Wright, P.E. Functional advantages of dynamic protein disorder. *FEBS Lett.* **2015**, *589*, 2433–2440. [CrossRef]
7. Uversky, V.N.; Oldfield, C.J.; Dunker, A.K. Intrinsically disordered proteins in human diseases: Introducing the D2 concept. *Annu. Rev. Biophys.* **2008**, *37*, 215–246. [CrossRef] [PubMed]
8. Borgia, A.; Borgia, M.B.; Bugge, K.; Kissling, V.M.; Heidarsson, P.O.; Fernandes, C.B.; Sottini, A.; Soranno, A.; Buholzer, K.J.; Nettels, D.; et al. Extreme disorder in an ultrahigh-affinity protein complex. *Nature* **2018**, *555*, 61–66. [CrossRef]
9. Tsytlonok, M.; Sanabria, H.; Wang, Y.; Felekyan, S.; Hemmen, K.; Phillips, A.; Yun, M.-K.; Waddell, B.; Park, C.-G.; Vaithiyalingam, S.; et al. Dynamic anticipation by Cdk2/Cyclin A-bound p27 mediates signal integration in cell cycle regulation. *arXiv*, 2018; arXiv:1812.07009.
10. Shoemaker, B.A.; Portman, J.J.; Wolynes, P.G. Speeding molecular recognition by using the folding funnel: The fly-casting mechanism. *Proc. Natl. Acad. Sci.* **2000**, *97*, 8868–8873. [CrossRef]
11. Hoffman, R.M.B.; Blumenschein, T.M.A.; Sykes, B.D. An interplay between protein disorder and structure confers the Ca2+ regulation of striated muscle. *J. Mol. Biol.* **2006**, *361*, 625–633. [CrossRef] [PubMed]
12. Metskas, L.A.; Rhoades, E. Conformation and Dynamics of the Troponin I C-Terminal Domain: Combining Single-Molecule and Computational Approaches for a Disordered Protein Region. *J. Am. Chem. Soc.* **2015**, *137*, 11962–11969. [CrossRef]
13. Podlaha, O.; Zhang, J. Positive selection on protein-length in the evolution of a primate sperm ion channel. *Proc. Natl. Acad. Sci. USA* **2003**, *100*, 12241–12246. [CrossRef]
14. Hoh, J.H. Functional protein domains from the thermally driven motion of polypeptide chains: A proposal. *Proteins* **1998**, *32*, 223–228. [CrossRef]
15. de Gennes, P.-G. Soft Matter (Nobel Lecture). *Angew. Chemie Int. Ed. English* **1992**, *31*, 842–845. [CrossRef]
16. Wiggins, P.A.; Nelson, P.C. Generalized theory of semiflexible polymers. *Phys. Rev. E* **2006**, *73*, 031906. [CrossRef] [PubMed]
17. Schuler, B.; Soranno, A.; Hofmann, H.; Nettels, D. Single-Molecule FRET Spectroscopy and the Polymer Physics of Unfolded and Intrinsically Disordered Proteins. *Annu. Rev. Biophys.* **2016**, *45*, 207–231. [CrossRef]
18. Vitalis, A.; Wang, X.; Pappu, R.V. Atomistic simulations of the effects of polyglutamine chain length and solvent quality on conformational equilibria and spontaneous homodimerization. *J. Mol. Biol.* **2008**, *384*, 279–297. [CrossRef] [PubMed]

19. Mao, A.H.; Crick, S.L.; Vitalis, A.; Chicoine, C.L.; Pappu, R.V. Net charge per residue modulates conformational ensembles of intrinsically disordered proteins. *Proc. Natl. Acad. Sci. USA* **2010**, *107*, 8183–8188. [CrossRef] [PubMed]
20. Fassolari, M.; Chemes, L.B.; Gallo, M.; Smal, C.; Sánchez, I.E.; de Prat-Gay, G. Minute time scale prolyl isomerization governs antibody recognition of an intrinsically disordered immunodominant epitope. *J. Biol. Chem.* **2013**, *288*, 13110–13123. [CrossRef]
21. Lin, Y.-H.; Brady, J.P.; Forman-Kay, J.D.; Chan, H.S. Charge pattern matching as a 'fuzzy' mode of molecular recognition for the functional phase separations of intrinsically disordered proteins. *New J. Phys.* **2017**, *19*, 115003. [CrossRef]
22. Das, S.; Amin, A.N.; Lin, Y.-H.; Chan, H.S. Coarse-grained residue-based models of disordered protein condensates: Utility and limitations of simple charge pattern parameters. *Phys. Chem. Chem. Phys.* **2018**, *20*, 28558–28574. [CrossRef] [PubMed]
23. Choi, U.B.; McCann, J.J.; Weninger, K.R.; Bowen, M.E. Beyond the Random Coil: Stochastic Conformational Switching in Intrinsically Disordered Proteins. *Structure* **2011**, *19*, 566–576. [CrossRef]
24. Lamboy, J.A.; Kim, H.; Lee, K.S.; Ha, T.; Komives, E.A. Visualization of the nanospring dynamics of the IkappaBalpha ankyrin repeat domain in real time. *Proc. Natl. Acad. Sci. USA* **2011**, *108*, 10178–10183. [CrossRef]
25. Lamboy, J.A.; Kim, H.; Dembinski, H.; Ha, T.; Komives, E.A. Single-molecule FRET reveals the native-state dynamics of the IκBα ankyrin repeat domain. *J. Mol. Biol.* **2013**, *425*, 2578–2590. [CrossRef]
26. Ferreon, A.C.M.; Gambin, Y.; Lemke, E.A.; Deniz, A.A. Interplay of alpha-synuclein binding and conformational switching probed by single-molecule fluorescence. *Proc. Natl. Acad. Sci.* **2009**, *106*, 5645–5650. [CrossRef] [PubMed]
27. Trexler, A.J.; Rhoades, E. α-Synuclein Binds Large Unilamellar Vesicles as an Extended Helix †. *Biochemistry* **2009**, *48*, 2304–2306. [CrossRef] [PubMed]
28. Moosa, M.M.; Ferreon, A.C.M.; Deniz, A.A. Forced Folding of a Disordered Protein Accesses an Alternative Folding Landscape. *ChemPhysChem* **2015**, *16*, 90–94. [CrossRef] [PubMed]
29. Darling, A.L.; Uversky, V.N. Intrinsic Disorder and Posttranslational Modifications: The Darker Side of the Biological Dark Matter. *Front. Genet.* **2018**, *9*, 158. [CrossRef] [PubMed]
30. Bah, A.; Forman-Kay, J.D. Modulation of Intrinsically Disordered Protein Function by Post-translational Modifications. *J. Biol. Chem.* **2016**, *291*, 6696–6705. [CrossRef]
31. Choi, U.B.; Xiao, S.; Wollmuth, L.P.; Bowen, M.E. Effect of Src kinase phosphorylation on disordered C-terminal domain of N-methyl-D-aspartic acid (NMDA) receptor subunit GluN2B protein. *J. Biol. Chem.* **2011**, *286*, 29904–29912. [CrossRef]
32. Wu, S.; Wang, D.; Liu, J.; Feng, Y.; Weng, J.; Li, Y.; Gao, X.; Liu, J.; Wang, W. The Dynamic Multisite Interactions between Two Intrinsically Disordered Proteins. *Angew. Chem. Int. Ed. Engl.* **2017**, *56*, 7515–7519. [CrossRef] [PubMed]
33. Mukhopadhyay, S.; Krishnan, R.; Lemke, E.A.; Lindquist, S.; Deniz, A.A. A natively unfolded yeast prion monomer adopts an ensemble of collapsed and rapidly fluctuating structures. *Proc. Natl. Acad. Sci.* **2007**, *104*, 2649–2654. [CrossRef]
34. Zheng, W.; Zerze, G.H.; Borgia, A.; Mittal, J.; Schuler, B.; Best, R.B. Inferring properties of disordered chains from FRET transfer efficiencies. *J. Chem. Phys.* **2018**, *148*, 123329. [CrossRef]
35. Uversky, V.N. Dancing Protein Clouds: The Strange Biology and Chaotic Physics of Intrinsically Disordered Proteins. *J. Biol. Chem.* **2016**, *291*, 6681–6688. [CrossRef]
36. Kramers, H.A. Brownian motion in a field of force and the diffusion model of chemical reactions. *Physica* **1940**, *7*, 284–304. [CrossRef]
37. Skinner, J.L.; Wolynes, P.G. Transition state and Brownian motion theories of solitons. *J. Chem. Phys.* **1980**, *73*, 4015–4021. [CrossRef]
38. Hänggi, P.; Talkner, P.; Borkovec, M. Reaction-rate theory: Fifty years after Kramers. *Rev. Mod. Phys.* **1990**, *62*, 251–341. [CrossRef]
39. Soranno, A.; Buchli, B.; Nettels, D.; Cheng, R.R.; Müller-Späth, S.; Pfeil, S.H.; Hoffmann, A.; Lipman, E.A.; Makarov, D.E.; Schuler, B. Quantifying internal friction in unfolded and intrinsically disordered proteins with single-molecule spectroscopy. *Proc. Natl. Acad. Sci. USA* **2012**, *109*, 17800–17806. [CrossRef] [PubMed]

40. Borgia, A.; Wensley, B.G.; Soranno, A.; Nettels, D.; Borgia, M.B.; Hoffmann, A.; Pfeil, S.H.; Lipman, E.A.; Clarke, J.; Schuler, B. Localizing internal friction along the reaction coordinate of protein folding by combining ensemble and single-molecule fluorescence spectroscopy. *Nat. Commun.* **2012**, *3*, 1195. [CrossRef] [PubMed]
41. Zheng, W.; Hofmann, H.; Schuler, B.; Best, R.B. Origin of Internal Friction in Disordered Proteins Depends on Solvent Quality. *J. Phys. Chem. B* **2018**, *122*, 11478–11487. [CrossRef]
42. Pirchi, M.; Ziv, G.; Riven, I.; Cohen, S.S.; Zohar, N.; Barak, Y.; Haran, G. Single-molecule fluorescence spectroscopy maps the folding landscape of a large protein. *Nat. Commun.* **2011**, *2*, 493. [CrossRef]
43. Weninger, K.; Qiu, R.; Ou, E.; Milikisiyants, S.; Sanabria, H.; Smirnova, T.I. smFRET and DEER Distance Measurements as Applied to Disordered and Structured Proteins. *Biophys. J.* **2016**, *110*, 559a. [CrossRef]
44. Kirkpatrick, T.R.; Wolynes, P.G. Stable and metastable states in mean-field Potts and structural glasses. *Phys. Rev. B. Condens. Matter* **1987**, *36*, 8552–8564. [CrossRef] [PubMed]
45. Kirkpatrick, T.R.; Thirumalai, D. Dynamics of the Structural Glass Transition and the *p*-Spin—Interaction Spin-Glass Model. *Phys. Rev. Lett.* **1987**, *58*, 2091–2094. [CrossRef] [PubMed]
46. Wolynes, P.G.; Lubchenko, V. *Structural Glasses and Supercooled Liquids: Theory, Experiment, and Applications*; Wiley: Hoboken, NJ, USA, 2012; ISBN 9780470452233.
47. Charbonneau, P.; Kurchan, J.; Parisi, G.; Urbani, P.; Zamponi, F. Fractal free energy landscapes in structural glasses. *Nat. Commun.* **2014**, *5*, 3725. [CrossRef] [PubMed]
48. Parisi, G. Order Parameter for Spin-Glasses. *Phys. Rev. Lett.* **1983**, *50*, 1946–1948. [CrossRef]
49. Choi, U.B.; Kazi, R.; Stenzoski, N.; Wollmuth, L.P.; Uversky, V.N.; Bowen, M.E. Modulating the Intrinsic Disorder in the Cytoplasmic Domain Alters the Biological Activity of the N-Methyl-d-aspartate-sensitive Glutamate Receptor. *J. Biol. Chem.* **2013**, *288*, 22506–22515. [CrossRef] [PubMed]
50. Monahan, Z.; Ryan, V.H.; Janke, A.M.; Burke, K.A.; Rhoads, S.N.; Zerze, G.H.; O'Meally, R.; Dignon, G.L.; Conicella, A.E.; Zheng, W.; et al. Phosphorylation of the FUS low-complexity domain disrupts phase separation, aggregation, and toxicity. *EMBO J.* **2017**, *36*, 2951–2967. [CrossRef] [PubMed]
51. Barnett, R.N.; Cleveland, C.L.; Joy, A.; Landman, U.; Schuster, G.B. Charge Migration in DNA: Ion-Gated Transport. *Science* **2001**, *294*, 567–571. [CrossRef]
52. Klenin, K.; Merlitz, H.; Langowski, J. A Brownian Dynamics Program for the Simulation of Linear and Circular DNA and Other Wormlike Chain Polyelectrolytes. *Biophys. J.* **1998**, *74*, 780–788. [CrossRef]
53. Murphy, M.C.; Rasnik, I.; Cheng, W.; Lohman, T.M.; Ha, T. Probing single-stranded DNA conformational flexibility using fluorescence spectroscopy. *Biophys. J.* **2004**, *86*, 2530–2537. [CrossRef]
54. Yedvabny, E.; Nerenberg, P.S.; So, C.; Head-Gordon, T. Disordered Structural Ensembles of Vasopressin and Oxytocin and Their Mutants. *J. Phys. Chem. B* **2015**, *119*, 896–905. [CrossRef]
55. Gruet, A.; Dosnon, M.; Vassena, A.; Lombard, V.; Gerlier, D.; Bignon, C.; Longhi, S. Dissecting Partner Recognition by an Intrinsically Disordered Protein Using Descriptive Random Mutagenesis. *J. Mol. Biol.* **2013**, *425*, 3495–3509. [CrossRef] [PubMed]
56. Babu, M.M. The contribution of intrinsically disordered regions to protein function, cellular complexity, and human disease. *Biochem. Soc. Trans.* **2016**, *44*, 1185–1200. [CrossRef]
57. Mohan, A.; Uversky, V.N.; Radivojac, P. Influence of Sequence Changes and Environment on Intrinsically Disordered Proteins. *PLoS Comput. Biol.* **2009**, *5*, e1000497. [CrossRef]
58. Davey, N.E.; Cyert, M.S.; Moses, A.M. Short linear motifs–ex nihilo evolution of protein regulation. *Cell Commun. Signal.* **2015**, *13*, 43. [CrossRef]
59. Fuxreiter, M.; Tompa, P.; Simon, I. Local structural disorder imparts plasticity on linear motifs. *Bioinformatics* **2007**, *23*, 950–956. [CrossRef]
60. Van Roey, K.; Dinkel, H.; Weatheritt, R.J.; Gibson, T.J.; Davey, N.E. The switches.ELM Resource: A Compendium of Conditional Regulatory Interaction Interfaces. *Sci. Signal.* **2013**, *6*, rs7. [CrossRef] [PubMed]
61. Diella, F.; Haslam, N.; Chica, C.; Budd, A.; Michael, S.; Brown, N.P.; Trave, G.; Gibson, T.J. Understanding eukaryotic linear motifs and their role in cell signaling and regulation. *Front. Biosci.* **2008**, *13*, 6580–6603. [CrossRef]
62. Akiva, E.; Friedlander, G.; Itzhaki, Z.; Margalit, H. A dynamic view of domain-motif interactions. *PLoS Comput. Biol.* **2012**, *8*, e1002341. [CrossRef]
63. Pancsa, R.; Fuxreiter, M. Interactions via intrinsically disordered regions: What kind of motifs? *IUBMB Life* **2012**, *64*, 513–520. [CrossRef]

64. Acharya, S.; Saha, S.; Ahmad, B.; Lapidus, L.J. Effects of Mutations on the Reconfiguration Rate of α-Synuclein. *J. Phys. Chem. B* **2015**, *119*, 15443–15450. [CrossRef]
65. Lesca, G.; Rudolf, G.; Bruneau, N.; Lozovaya, N.; Labalme, A.; Boutry-Kryza, N.; Salmi, M.; Tsintsadze, T.; Addis, L.; Motte, J.; et al. GRIN2A mutations in acquired epileptic aphasia and related childhood focal epilepsies and encephalopathies with speech and language dysfunction. *Nat. Genet.* **2013**, *45*, 1061–1066. [CrossRef]
66. Lemke, J.R.; Lal, D.; Reinthaler, E.M.; Steiner, I.; Nothnagel, M.; Alber, M.; Geider, K.; Laube, B.; Schwake, M.; Finsterwalder, K.; et al. Mutations in GRIN2A cause idiopathic focal epilepsy with rolandic spikes. *Nat. Genet.* **2013**, *45*, 1067–1072. [CrossRef]
67. Weninger, K.; Bowen, M.E.; Choi, U.B.; Chu, S.; Brunger, A.T. Accessory Proteins Stabilize the Acceptor Complex for Synaptobrevin, the 1:1 Syntaxin/SNAP-25 Complex. *Structure* **2008**, *16*, 308–320. [CrossRef]
68. Bah, A.; Vernon, R.M.; Siddiqui, Z.; Krzeminski, M.; Muhandiram, R.; Zhao, C.; Sonenberg, N.; Kay, L.E.; Forman-Kay, J.D. Folding of an intrinsically disordered protein by phosphorylation as a regulatory switch. *Nature* **2015**, *519*, 106–109. [CrossRef]
69. Muller, P.; Chan, J.M.; Simoncik, O.; Fojta, M.; Lane, D.P.; Hupp, T.; Vojtesek, B. Evidence for allosteric effects on p53 oligomerization induced by phosphorylation. *Protein Sci.* **2018**, *27*, 523–530. [CrossRef] [PubMed]
70. Valk, E.; Venta, R.; Ord, M.; Faustova, I.; Kõivomägi, M.; Loog, M. Multistep phosphorylation systems: Tunable components of biological signaling circuits. *Mol. Biol. Cell* **2014**, *25*, 3456–3460. [CrossRef] [PubMed]
71. Kulkarni, P.; Solomon, T.L.; He, Y.; Chen, Y.; Bryan, P.N.; Orban, J. Structural metamorphism and polymorphism in proteins on the brink of thermodynamic stability. *Protein Sci.* **2018**. [CrossRef] [PubMed]
72. Galea, C.A.; Nourse, A.; Wang, Y.; Sivakolundu, S.G.; Heller, W.T.; Kriwacki, R.W. Role of intrinsic flexibility in signal transduction mediated by the cell cycle regulator, p27 Kip1. *J. Mol. Biol.* **2008**, *376*, 827–838. [CrossRef]
73. Iakoucheva, L.M.; Radivojac, P.; Brown, C.J.; O'Connor, T.R.; Sikes, J.G.; Obradovic, Z.; Dunker, A.K. The importance of intrinsic disorder for protein phosphorylation. *Nucleic Acids Res.* **2004**, *32*, 1037–1049. [CrossRef] [PubMed]
74. Xie, H.; Vucetic, S.; Iakoucheva, L.M.; Oldfield, C.J.; Dunker, A.K.; Obradovic, Z.; Uversky, V.N. Functional anthology of intrinsic disorder. 3. Ligands, post-translational modifications, and diseases associated with intrinsically disordered proteins. *J. Proteome Res.* **2007**, *6*, 1917–1932. [CrossRef] [PubMed]
75. Collins, M.O.; Yu, L.; Campuzano, I.; Grant, S.G.N.; Choudhary, J.S. Phosphoproteomic analysis of the mouse brain cytosol reveals a predominance of protein phosphorylation in regions of intrinsic sequence disorder. *Mol. Cell. Proteomics* **2008**, *7*, 1331–1348. [CrossRef] [PubMed]
76. Traynelis, S.F.; Wollmuth, L.P.; McBain, C.J.; Menniti, F.S.; Vance, K.M.; Ogden, K.K.; Hansen, K.B.; Yuan, H.; Myers, S.J.; Dingledine, R. Glutamate receptor ion channels: Structure, regulation, and function. *Pharmacol. Rev.* **2010**, *62*, 405–496. [CrossRef] [PubMed]
77. Kulkarni, P.; Dunker, A.K.; Weninger, K.; Orban, J. Prostate-associated gene 4 (PAGE4), an intrinsically disordered cancer/testis antigen, is a novel therapeutic target for prostate cancer. *Asian J. Androl.* **2016**, *18*, 695–703. [CrossRef]
78. Kulkarni, P.; Jolly, M.K.; Jia, D.; Mooney, S.M.; Bhargava, A.; Kagohara, L.T.; Chen, Y.; Hao, P.; He, Y.; Veltri, R.W.; et al. Phosphorylation-induced conformational dynamics in an intrinsically disordered protein and potential role in phenotypic heterogeneity. *Proc. Natl. Acad. Sci. USA* **2017**, *114*, E2644–E2653. [CrossRef]
79. Salgia, R.; Jolly, M.K.; Dorff, T.; Lau, C.; Weninger, K.; Orban, J.; Kulkarni, P. Prostate-Associated Gene 4 (PAGE4): Leveraging the Conformational Dynamics of a Dancing Protein Cloud as a Therapeutic Target. *J. Clin. Med.* **2018**, *7*, 156. [CrossRef] [PubMed]
80. Jolly, M.K.; Kulkarni, P.; Weninger, K.; Orban, J.; Levine, H. Phenotypic Plasticity, Bet-Hedging, and Androgen Independence in Prostate Cancer: Role of Non-Genetic Heterogeneity. *Front. Oncol.* **2018**, *8*, 50. [CrossRef]
81. Zeng, Y.; He, Y.; Yang, F.; Mooney, S.M.; Getzenberg, R.H.; Orban, J.; Kulkarni, P. The Cancer/Testis Antigen Prostate-associated Gene 4 (PAGE4) Is a Highly Intrinsically Disordered Protein. *J. Biol. Chem.* **2011**, *286*, 13985–13994. [CrossRef]
82. Rajagopalan, K.; Qiu, R.; Mooney, S.M.; Rao, S.; Shiraishi, T.; Sacho, E.; Huang, H.; Shapiro, E.; Weninger, K.R.; Kulkarni, P. The Stress-response protein prostate-associated gene 4, interacts with c-Jun and potentiates its transactivation. *Biochim. Biophys. Acta* **2014**, *1842*, 154–163. [CrossRef] [PubMed]

83. Lin, X.; Kulkarni, P.; Bocci, F.; Schafer, N.; Roy, S.; Tsai, M.-Y.; He, Y.; Chen, Y.; Rajagopalan, K.; Mooney, S.; et al. Structural and Dynamical Order of a Disordered Protein: Molecular Insights into Conformational Switching of PAGE4 at the Systems Level. *Biomolecules* **2019**, *9*, 77. [CrossRef] [PubMed]
84. Lin, X.; Roy, S.; Jolly, M.K.; Bocci, F.; Schafer, N.P.; Tsai, M.-Y.; Chen, Y.; He, Y.; Grishaev, A.; Weninger, K.; et al. PAGE4 and Conformational Switching: Insights from Molecular Dynamics Simulations and Implications for Prostate Cancer. *J. Mol. Biol.* **2018**, *430*, 2422–2438. [CrossRef]
85. Mooney, S.M.; Qiu, R.; Kim, J.J.; Sacho, E.J.; Rajagopalan, K.; Johng, D.; Shiraishi, T.; Kulkarni, P.; Weninger, K.R. Cancer/testis antigen PAGE4, a regulator of c-Jun transactivation, is phosphorylated by homeodomain-interacting protein kinase 1, a component of the stress-response pathway. *Biochemistry* **2014**, *53*, 1670–1679. [CrossRef]
86. He, Y.; Chen, Y.; Mooney, S.M.; Rajagopalan, K.; Bhargava, A.; Sacho, E.; Weninger, K.; Bryan, P.N.; Kulkarni, P.; Orban, J. Phosphorylation-induced Conformational Ensemble Switching in an Intrinsically Disordered Cancer/Testis Antigen. *J. Biol. Chem.* **2015**, *290*, 25090–25102. [CrossRef]
87. Shin, Y.; Brangwynne, C.P. Liquid phase condensation in cell physiology and disease. *Science* **2017**, *357*, eaaf4382. [CrossRef] [PubMed]
88. Harmon, T.S.; Holehouse, A.S.; Rosen, M.K.; Pappu, R.V. Intrinsically disordered linkers determine the interplay between phase separation and gelation in multivalent proteins. *Elife* **2017**, *6*. [CrossRef]
89. LeBlanc, S.; Kulkarni, P.; Weninger, K. Single Molecule FRET: A Powerful Tool to Study Intrinsically Disordered Proteins. *Biomolecules* **2018**, *8*, 140. [CrossRef] [PubMed]
90. Sakon, J.J.; Weninger, K.R. Detecting the conformation of individual proteins in live cells. *Nat. Methods* **2010**, *7*, 203–205. [CrossRef]
91. Aigrain, L.; Crawford, R.; Torella, J.; Plochowietz, A.; Kapanidis, A. Single-molecule FRET measurements in bacterial cells. *FEBS J.* **2012**, *279*, 513.
92. König, I.; Zarrine-Afsar, A.; Aznauryan, M.; Soranno, A.; Wunderlich, B.; Dingfelder, F.; Stüber, J.C.; Plückthun, A.; Nettels, D.; Schuler, B. Single-molecule spectroscopy of protein conformational dynamics in live eukaryotic cells. *Nat. Methods* **2015**, *12*, 773–779. [CrossRef]
93. Elbaum-Garfinkle, S.; Kim, Y.; Szczepaniak, K.; Chen, C.C.-H.; Eckmann, C.R.; Myong, S.; Brangwynne, C.P. The disordered P granule protein LAF-1 drives phase separation into droplets with tunable viscosity and dynamics. *Proc. Natl. Acad. Sci.* **2015**, *112*, 7189–7194. [CrossRef] [PubMed]
94. Uversky, V.N. Intrinsically Disordered Proteins and Their "Mysterious" (Meta)Physics. *Front. Phys.* **2019**, *7*, 10. [CrossRef]
95. Rauscher, S.; Gapsys, V.; Gajda, M.J.; Zweckstetter, M.; de Groot, B.L.; Grubmüller, H. Structural Ensembles of Intrinsically Disordered Proteins Depend Strongly on Force Field: A Comparison to Experiment. *J. Chem. Theory Comput.* **2015**, *11*, 5513–5524. [CrossRef] [PubMed]
96. Huang, J.; Rauscher, S.; Nawrocki, G.; Ran, T.; Feig, M.; de Groot, B.L.; Grubmüller, H.; MacKerell, A.D. CHARMM36m: An improved force field for folded and intrinsically disordered proteins. *Nat. Methods* **2017**, *14*, 71–73. [CrossRef] [PubMed]
97. Lindorff-Larsen, K.; Trbovic, N.; Maragakis, P.; Piana, S.; Shaw, D.E. Structure and Dynamics of an Unfolded Protein Examined by Molecular Dynamics Simulation. *J. Am. Chem. Soc.* **2012**, *134*, 3787–3791. [CrossRef]
98. Robustelli, P.; Piana, S.; Shaw, D.E. Developing a molecular dynamics force field for both folded and disordered protein states. *Proc. Natl. Acad. Sci.* **2018**, *115*, E4758–E4766. [CrossRef] [PubMed]
99. Fuertes, G.; Banterle, N.; Ruff, K.M.; Chowdhury, A.; Mercadante, D.; Koehler, C.; Kachala, M.; Estrada Girona, G.; Milles, S.; Mishra, A.; et al. Decoupling of size and shape fluctuations in heteropolymeric sequences reconciles discrepancies in SAXS vs. FRET measurements. *Proc. Natl. Acad. Sci. USA* **2017**, *114*, E6342–E6351. [CrossRef]
100. Merchant, K.A.; Best, R.B.; Louis, J.M.; Gopich, I.V.; Eaton, W.A. Characterizing the unfolded states of proteins using single-molecule FRET spectroscopy and molecular simulations. *Proc. Natl. Acad. Sci.* **2007**, *104*, 1528–1533. [CrossRef]
101. Best, R.B. Computational and theoretical advances in studies of intrinsically disordered proteins. *Curr. Opin. Struct. Biol.* **2017**, *42*, 147–154. [CrossRef]
102. Soranno, A.; Holla, A.; Dingfelder, F.; Nettels, D.; Makarov, D.E.; Schuler, B. Integrated view of internal friction in unfolded proteins from single-molecule FRET, contact quenching, theory, and simulations. *Proc. Natl. Acad. Sci. USA* **2017**, *114*, E1833–E1839. [CrossRef]

103. Zheng, W.; Borgia, A.; Buholzer, K.; Grishaev, A.; Schuler, B.; Best, R.B. Probing the Action of Chemical Denaturant on an Intrinsically Disordered Protein by Simulation and Experiment. *J. Am. Chem. Soc.* **2016**, *138*, 11702–11713. [CrossRef] [PubMed]
104. Ferrie, J.J.; Haney, C.M.; Yoon, J.; Pan, B.; Lin, Y.-C.; Fakhraai, Z.; Rhoades, E.; Nath, A.; Petersson, E.J. Using a FRET Library with Multiple Probe Pairs To Drive Monte Carlo Simulations of α-Synuclein. *Biophys. J.* **2018**, *114*, 53–64. [CrossRef] [PubMed]
105. Jeschke, G. Ensemble models of proteins and protein domains based on distance distribution restraints. *Proteins Struct. Funct. Bioinform.* **2016**, *84*, 544–560. [CrossRef] [PubMed]
106. Nath, A.; Sammalkorpi, M.; DeWitt, D.C.; Trexler, A.J.; Elbaum-Garfinkle, S.; O'Hern, C.S.; Rhoades, E. The conformational ensembles of α-synuclein and tau: Combining single-molecule FRET and simulations. *Biophys. J.* **2012**, *103*, 1940–1949. [CrossRef] [PubMed]
107. Jao, C.C.; Hegde, B.G.; Chen, J.; Haworth, I.S.; Langen, R. Structure of membrane-bound α-synuclein from site-directed spin labeling and computational refinement. *Proc. Natl. Acad. Sci.* **2008**, *105*, 19666–19671. [CrossRef] [PubMed]
108. Tsafou, K.; Tiwari, P.B.; Forman-Kay, J.D.; Metallo, S.J.; Toretsky, J.A. Targeting Intrinsically Disordered Transcription Factors: Changing the Paradigm. *J. Mol. Biol.* **2018**, *430*, 2321–2341. [CrossRef] [PubMed]
109. Zhang, Z.; Boskovic, Z.; Hussain, M.M.; Hu, W.; Inouye, C.; Kim, H.-J.; Abole, A.K.; Doud, M.K.; Lewis, T.A.; Koehler, A.N.; et al. Chemical perturbation of an intrinsically disordered region of TFIID distinguishes two modes of transcription initiation. *Elife* **2015**, *4*. [CrossRef] [PubMed]

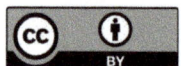

© 2019 by the authors. Licensee MDPI, Basel, Switzerland. This article is an open access article distributed under the terms and conditions of the Creative Commons Attribution (CC BY) license (http://creativecommons.org/licenses/by/4.0/).

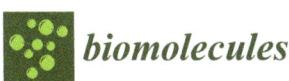

Article

Electrostatics of Tau Protein by Molecular Dynamics

Tarsila G. Castro [1,2], Florentina-Daniela Munteanu [1] and Artur Cavaco-Paulo [1,2,*]

1. Aurel Vlaicu University of Arad, Str. Elena Drăgoi 2-4, RO-310330 Arad, Romania; castro.tarsila@ceb.uminho.pt (T.G.C.); florentina.munteanu@uav.ro (F.-D.M.)
2. Centre of Biological Engineering, University of Minho, Campus de Gualtar, 4710-057, Braga, Portugal
* Correspondence: artur@deb.uminho.pt; Tel.: +351-253-604-409

Received: 18 February 2019; Accepted: 20 March 2019; Published: 23 March 2019

Abstract: Tau is a microtubule-associated protein that promotes microtubule assembly and stability. This protein is implicated in several neurodegenerative diseases, including Alzheimer's. To date, the three-dimensional (3D) structure of tau has not been fully solved, experimentally. Even the most recent information is sometimes controversial in regard to how this protein folds, interacts, and behaves. Predicting the tau structure and its profile sheds light on the knowledge about its properties and biological function, such as the binding to microtubules (MT) and, for instance, the effect on ionic conductivity. Our findings on the tau structure suggest a disordered protein, with discrete portions of well-defined secondary structure, mostly at the microtubule binding region. In addition, the first molecular dynamics simulation of full-length tau along with an MT section was performed, unveiling tau structure when associated with MT and interaction sites. Electrostatics and conductivity were also examined to understand how tau affects the ions in the intracellular fluid environment. Our results bring a new insight into tau and tubulin MT proteins, their characteristics, and the structure–function relationship.

Keywords: tau; microtubules; electrostatics; diffusion; protein structure prediction; molecular modelling; molecular dynamics; tau–microtubule association

1. Introduction

Tau is an intrinsically disordered protein (IDP) that stabilizes and promotes the assembly of microtubules (MTs) in neurons (Figure 1); it is, therefore, a microtubule-associated protein (MAP) [1]. Tau is involved in cell polarity and, as it is distributed along the axons, is responsible for the maintenance of neuron structure and healthy function [2,3]. Structurally, tau is also considered as a spacer between adjacent MTs, although that is not its main function [4].

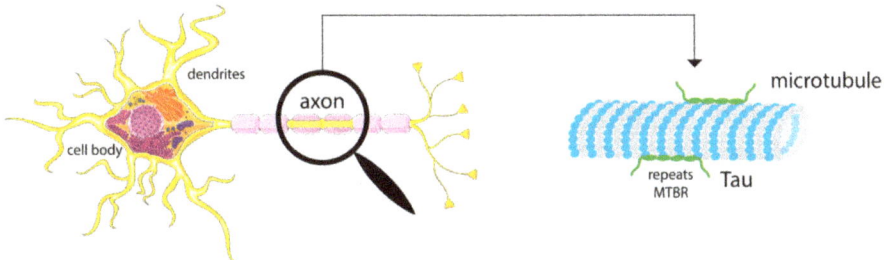

Figure 1. Graphical representation of a neuron, highlighting a microtubule present in the axon and the interaction with the tau protein, through the four repeats at the microtubule binding region (MTBR). Adapted from Servier Medical Art [5].

The adult largest tau isoform has 441 amino acids, comprising a projection domain with two amino-terminal inserts N, encoded by exons 2 and 3, a proline-rich region and the microtubule binding region (MTBR), with four imperfect repeats (Figure 2). This isoform is commonly cited as 2N4RTau, isoform-F, htau40 and Tau-4, and is the largest one in the human central nervous system (CNS), which has five other isoforms [6].

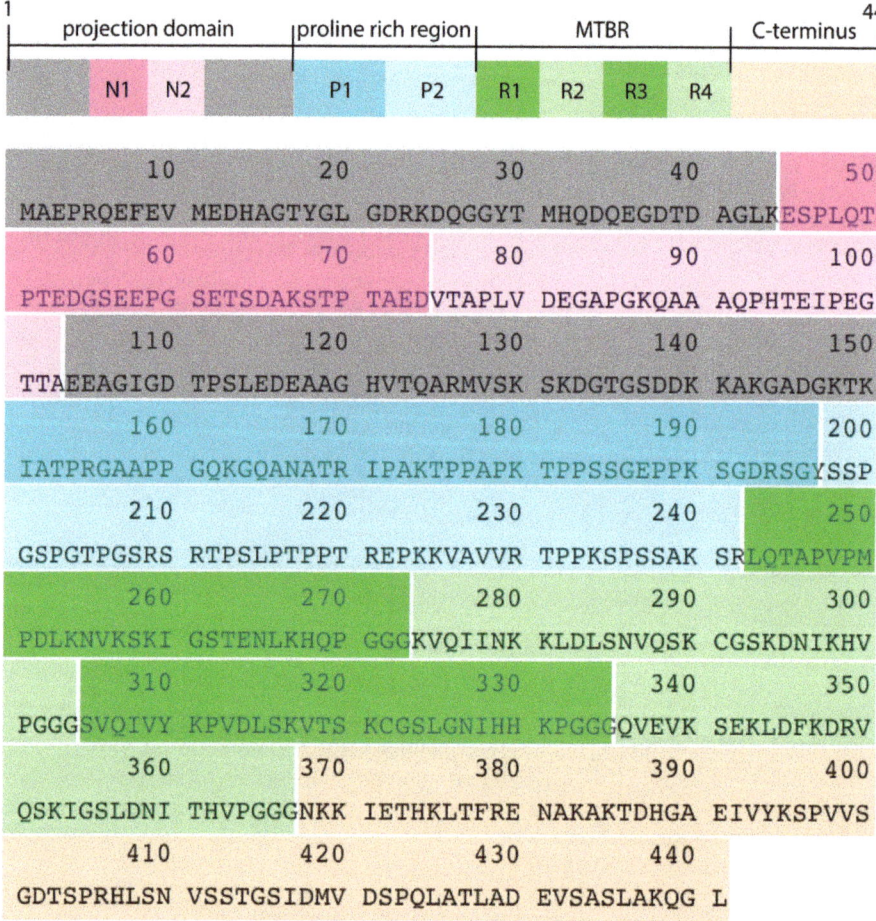

Figure 2. Primary sequence and regions of 2N4RTau isoform, comprising 441 amino acids. N1 and N2 correspond to the two N terminal inserts, P1 and P2 are the proline-rich regions, and R1 to R4 are the four imperfect repeats responsible for the binding to the microtubule.

Besides the relevant structural support function, that comes from the interaction between tau and the tubulin MTs, tau plays an important role in nervous system diseases. If hyperphosphorylated, tau does not perform its normal function, but aggregates in paired helical filaments (PHF) [7,8] which inhibits the MT assembly. The PHFs cause tau lesions found in Alzheimer's disease (AD) brains and in other types of dementia [9–12].

Several post-translational modifications can occur in tau, namely, phosphorylation, glycosylation, nitration, glycation, ubiquitination, among others [13,14]. The degree of these modifications is what will lead to a normal or pathological functioning. In particular, tau phosphorylation is the most studied alteration, as it is established that the abnormal hyperphosphorylation is associated with AD [15,16], a dementia that currently has no cure.

To date, tau's complete structure has not been fully solved experimentally. Only portions of the canonical sequence are known, or hyperphosphorylated sections, as listed in UniProt (Universal Protein resource) [17] and in the RCSB PDB (Research Collaboratory for Structural Bioinformatics Protein Data Bank) [18]. This fact hinders a more complete understanding of the structure–function relationship for this protein. Indeed, the information concerning tau structure bound to MT is controversial [19–21], even in the most recent papers on the subject [22,23].

Our work sheds light on the tau three-dimensional (3D) structure. We performed the complete modelling of the 2N4RTau isoform, using protein structure prediction (PSP) techniques, and submitted the obtained model to molecular dynamics (MD) simulations in order to characterize the following: tau profile in neuron fluid, its interactions and structure when associated with MT, the effect of tau on ions' diffusion and conductivity, among other properties.

2. Materials and Methods

2.1. Tau Structure Prediction

Tau conformation was predicted using the I-TASSER (Iterative Threading ASSEmbly Refinement) server, a method to predict protein structure and function that uses a multiple threading approach based on templates from the Protein Data Bank (PDB) [24]. The I-TASSER is consistently considered the best server for PSP in community-wide CASP (Critical Assessment of protein Structure Prediction) experiments [25,26]. The threading templates used to predict tau structure were the proteins with the following codes: 2nbi, 3zue, 2mz7, 1w0r, 4dur, and 1ziw. 2nbi corresponds to pleuralin-1, a structural protein that shares 19% of sequence identity with tau. 3zue is a virus capsid protein presenting 22% of overall sequence identity with tau. 2mz7 is the only template that matches an NMR tau structure (amino acids 267–312) [21], and fulfil 10% of similarity. 1w0r is properdin, a glycoprotein with 20% of sequence alignment with tau. 4dur corresponds to the X-ray structure of type II human plasminogen, a hydrolase that shares 17% of similarity with tau, and 1ziw is the human toll-like receptor 3, making a total of 17% of identity with tau.

The I-TASSER server starts the modelling from the structure templates mentioned above, identified with LOMETS (Local Meta-Threading-Server), but other procedures and programs take place to generate the final five hit models. From this list we chose the one with the best C-score. The model was predicted in 2017 with the template structures available that year.

2.2. System Setup

Three types of systems were designed to study tau (Figure 3). The first one was a simulation box composed only of neuronal intracellular fluid as control (Figure 3a). The second was a simulation box containing the predicted tau structure in the neuronal fluid (Figure 3b), and the third contained tau next to a tubulin wall (an MT section (PDB ID: 5JCO)) in the fluid (Figure 3c). The second and third systems are hereinafter referred as tau in fluid and Tau::MT in fluid. For tau in the fluid, the protein was centered in the box, but in the case of Tau::MT systems, the tubulin wall was placed at one of the walls of the box and tau randomly near to MT, as shown in Figure 3.

The fluid inside the neurons was composed of water, a high concentration of potassium and proteins with negative character, and a discrete concentration of sodium and chloride among other ions [27]. In the simulations performed, we fixed the concentration of K^+ and Na^+ to the reported values [27–29]: 140 mM for K^+ and 5–15 mM for Na^+ at the neuron resting state. These cations are the ions involved in the transmission of electrical signals in these cells and, most importantly, the probability of being affected by the negatively charged MT wall and by tau is high.

As it was not feasible to simulate explicitly all cytoplasmic proteins in neuronal fluid, since it would require a greater computational power, we decided to replace the negative contribution from these proteins for Cl$^-$. The final balance of charges, in the simulation boxes, would be the same using negatively charged proteins or Cl$^-$ ions. In addition, as described below, we used particle mesh Ewald (PME) for electrostatic treatment and periodic boundary conditions (PBC) in our simulations, therefore the simulation only formally converges if the net electric charge is zero. That is why the addition of ions to achieve neutrality is a common procedure in MD simulations.

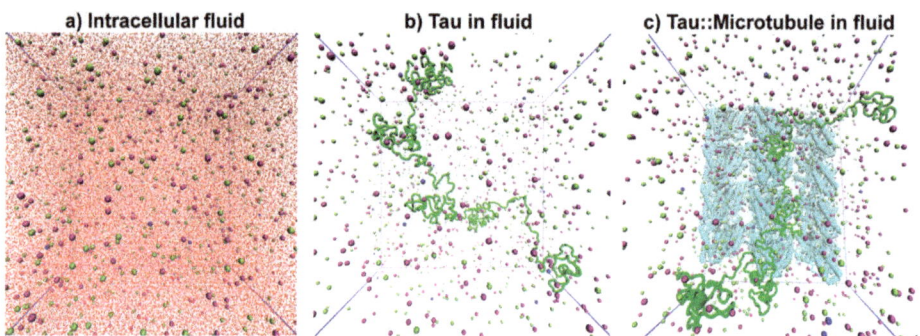

Figure 3. Front view snapshots of the systems under simulation: (**a**) Intracellular fluid, (**b**) tau in fluid, and (**c**) tau::microtubule wall in fluid. Water molecules were omitted in (**b**) and (**c**) to allow better visualization. Tau is represented in green, microtubule in cyan, K$^+$ in purple, Na$^+$ in blue, and Cl$^-$ in green spheres.

In all three cases, a simulation box with an approximate volume of 7200 nm^3 was necessary. The final number of simple point-charge (SPC) water molecules depended on the volume occupied by tau or the pair Tau::MT.

2.3. Molecular Dynamics Simulations

Molecular dynamics simulations were performed on the systems described above, to understand tau structure and properties.

Two stages of energy minimization were performed using a maximum of 50,000 steps: the first using the steepest descent method and the second with the conjugate gradient algorithm [30]. Initialization steps using canonical (NVT, constant number of particles, volume and temperature) and isothermal-isobaric (NPT, constant number of particles, pressure and temperature) ensembles were performed applying position restraints (with force constant of 1000 kJ·mol^{-1}·nm^{-2}) to all heavy atoms in the NVT procedure, and to the main chain at the NPT initialization step, during 100 ps each. In the control situation (fluid), no position restraints were applied. The temperature was maintained constant at 310 K with V-rescale algorithm [31] and the pressure was regulated at 1 atm with the Parrinello–Rahman barostat [32]. The following coupling constants were considered: τ_T = 0.10 ps and τ_P = 2.0 ps. Subsequently, all systems were submitted to MD simulations: the fluid during 10 ns, tau in fluid during 60 ns, and Tau::MT in fluid for 70 ns, all using the NPT ensemble, without position restraints. Three replicates of each system were run to guarantee a better sampling of conformation states for these very large proteins under study.

All MD simulations were performed using the computational package GROMACS 5.1.4 version [30,33], within the GROMOS 54a7 force field (FF) [34,35]. The Lennard-Jones interactions were truncated at 1.4 nm and we used the particle mesh Ewald (PME) [36] method for electrostatic interactions, with a cut-off of 1.4 nm. The algorithm LINCS [37] was used to constrain the chemical bonds of the proteins and the algorithm SETTLE [38] in the case of water. Parameters for K$^+$ in the scope of G54a7 FF were obtained from the paper of Cordomí et al. [39].

2.4. Analysis

From the MD simulations, we analyzed the trajectories looking at the root-mean-square deviation (RMSD) to determine when the systems were at equilibrium. Based on the RMSD results, the following analyses were performed from 30 ns.

Root-mean-square fluctuation (RMSF) analysis and CLUSTER analysis with the single-linkage method were used to understand regions and amino acids with greater flexibility and to determine the middle structure of each tau replicate, respectively. This technique adds structures that are below an RMSD cut-off, generating more or less populated clusters and, within the largest cluster, it finds a middle structure that is the most representative of the whole simulation. Radial distribution functions (RDF) were calculated for the positive ions around the tau surface.

GROMACS' mean square displacement (MSD) was used to calculate the ions' mean square displacement in all systems. To calculate the diffusion coefficient (D_i) of the particles, one can use the Einstein relation [40], illustrated in Equation 1, where r_i corresponds to the particle center of mass position at a certain time t:

$$D_i = \lim_{t \to \infty} \frac{1}{6t} \langle \| r_i(t) - r_i(0) \|^2 \rangle. \tag{1}$$

From the D_i obtained with this analysis, it is possible to calculate the molar conductivity, as demonstrated in Equation 2. The Nernst–Einstein equation (2) establishes the relationship between the molar limiting conductivity $\Lambda_{m,i}$ and the diffusion coefficient Di for any given ion i, at a certain temperature (T). In the equation, z corresponds to the charge of the ion i, F corresponds to Faraday's constant, and R is the gas constant. Here, our conductivity calculation is an approximation, since our systems do not represent an infinite dilution of the ions (non-interacting ions). We disregarded the ion–ion correction factor to use Equation (2) directly:

$$\Lambda^{\circ}_{m,i} = z_i^2 D_i \left(\frac{F^2}{RT} \right). \tag{2}$$

The MSD was calculated for the total simulation time but considering time intervals of about 10 ns. We chose to do this because this analysis requires a large memory capacity for large systems and to ensure reliable MSD data, resulting in a linear MSD(t) plot for each "-b to -e" time interval option. All analysis programs used are available in the GROMACS 5.1.4 package [29,32].

The analyses of the electrostatic potential of the predicted tau structure and the microtubule section (5JCO) were performed using the PDB2PQR server [41] and the APBS (Adaptive Poisson-Boltzmann Solver) plugin in PyMOL molecular visualization program [42–44]. For the microtubule we calculated the electrostatic surface for a tubulin heterodimer, since it is representative of the whole structure.

All figures presenting molecular structures were made with PyMOL and VMD (Visual Molecular Dynamics) software [45].

3. Results and Discussion

3.1. Tau Structure Prediction and Validation

Tau conformation was predicted with the I-TASSER server (Figure 4a). This method generates five hit models, from which we chose the one with the best C-score. The predicted tau is an elongated structure with only two small portions presenting a well-defined secondary structure (SS). The lack of SS is consistent with what is cited in the literature, which describes tau as an intrinsically disordered protein [46,47]. This extended form is important to the tau function, as it allows a proper exposure, flexibility, and contact of the MTBR residues with tubulin MT [48].

Some authors describe how the MTBR can gain some helical SS when interactions take place with MTs or actin filaments [19,49]. Recently, Zabik et al. [23] performed NMR studies in tau peptide fragments and in full-length tau, but tau easily forms oligomers, influencing tau 3D structure. Moreover, tau in solution adopts a more compact conformation, with N- and C- termini interacting and inducing a paperclip structure (i.e., a folding over the MTBR that approximates the terminals). This conformation contrasts with the extended conformation required for interaction with MT but is the most typical in solution [23,50–52]. To address both situations, tau in intracellular solution and tau bound to MTs, we simulated these two systems to disclose the tau structure in different contexts.

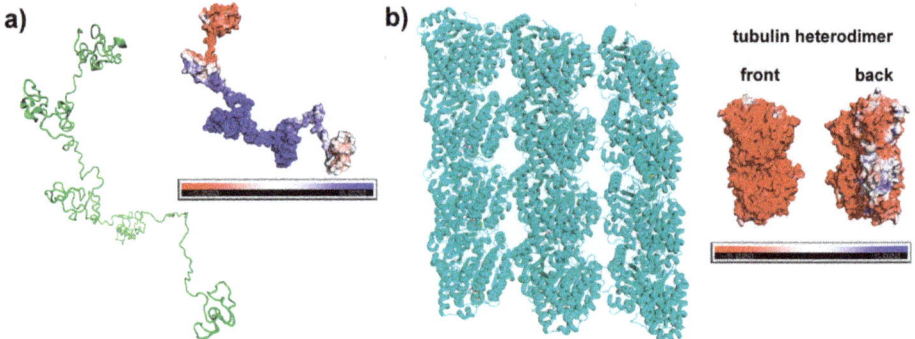

Figure 4. (a) Predicted structure of tau using I-TASSER and (b) 5JCO microtubule section from Protein Data Bank (PDB). Both structures are side by side to its electrostatic potential surface, which in red represents the negative potential values and in blue, the positive potential values. The electrostatic potential (k_b T e_c^{-1}) was calculated using APBS-PDB2PQR software. For the microtubule, the calculation was made using a tubulin heterodimer.

Predicted tau presents an electrostatic surface highly positive in the central region and a negatively charged patch at the N-terminal. Tau electrostatics reinforces the approximation between terminals that occurs in solution, folding over the middle domain of tau and resulting in a paperclip conformation.

In the case of tubulin heterodimer, the constituents of a microtubule, the surface is predominantly negative with few neutral or positive patches on the back (microtubule interior). The electrostatic surface that we calculated is very similar to the one presented by Baker et al. for a larger microtubule structure [43].

Root-mean-square deviation is the most used analysis to monitor the structural behavior of a protein—either to see the maintenance of a tertiary structure (protein stability in a medium) or to follow the equilibration of a sampled conformation (the folding). In the case of the tau protein, we started from a model structure that needed to be equilibrated in its most typical environment, that is, embedded in the neuronal fluid, interacting or not with MTs. A large structural deviation was expected at the beginning of the simulation as well as a conformational variety. Our systems, tau in fluid and Tau::MT in fluid, took about 30 ns to reach equilibration (Figure 5a,b) and to start sampling conformations more similar among each other.

The RMSF provides an insight into tau residue mobility, indicating the more rigid and more flexible regions. In fluid (Figure 6a), tau is more flexible at the N-termini region and projection domain. From the proline-rich region, it becomes less fluctuating. When near to the MT wall (Figure 6b), the amount of interactions between tau and MT (electrostatics, van der Waals and hydrogen bonds), which must form and break repeatedly, induces a more pronounced fluctuation throughout the tau structure, with proline-rich region and MTBR being the most rigid regions for replicates 1 and 2. This fact is in agreement with the strongest interaction of MTBR with the MT wall, reducing the mobility of this area.

The cluster analyses were employed from 30 to 60/70 ns to determine the middle conformation of each replicate (Figure 7a,b). Middle structures for tau in fluid also have helical SS in MTBR, namely, replicate 1: amino acids 275–277 and 315–318; replicate 2: amino acids 315–319; and replicate 3: amino acids 253–259, 269–273, 280–282, and 359–362. However, these structures seem to fold over themselves, becoming more compact and less exposed, agreeing with tau NMR prediction in solution [23]. Visually, the structures obtained for Tau::MT in fluid are more similar and extended. In fact, all three present helical content in MTBR, namely, replicate 1: amino acids 274–277 and 305–310; replicate 2: amino acids 256–260 and 357–362; and replicate 3: amino acids 253–257 and 350–354. In addition, for tau from Tau::MT replicates, we observed a more extended structure with N- and C-termini far from each other.

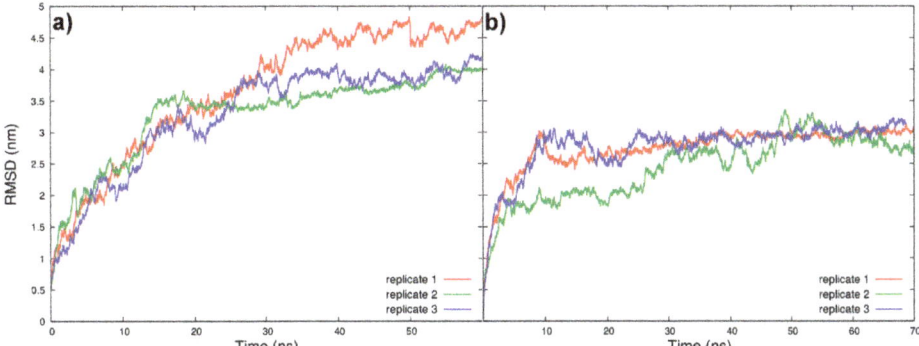

Figure 5. Backbone root-mean-square deviation (RMSD) of tau, fitting the backbone, for all tau replicates (**a**) in fluid and (**b**) when associated with microtubule, from the initial predicted model.

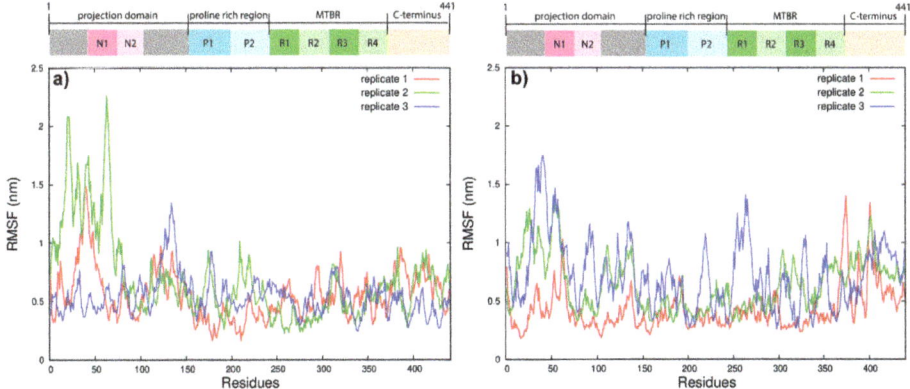

Figure 6. Residue root-mean-square fluctuation (RMSF) (**a**) of each tau replicate in fluid and (**b**) of tau::microtubule pair in fluid.

To better understand the interaction between tau and the tubulin MT wall, the middle conformations for the pair Tau::MT were also calculated. Figure 7c shows these pairs highlighting the N-terminal, proline-rich region, MTBR, and C-terminal with the color scheme proposed in Figure 2.

Replicates 2 and 3 interact with parts of two tubulin heterodimers and the N-termini are further apart from the tubulin wall than in the case of replicate 1. There is no consensus on the type of tubulin (α or β) to which tau binds preferentially, on the number of units [48,53], or even if the interaction is longitudinal or lateral [54]. More recently, Kellogg et al. [22] proposed an atomic model of tau bound to MT, suggesting that each tau repeat spans over three tubulin monomers as a continuous stretch, even more extended than our middle structures and reaching a higher number of tubulin monomers. The determination of the interaction mode between tau and MT has to take into account the highly dynamic behavior of tau and its ability to disconnect from one MT to connect to another in the neighborhood, in a kiss-and-hop mechanism, as cited by Janning et al. [55], suggesting that tau binding might be slightly different in interactions each time.

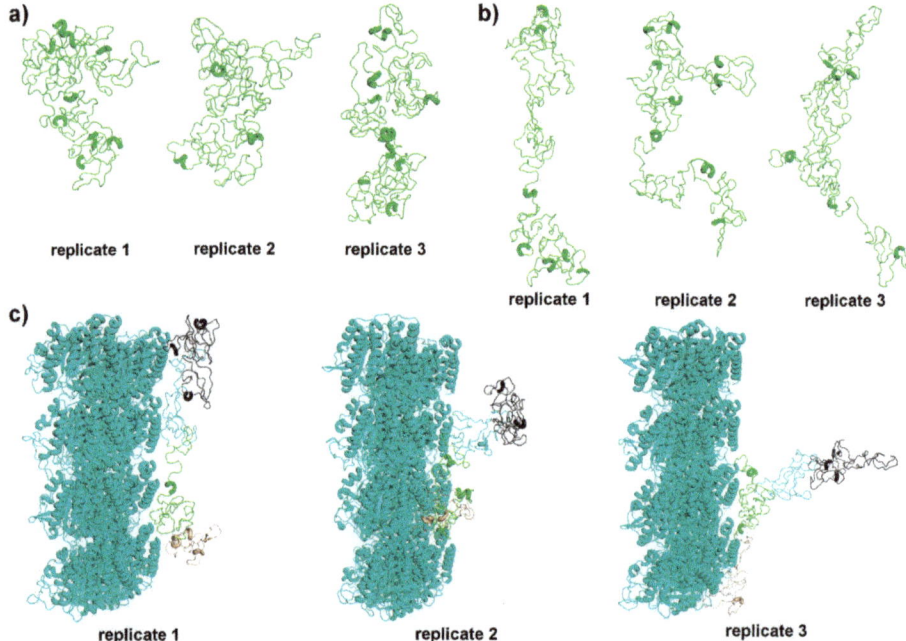

Figure 7. (**a**) Middle structures of tau in fluid, (**b**) middle structures of tau when associated with microtubules, with N-termini oriented to the top, and (**c**) tau::microtubule middle structures, with a color scheme following Figure 2: grey for N-terminal, cyan for proline-rich domain, green representing the MTBR, and beige for C-terminal. (**c**) Microtubule wall is represented in cyan cartoon and (**a**,**b**) tau is represented in green cartoon.

Electrostatic interactions and hydrogen bonds take place in all three replicates associated with MT, although for replicate 3, only the MTBR (Thr263, Lys281, and Lys290) and C-termini interact. Tau replicate 1 interacts along all its structure, with important interactions at the proline-rich region and MTBR (Ser202, Lys224, Arg230, Ser237, Ser241, Val306, Ser316, and Lys317). Replicate 2 interacts a little less with the proline-rich region (Ser202, Val228, and Lys240), much with the MTBR (Arg242, Lys274, Lys 280, His268, Gln288, Cys291, Gly308, and Leu315) and through the C-termini. It has to be stressed that the amino acids cited above are mostly polar and many of them positively charged, resulting in a good binding to the acidic C-terminal of tubulins (cyan helices, near tau, in Figure 7c).

Structurally, tau 3D structure, when tau interacts with MTs, is more extended than tau in solution, with the termini far from each other. If oriented to the same direction, all three replicates are quite similar (Figure 7b), which is a very good result for a simulation of a very dynamic IDP, under the interaction forces from the MT wall. In addition, we observed that tau replicates sample helical portions at the MTBR, as predicted or suggested in some works [19,46]. It is important to note that at the end of each MTBR repeat, there is a PGGG motif. Proline is a helical breaker and glycine, due to the absence of a side chain, is highly flexible and rarely found in helices. This motif should correspond to an extended or bended region that will connect the four repeats. In fact, in our simulations, PGGG does not sample secondary structure, and its inherent flexibility causes repeats not to be completely extended along the MT wall, but to approach one another.

3.2. Tau Effect on Ionic Diffusion and Conductivity

To analyze the ions' behavior, the RDF and the diffusion coefficients were studied. This is important to understand the role of tau or Tau::MT pair in the distribution of the ions present in the intracellular fluid. The RDF describes how the density of a particle varies as a function of distance from a reference molecule. Following this rationale, we can perceive how the K$^+$ and Na$^+$ ions interact with tau and MT.

Figure 8 shows the RDF graphs for K$^+$ and Na$^+$ ions for all three replicates of tau in fluid (Figure 8a–c) and Tau::MT in fluid (Figure 8d–f). This analysis helps to understand the role of the electrostatic interaction with the proteins, in the ions' mobility through the fluid. In all cases, K$^+$ has a higher probability of being closer to the tau negative area (N-termini) than Na$^+$. Note that the concentration of both ions is very different (interfering with the probability), namely, 140 mM for K$^+$ and around 5 mM for Na$^+$, yet sodium is lighter than potassium and could be more mobile and interact with tau more often, but an interaction preference with K$^+$ is perceived. In this analysis, we focus on the ions' distribution up to 1 nm from the protein surface. Naturally, the ions also populate the bulk water, corresponding to a high probability far from protein, but we neglected the distribution in this area. If tau N-terminal retains K$^+$, it can keep these ions further away from the cell membrane inner face, increasing the membrane potential.

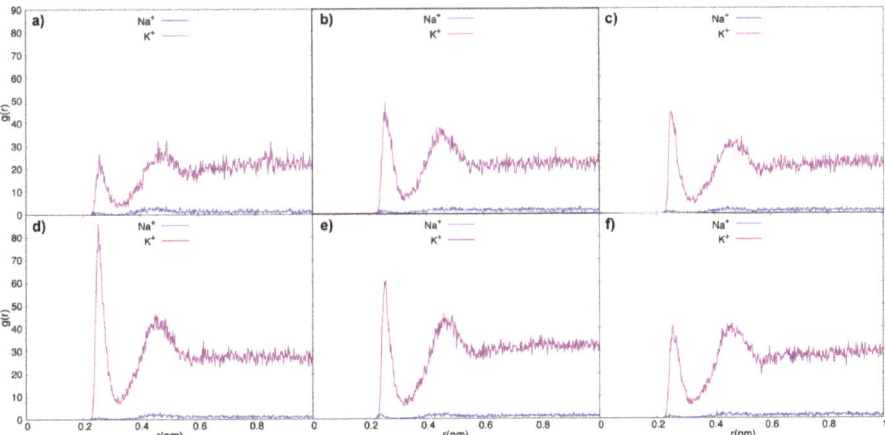

Figure 8. Radial distribution functions (g(r)) of K$^+$ and Na$^+$ ions in the vicinity of the tau surface, for tau replicates in fluid (**a–c**) and tau::microtubule replicates (**d–f**). Purple trace for potassium and blue trace for sodium.

The ion's diffusion coefficients were calculated for K$^+$, Na$^+$, and Cl$^-$ (Figure 9). Chloride is used for two reasons: to mimic the negative contribution from cytoplasmic proteins and to neutralize the simulation box. In fact, Cl$^-$ is more mobile than the proteins in neuronal cytoplasm, but tau and MT should be less sensitive to this negative ion, especially MT due to its electrostatics. Therefore, the interaction pattern of Na$^+$ and K$^+$ with tau and MT proteins is probably little influenced by chloride in our simulations.

Experimentally, the ions' diffusion and conductivity are always expressed at 25 °C, not at 37 °C. In addition, this calculation is made at infinite dilution, so in our systems we have to consider the concentration effect, which makes a direct comparison to experimental values difficult. However, the trend of Na$^+$ < K$^+$ < Cl$^-$ in terms of diffusion and conductivity is expected in all simulated systems.

In the first simulation, the intracellular fluid, the ions were free to move around the simulation box, respecting the intracellular concentration and in the presence of chloride ions to neutralize the system. We observed that the diffusion (Figure 9) follow the expected trend of Na$^+$ < K$^+$ < Cl$^-$ found in many ionic solutions [56].

Looking at the ions in the system tau in fluid, we emphasize that the presence of tau does not decrease the ions' diffusion. All three ions maintain the diffusion rate, if we consider the estimated error (Figure 9). In contrast, when tau is directly associated with the MT (Tau::MT replicates), there is a decrease in the diffusion. It was reported that tau diffusion along an MT lattice is influenced by the ionic strength and pH, especially by K$^+$ [57]. This suggests that when tau is near or attached to the MT, the ions' diffusion through the fluid should decrease as the ions are participating in the protein diffusion process.

To circumvent the direct contribution of MT in ionic diffusion, we simulated a tau middle structure (from Tau::MT replicate 2) attached to the box wall, and constraining the MTBR. Thus, we obtained the expected structure when tau interacts with the tubulin wall, but only the tau effect on the conductivity is observed.

A simulation box with the same volume and ion concentrations was modelled during 12 ns (Figure 10). We observed, in this case, that tau increases the diffusion of the Na$^+$ cation, possibly making this ion more available in the fluid to move through the sodium channels and across the membrane, as the probability of tau to retain K$^+$ is much bigger than to retain Na$^+$ (radial distribution functions in Figure 8). The diffusion of K$^+$ is once again similar to the one calculated in the intracellular fluid, reinforcing the statement that tau is a protein that does not prevent the normal movement of this ion and the consequent concentration balance in the interior and exterior of the cell.

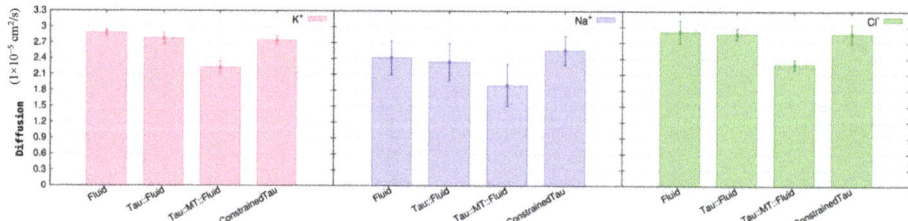

Figure 9. K$^+$, Na$^+$, and Cl$^-$ diffusion, D$_i$ (1×10^{-5} cm^2/s), in the different systems under study: Neuron intracellular fluid (Fluid), tau in fluid (Tau::fluid), tau::microtubule in fluid (Tau::MT::Fluid) and constrained tau in fluid (ConstrainedTau).

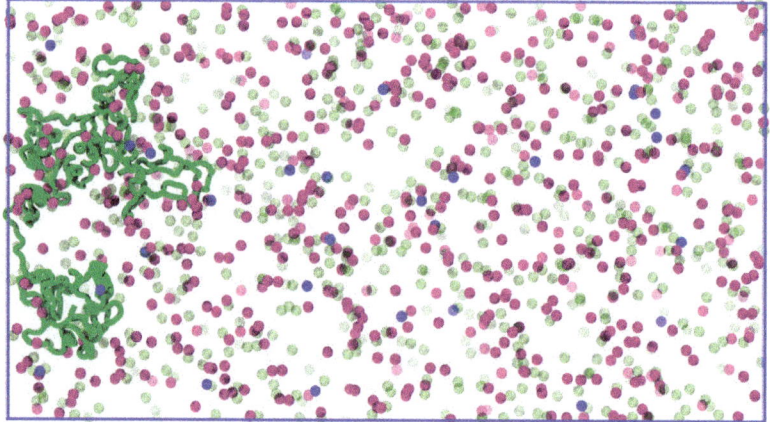

Figure 10. Orthographic view of constrained tau to the box wall. Tau is represented in green cartoon, K$^+$ in purple, Na$^+$ in blue, and Cl$^-$ in green transparent spheres.

Predictions for ion membrane diffusion in neurons indicate a D$_K^+$ of 1.96 cm^2/s and a D$_{Na}^+$ of 1.33 cm^2/s [58]. In addition, the potassium diffusive coupling has been reviewed in neural network processes [59], but less information is mentioned for the behavior of the ions in the axonal region, that is, when exclusively embedded in the intracellular medium. Our results for K$^+$ and Na$^+$ diffusions are slightly higher than the cited literature for transmembrane diffusion, but they result in almost the same difference between these ions.

Looking now to the calculated conductivities (Table 1), we observe very similar conductivity values in all systems, except for Tau::MT in fluid. In general, proteins affect the conductivity in two ways: by carrying a charge and by influencing viscosity. Therefore, it is acceptable that the MT, a bulky and negatively charged protein wall, has the effect of diminishing the global conductivity. The MT has a very negative electrostatic profile that retains the cations, decreasing the diffusion and the conductivity.

Table 1. Calculated conductivity (Λ_i) at 310 K, for each ion type in fluid, in all systems.

System	Ion	Average Conductivity (Λ_i) (S·cm^2/mol)
Intracellular fluid	K$^+$	104.21 ± 2.351
	Na$^+$	87.26 ± 11.621
	Cl$^-$	105.35 ± 7.728
Tau in fluid	K$^+$	100.53 ± 3.904
	Na$^+$	84.60 ± 12.674
	Cl$^-$	103.87 ± 3.667
Tau::MT in fluid	K$^+$	80.39 ± 4.117
	Na$^+$	68.67 ± 14.327
	Cl$^-$	82.93 ± 3.398
Constrained Tau in fluid	K$^+$	99.24 ± 2.914
	Na$^+$	92.40 ± 10.121
	Cl$^-$	103.88 ± 6.523

Our findings indicate that tau in its dephosphorylated form (i.e., when performing its normal function, with the proper conformation in solution and/or associated with MT) maintains the normal K$^+$ diffusion and discreetly increases Na$^+$ diffusion, which, in fact, must be more available to leave the inside of the neuron. The biological relevance of this finding is still unclear, but tau may have a role in the electrical signal transmission along the axon.

4. Discussion

The present study unveils tau's structural preferences and electrostatics, when this protein is free in solution (intracellular fluid) or bound to microtubule in neuron fluid. The electrostatic potential surface of tau (Figure 4) reveals a dipolar protein, where the proline-rich region and MTBR are predominantly composed of basic amino acids (positive charge from side-chains). On the other hand, the N-terminal is acidic, with several amino acids negatively charged at physiological pH. Looking at the tubulin MT potential surface, a very negative electrostatic potential can be observed, especially for the exterior (front), indicating that the binding of tau to its wall will occur through the positive region of this protein, and the N-terminal will tend to move away from the wall, as much as possible. In fact, it is widely reported that the binding occurs between tau MTBR and MT, and the electrostatic distribution of both proteins indicates that this is the best choice to prevent repulsion.

The work of Guo et al. [60] (and references therein) summarizes tau's structural basis and points to a paperclip conformation in solution [50], where the terminals are in close proximity, as we verified with our simulations. Kellogg et al. provided, in their work published last year, a near-atomic model of Tau::MT interactions [22]. In contrast to the paperclip model, observed in solution, they determined that tau is in an extended form, in which each MTBR repeat interacts with one tubulin dimer and with its interface to the next tubulin. This configuration separates the terminals, which agrees with what we see for tau in our Tau::MT simulations (Figure 5), although we sampled a less elongated MTBR. Under dynamics, the PGGG motif localized in each repeat causes consecutives bends that result in a folded MTBR, thus our simulated model interacts with a small number of tubulin monomers. Summing up, structurally, when we simulate our tau model, it behaves as expected in solution, as a paperclip, and shares similarities with the findings of Kellogg, such as the distance between terminals.

Tau performs other important functions in the intracellular neuron environment, besides the well-known functions in MT binding and stabilization [60]. Interestingly, with the exception of the C-termini, each tau domain can be related with the interaction to other proteins. The N-terminal has been involved in the inhibition of axoplasmic transport through a signaling cascade [61] and in interactions with proteins at the neuron plasma membrane [62]. The proline-rich region also interacts with several proteins, specially the Src family of protein kinases [63]. The MTBR has been also associated with an interaction with the lipid membranes [64].

The tau localization in neurons is also an important factor for tau interaction and function. Tau is mainly located in axons [63] and in a much smaller amount in somatodendritic compartments [65–67]. Guo et al. [60] summarizes the presence of tau in different neuron locations, but we highlight here the association with neuronal membranes, which is required for tau participation in intracellular signaling pathways [68,69]. It is also in the membrane that the propagation of electrical impulse occurs, through the flow of positively charged ions. The action potential is maintained due to a concentration difference of certain ions. Potassium has a higher concentration inside the cell, and sodium has a higher concentration on the outside. The flux of these ions, using sodium and potassium channels at the membrane, guarantees the process of polarization/depolarization and maintains an ionic balance. Our simulations used concentrations of Na^+ and K^+ typical for the resting state.

Tau has been reported as a protein that interacts with many others and also with the cell membrane, inside the neuron [47,60,63]. However, little information is provided concerning the effect of this protein on sodium and potassium ions [57,70]. Our simulations point to a possible novel function or role: due to its polar profile, tau may also play a role in the normal flow of the ions present in the intracellular fluid, as it is highly localized in the axon. The axon propagates the signal, like a wire, and this occurs due to the potential difference maintained by the flow of ions in the axon membrane [71].

Recently, the behavior of tau near a membrane was evaluated. Patel et al. [72] thought that once tau aggregates in a similar way to amyloid peptides, it would be valid to look at its behavior when close to the cell membrane. A tendency for the formation of ion channels, which allow the passage of nonspecific ions, was observed. This fact reinforces the role of tau in the balance of K^+ and Na^+ ions within the neuron and in the electrical signal propagation between cells. Our work paves the way to disclose these interactions.

K^+ and Na^+ imbalances in neurons were observed in Alzheimer's disease brains [70]. This fact could arise from the malfunctioning of several proteins, including tau, which causes changes at the structural and signaling level, affecting the normal concentrations of these ions.

Globally, tau has a basic character with a higher content of positively charged amino acids, but among the 27% of charged residues, there are also negatively charged amino acids, which results in a predominantly negative area, the N-terminal (Figure 4). Tau is, therefore, able to interact with ions in an attractive or repulsive manner. In particular, the acidic N-terminal is prone to attracting cations, since it is the tau acidic area and the portion that will interact less with MT, also negatively charged. In fact, RDF and diffusion analyses have suggested that tau retains K^+ near its surface, but maintaining a normal diffusion, and increases Na^+ mobility, which is less probable to be near tau.

5. Conclusions

Tau modelling and simulations disclose many properties concerning tau structure and function. First, the prediction of a tau 3D structure leads to a model that was equilibrated in solution—intracellular ionic fluid—and associated with an MT wall. In both cases, the secondary structure features observed for the middle conformations are in agreement with experimental estimates: tau in fluid is more compact, with N^- and C^- termini closer to each other, and with some helical SS at

MTBR. Tau in Tau::MT systems is in an extended conformation, with helical portions at the MTBR and with the terminals far from each other.

In terms of interactions, tau interacts with two tubulin heterodimers on average, through hydrogen bonds and electrostatic interactions, mostly established between the basic region of tau and the acidic C-termini of tubulins. Kellogg et al. [22] suggested a more elongated MTBR able to interact with a higher number of tubulin dimers. However, we observed a less extended tau MTBR, due to the great dynamics of this protein.

Concerning the effect of tau on ions, we observed a preference for interacting with K^+ cations, through the negatively charged N-terminal. More importantly, tau maintains the normal ion diffusion, being a key factor to cell conductivity and signaling. Tau also increases the conductivity of Na^+ ions, in comparison with the fluid control, in the surrounding environment.

The maintenance of a normal tau structure–function relationship results in a normal interaction with the ions, keeping K^+ close to the tau surface and Na^+ ions more available to leave the cell, as expected, to maintain the intracellular concentration balance of both ions at the axon resting state. Our findings about diffusion and conductivity are a starting point to understand, at the molecular level, the participation of tau in the electrical signal propagation across healthy neurons.

In future work, we intend to study different degrees of phosphorylation in our tau model, to evaluate what it will entail in the structure, in the interaction with MTs, and in the ions' diffusion.

Author Contributions: Conceptualization, A.C.-P.; Investigation, T.C.; Methodology, T.C.; Supervision, A.C.-P.; Writing—original draft, T.C.; Writing—review and editing, F.M. and A.C.-P. All authors discussed the results and commented on the manuscript. All authors read and approved the final manuscript.

Funding: All authors thank the European Union through the European Regional Development Fund (ERDF) under the Competitiveness Operational Program (*BioCell-NanoART = Novel Bio-inspired Cellular Nano-architectures*, POC-A1.1.4-E-2015 nr. 30/01.09.2016). Artur Cavaco-Paulo thanks the support received from the Portuguese Foundation for Science and Technology (FCT) through the strategic funding of UID/BIO/04469/2019 unit and BioTecNorte Operation (NORTE-01-0145-FEDER-000004) funded by the European Regional Development Fund under the scope of Norte2020—Programa Operacional Regional do Norte.

Acknowledgments: Access to computing resources funded by the Project "Search-ON2: Revitalization of HPC infrastructure of UMinho" (NORTE-07-0162-FEDER-000086), co-founded by the North Portugal Regional Operational Programme (ON.2 –O Novo Norte), under the National Strategic Reference Framework (NSRF), through the European Regional Development Fund (ERDF), is gratefully acknowledged. We express our deepest appreciation to Teresa Matamá for valuable advice and discussion on neuron physiology.

Conflicts of Interest: The authors declare no conflict of interest.

References

1. Weingarten, M.D.; Lockwood, A.H.; Hwo, S.Y.; Kirschner, M.W. A protein factor essential for microtubule assembly. *Proc. Natl. Acad. Sci. USA* **1975**, *72*, 1858–1862. [CrossRef]
2. Drubin, D.G.; Kirschner, M.W. Tau protein function in living cells. *J. Cell Biol.* **1986**, *103*, 2739–2746. [CrossRef] [PubMed]
3. Himmler, A.; Drechsel, D.; Kirschner, M.W.; Martin, D.W. Tau consists of a set of proteins with repeated C-terminal microtubule-binding domains and variable N-terminal domains. *Mol. Cell. Biol.* **1989**, *9*, 1381–1388. [CrossRef]
4. Chen, J.; Kanai, Y.; Cowan, N.J.; Hirokawa, N. Projection domains of MAP2 and tau determine spacings between microtubules in dendrites and axons. *Nature* **1992**, *360*, 674–677. [CrossRef]
5. Servier Medical Art by Servier (https://smart.servier.com/), licensed under a Creative Commons Attribution 3.0 Unported License (https://creativecommons.org/licenses/by/3.0/).
6. Andreadis, A. Tau gene alternative splicing: Expression patterns, regulation and modulation of function in normal brain and neurodegenerative diseases. *Biochim. Biophys. Acta (BBA) Mol. Basis Dis.* **2005**, *1739*, 91–103. [CrossRef]
7. Despres, C.; Byrne, C.; Qi, H.; Cantrelle, F.-X.; Huvent, I.; Chambraud, B.; Baulieu, E.-E.; Jacquot, Y.; Landrieu, I.; Lippens, G.; et al. Identification of the Tau phosphorylation pattern that drives its aggregation. *Proc. Natl. Acad. Sci. USA* **2017**, *114*, 9080–9085. [CrossRef]

8. Morishima-Kawashima, M.; Hasegawa, M.; Takio, K.; Suzuki, M.; Yoshida, H.; Watanabe, A.; Titani, K.; Ihara, Y. Hyperphosphorylation of Tau in PHF. *Neurobiol. Aging* **1995**, *16*, 365–371. [CrossRef]
9. Gong, C.X.; Iqbal, K. Hyperphosphorylation of microtubule-associated protein tau: A promising therapeutic target for Alzheimer disease. *Curr. Med. Chem.* **2008**, *15*, 2321–2328. [CrossRef]
10. Šimić, G.; Babić Leko, M.; Wray, S.; Harrington, C.; Delalle, I.; Jovanov-Milošević, N.; Bažadona, D.; Buée, L.; de Silva, R.; Di Giovanni, G.; et al. Tau protein hyperphosphorylation and aggregation in Alzheimer's disease and other tauopathies, and possible neuroprotective strategies. *Biomolecules* **2016**, *6*, 6. [CrossRef] [PubMed]
11. Kolarova, M.; García-Sierra, F.; Bartos, A.; Ricny, J.; Ripova, D. Structure and pathology of tau protein in Alzheimer disease. *Int. J. Alzheimers Dis.* **2012**, *2012*, 1–13. [CrossRef] [PubMed]
12. Kontaxi, C.; Piccardo, P.; Gill, A.C. Lysine-directed post-translational modifications of tau protein in Alzheimer's disease and related tauopathies. *Front. Mol. Biosci.* **2017**, *4*, 56. [CrossRef]
13. Gong, C.X.; Liu, F.; Grundke-Iqbal, I.; Iqbal, K. Post-translational modifications of tau protein in Alzheimer's disease. *J. Neural Transm. (Vienna)* **2005**, *112*, 813–838. [CrossRef]
14. Pevalova, M.; Filipcik, P.; Novak, M.; Avila, J.; Iqbal, K. Post-translational modifications of tau protein. *Bratisl. Lek. Listy* **2006**, *107*, 346–353.
15. Grundke-Iqbal, I.; Iqbal, K.; Quinlan, M.; Tung, Y.C.; Zaidi, M.S.; Wisniewski, H.M. Microtubule-associated protein tau. A component of Alzheimer paired helical filaments. *J. Biol. Chem.* **1986**, *261*, 6084–6089.
16. Grundke-Iqbal, I.; Iqbal, K.; Tung, Y.C.; Quinlan, M.; Wisniewski, H.M.; Binder, L.I. Abnormal phosphorylation of the microtubule-associated protein tau (tau) in Alzheimer cytoskeletal pathology. *Proc. Natl. Acad. Sci. USA* **1986**, *83*, 4913–4917. [CrossRef]
17. Bateman, A.; Martin, M.J.; O'Donovan, C.; Magrane, M.; Alpi, E.; Antunes, R.; Bely, B.; Bingley, M.; Bonilla, C.; Britto, R.; et al. UniProt: The universal protein knowledgebase. *Nucleic Acids Res.* **2017**, *45*, D158–D169.
18. Berman, H.M.; Westbrook, J.; Feng, Z.; Gilliland, G.; Bhat, T.N.; Weissig, H.; Shindyalov, I.N.; Bourne, P.E. The protein data bank. *Nucleic Acids Res.* **2000**, *28*, 235–242. [CrossRef]
19. Li, X.-H.; Culver, J.A.; Rhoades, E. Tau binds to multiple tubulin dimers with helical structure. *J. Am. Chem. Soc.* **2015**, *137*, 9218–9221. [CrossRef]
20. Kar, S.; Fan, J.; Smith, M.J.; Goedert, M.; Amos, L.A. Repeat motifs of tau bind to the insides of microtubules in the absence of taxol. *EMBO J.* **2003**, *22*, 70–77. [CrossRef]
21. Kadavath, H.; Jaremko, M.; Jaremko, Ł.; Biernat, J.; Mandelkow, E.; Zweckstetter, M. Folding of the tau protein on microtubules. *Angew. Chem. Int. Ed.* **2015**, *54*, 10347–10351. [CrossRef]
22. Kellogg, E.H.; Hejab, N.M.A.; Poepsel, S.; Downing, K.H.; DiMaio, F.; Nogales, E. Near-atomic model of microtubule–Tau interactions. *Science* **2018**, *360*, 1242–1246. [CrossRef]
23. Zabik, N.L.; Imhof, M.M.; Martic-Milne, S. Structural evaluations of tau protein conformation: Methodologies and approaches. *Biochem. Cell Biol.* **2017**, *95*, 338–349. [CrossRef]
24. Zhang, Y. Progress and challenges in protein structure prediction. *Curr. Opin. Struct. Biol.* **2008**, *18*, 342–348. [CrossRef]
25. Moult, J.; Fidelis, K.; Kryshtafovych, A.; Schwede, T.; Tramontano, A. Critical assessment of methods of protein structure prediction (CASP)—Round x: Critical Assessment of structure prediction. *Proteins Str. Funct. Bioinform.* **2014**, *82*, 1–6. [CrossRef]
26. Zhang, C.; Mortuza, S.M.; He, B.; Wang, Y.; Zhang, Y. Template-based and free modeling of I-TASSER and QUARK pipelines using predicted contact maps in CASP12. *Proteins Struct. Funct. Bioinform.* **2018**, *86*, 136–151. [CrossRef]
27. Izhikevich, E.M. *Dynamical Systems in Neuroscience: The Geometry of Excitability and Bursting*; MIT Press: Cambridge, MA, USA, 2005.
28. Barreto, E.; Cressman, J.R. Ion concentration dynamics as a mechanism for neuronal bursting. *J. Biol. Phys.* **2011**, *37*, 361–373. [CrossRef]
29. Raimondo, J.V.; Burman, R.J.; Katz, A.A.; Akerman, C.J. Ion dynamics during seizures. *Front. Cell. Neurosci.* **2015**, *9*, 419. [CrossRef]
30. Abraham, M.J.; van der Spoel, D.; Lindahl, E.; Hess, B. *Development Team GROMACS User Manual Version 5.1.5*; GROMACS, Groningen University: Groningen, The Netherlands, 2017.
31. Bussi, G.; Donadio, D.; Parrinello, M. Canonical sampling through velocity rescaling. *J. Chem. Phys.* **2007**, *126*, 014101. [CrossRef]

32. Martoňák, R.; Laio, A.; Parrinello, M. Predicting crystal structures: The Parrinello-Rahman method revisited. *Phys. Rev. Lett.* **2003**, *90*, 4. [CrossRef]
33. Berendsen, H.J.C.; van der Spoel, D.; van Drunen, R. GROMACS: A message-passing parallel molecular dynamics implementation. *Comput. Phys. Commun.* **1995**, *91*, 43–56. [CrossRef]
34. Huang, W.; Lin, Z.; van Gunsteren, W.F. Validation of the GROMOS 54A7 force field with respect to β-peptide folding. *J. Chem. Theory Comput.* **2011**, *7*, 1237–1243. [CrossRef]
35. Schmid, N.; Eichenberger, A.P.; Choutko, A.; Riniker, S.; Winger, M.; Mark, A.E.; van Gunsteren, W.F. Definition and testing of the GROMOS force-field versions 54A7 and 54B7. *Eur. Biophys. J.* **2011**, *40*, 843. [CrossRef]
36. Darden, T.; York, D.; Pedersen, L. Particle mesh Ewald: An N·log (N) method for Ewald sums in large systems. *J. Chem. Phys.* **1993**, *98*, 10089–10092. [CrossRef]
37. Hess, B. P-LINCS: A parallel linear constraint solver for molecular simulation. *J. Chem. Theory Comput.* **2008**, *4*, 116–122. [CrossRef]
38. Miyamoto, S.; Kollman, P.A. Settle: An analytical version of the SHAKE and RATTLE algorithm for rigid water models. *J. Comput. Chem.* **1992**, *13*, 952–962. [CrossRef]
39. Cordomí, A.; Edholm, O.; Perez, J.J. Effect of force field parameters on sodium and potassium ion binding to dipalmitoyl phosphatidylcholine bilayers. *J. Chem. Theory Comput.* **2009**, *5*, 2125–2134. [CrossRef]
40. Allen, M.P.; Tildesley, D.J. *Computer Simulations of Liquids*; Oxford Science Publications: Oxford, UK, 1987.
41. Dolinsky, T.J.; Nielsen, J.E.; McCammon, J.A.; Baker, N.A. PDB2PQR: An automated pipeline for the setup of Poisson-Boltzmann electrostatics calculations. *Nucleic Acids Res.* **2004**, *32*, W665–W667. [CrossRef]
42. Jurrus, E.; Engel, D.; Star, K.; Monson, K.; Brandi, J.; Felberg, L.E.; Brookes, D.H.; Wilson, L.; Chen, J.; Liles, K.; et al. Improvements to the APBS biomolecular solvation software suite. *Protein Sci.* **2018**, *27*, 112–128. [CrossRef]
43. Baker, N.A.; Sept, D.; Joseph, S.; Holst, M.J.; McCammon, J.A. Electrostatics of nanosystems: Application to microtubules and the ribosome. *Proc. Natl. Acad. Sci. USA* **2001**, *98*, 10037–10041. [CrossRef]
44. PyMOL; *The PyMOL Molecular Graphics System, Version 2.0 Schrödinger*; DeLano Scientific LLC: Portland, OR, USA, 2000.
45. Humphrey, W.; Dalke, A.; Schulten, K. VMD: Visual molecular dynamics. *J. Mol. Graph.* **1996**, *14*, 33–38. [CrossRef]
46. Luo, Y.; Ma, B.; Nussinov, R.; Wei, G. Structural insight into tau protein's paradox of intrinsically disordered behavior, self-acetylation activity, and aggregation. *J. Phys. Chem. Lett.* **2014**, *5*, 3026–3031. [CrossRef]
47. Avila, J.; Jiménez, J.S.; Sayas, C.L.; Bolós, M.; Zabala, J.C.; Rivas, G.; Hernández, F. Tau structures. *Front. Ag. Neurosci.* **2016**, *8*, 262. [CrossRef]
48. Melo, A.M.; Coraor, J.; Alpha-Cobb, G.; Elbaum-Garfinkle, S.; Nath, A.; Rhoades, E. A functional role for intrinsic disorder in the tau-tubulin complex. *Proc. Natl. Acad. Sci. USA* **2016**, *113*, 14336–14341. [CrossRef]
49. Cabrales Fontela, Y.; Kadavath, H.; Biernat, J.; Riedel, D.; Mandelkow, E.; Zweckstetter, M. Multivalent cross-linking of actin filaments and microtubules through the microtubule-associated protein Tau. *Nat. Commun.* **2017**, *8*, 1981. [CrossRef]
50. Jeganathan, S.; von Bergen, M.; Brutlach, H.; Steinhoff, H.-J.; Mandelkow, E. Global hairpin folding of tau in solution. *Biochemistry* **2006**, *45*, 2283–2293. [CrossRef]
51. Andronesi, O.C.; von Bergen, M.; Biernat, J.; Seidel, K.; Griesinger, C.; Mandelkow, E.; Baldus, M. Characterization of Alzheimer's-like paired helical filaments from the core domain of tau protein using solid-state NMR spectroscopy. *J. Am. Chem. Soc.* **2008**, *130*, 5922–5928. [CrossRef]
52. Mukrasch, M.D.; Bibow, S.; Korukottu, J.; Jeganathan, S.; Biernat, J.; Griesinger, C.; Mandelkow, E.; Zweckstetter, M. Structural polymorphism of 441-residue tau at single residue resolution. *PLoS Biol.* **2009**, *7*, e1000034. [CrossRef]
53. Kadavath, H.; Hofele, R.V.; Biernat, J.; Kumar, S.; Tepper, K.; Urlaub, H.; Mandelkow, E.; Zweckstetter, M. Tau stabilizes microtubules by binding at the interface between tubulin heterodimers. *Proc. Natl. Acad. Sci. USA* **2015**, *112*, 7501–7506. [CrossRef]
54. Duan, A.R.; Jonasson, E.M.; Alberico, E.O.; Li, C.; Scripture, J.P.; Miller, R.A.; Alber, M.S.; Goodson, H.V. Interactions between tau and different conformations of tubulin: Implications for tau function and mechanism. *J. Mol. Biol.* **2017**, *429*, 1424–1438. [CrossRef]

55. Janning, D.; Igaev, M.; Sündermann, F.; Brühmann, J.; Beutel, O.; Heinisch, J.J.; Bakota, L.; Piehler, J.; Junge, W.; Brandt, R. Single-molecule tracking of tau reveals fast kiss-and-hop interaction with microtubules in living neurons. *Mol. Biol. Cell* **2014**, *25*, 3541–3551. [CrossRef]
56. Vanýsek, P. *Ionic Conductivity and Diffusion at Infinite Dilution, Handbook of Chemistry and Physics*, 93th ed.; CRC Press: Boca Raton, FL, USA, 1992.
57. Hinrichs, M.H.; Jalal, A.; Brenner, B.; Mandelkow, E.; Kumar, S.; Scholz, T. Tau protein diffuses along the microtubule lattice. *J. Biol. Chem.* **2012**, *287*, 38559–38568. [CrossRef]
58. Qian, N.; Sejnowski, T.J. Electrodiffusion model of electrical conduction in neuronal processes. In *Cellular Mechanisms of Conditioning and Behavioral Plasticity*; Woody, C.D., Alkon, D.L., McGaugh, J.L., Eds.; Springer: Boston, MA, USA, 1988; pp. 237–244. ISBN 978-1-4757-9612-4.
59. Durand, D.M.; Park, E.-H.; Jensen, A.L. Potassium diffusive coupling in neural networks. *Philos. Trans. R. Soc. Lond. B Biol. Sci.* **2010**, *365*, 2347–2362. [CrossRef]
60. Guo, T.; Noble, W.; Hanger, D.P. Roles of tau protein in health and disease. *Acta Neuropathol.* **2017**, *133*, 665–704. [CrossRef]
61. Kanaan, N.M.; Morfini, G.A.; LaPointe, N.E.; Pigino, G.F.; Patterson, K.R.; Song, Y.; Andreadis, A.; Fu, Y.; Brady, S.T.; Binder, L.I. Pathogenic forms of tau inhibit kinesin-dependent axonal transport through a mechanism involving activation of axonal phosphotransferases. *J. Neurosci.* **2011**, *31*, 9858–9868. [CrossRef]
62. Brandt, R.; Léger, J.; Lee, G. Interaction of tau with the neural plasma membrane mediated by tau's amino-terminal projection domain. *J. Cell Biol.* **1995**, *131*, 1327–1340. [CrossRef]
63. Morris, M.; Maeda, S.; Vossel, K.; Mucke, L. The many faces of tau. *Neuron* **2011**, *70*, 410–426. [CrossRef]
64. Georgieva, E.R.; Xiao, S.; Borbat, P.P.; Freed, J.H.; Eliezer, D. Tau binds to lipid membrane surfaces via short amphipathic helices located in its microtubule-binding repeats. *Biophys. J.* **2014**, *107*, 1441–1452. [CrossRef]
65. Ittner, L.M.; Ke, Y.D.; Delerue, F.; Bi, M.; Gladbach, A.; van Eersel, J.; Wölfing, H.; Chieng, B.C.; Christie, M.J.; Napier, I.A.; et al. Dendritic function of tau mediates amyloid-β toxicity in Alzheimer's disease mouse models. *Cell* **2010**, *142*, 387–397. [CrossRef]
66. Tashiro, K.; Hasegawa, M.; Ihara, Y.; Iwatsubo, T. Somatodendritic localization of phosphorylated tau in neonatal and adult rat cerebral cortex. *NeuroReport* **1997**, *8*, 2797–2801. [CrossRef]
67. Kimura, T.; Whitcomb, D.J.; Jo, J.; Regan, P.; Piers, T.; Heo, S.; Brown, C.; Hashikawa, T.; Murayama, M.; Seok, H.; et al. Microtubule-associated protein tau is essential for long-term depression in the hippocampus. *Philos. Trans. R. Soc. Lond. B Biol. Sci.* **2014**, *369*, 20130144. [CrossRef]
68. Pooler, A.M.; Hanger, D.P. Functional implications of the association of tau with the plasma membrane. *Biochem. Soc. Trans.* **2010**, *38*, 1012–1015. [CrossRef]
69. Kim, W.; Lee, S.; Jung, C.; Ahmed, A.; Lee, G.; Hall, G.F. Interneuronal transfer of human tau between lamprey central neurons in situ. *J. Alzheimers Dis.* **2010**, *19*, 647–664. [CrossRef]
70. Vitvitsky, V.M.; Garg, S.K.; Keep, R.F.; Albin, R.L.; Banerjee, R. Na$^+$ and K$^+$ ion imbalances in Alzheimer's disease. *Biochim. Biophys. Acta (BBA) Mol. Basis Dis.* **2012**, *1822*, 1671–1681. [CrossRef]
71. Hodgkin, A.L.; Huxley, A.F. A quantitative description of membrane current and its application to conduction and excitation in nerve. *J. Phys.* **1952**, *117*, 500–544. [CrossRef]
72. Patel, N.; Ramachandran, S.; Azimov, R.; Kagan, B.L.; Lal, R. Ion Channel formation by tau protein: implications for Alzheimer's disease and tauopathies. *Biochemistry* **2015**, *54*, 7320–7325. [CrossRef]

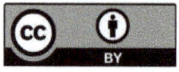

© 2019 by the authors. Licensee MDPI, Basel, Switzerland. This article is an open access article distributed under the terms and conditions of the Creative Commons Attribution (CC BY) license (http://creativecommons.org/licenses/by/4.0/).

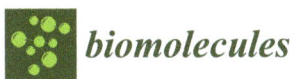

Review

Recent Advances in Computational Protocols Addressing Intrinsically Disordered Proteins

Supriyo Bhattacharya [1,*] and Xingcheng Lin [2,3]

1. Division of Research Informatics, Beckman Research Institute at City of Hope National Medical Center, Duarte, CA 91010, USA
2. Center for Theoretical Biological Physics, Rice University, Houston, TX 77030, USA; xclin@mit.edu
3. Department of Chemistry, Massachusetts Institute of Technology, Cambridge, MA 02139, USA
* Correspondence: sbhattach@coh.org; Tel.: +1-626-218-4837

Received: 5 March 2019; Accepted: 10 April 2019; Published: 11 April 2019

Abstract: Intrinsically disordered proteins (IDP) are abundant in the human genome and have recently emerged as major therapeutic targets for various diseases. Unlike traditional proteins that adopt a definitive structure, IDPs in free solution are disordered and exist as an ensemble of conformations. This enables the IDPs to signal through multiple signaling pathways and serve as scaffolds for multi-protein complexes. The challenge in studying IDPs experimentally stems from their disordered nature. Nuclear magnetic resonance (NMR), circular dichroism, small angle X-ray scattering, and single molecule Förster resonance energy transfer (FRET) can give the local structural information and overall dimension of IDPs, but seldom provide a unified picture of the whole protein. To understand the conformational dynamics of IDPs and how their structural ensembles recognize multiple binding partners and small molecule inhibitors, knowledge-based and physics-based sampling techniques are utilized in-silico, guided by experimental structural data. However, efficient sampling of the IDP conformational ensemble requires traversing the numerous degrees of freedom in the IDP energy landscape, as well as force-fields that accurately model the protein and solvent interactions. In this review, we have provided an overview of the current state of computational methods for studying IDP structure and dynamics and discussed the major challenges faced in this field.

Keywords: intrinsically disordered protein; conformational ensemble; nuclear magnetic resonance; replica exchange molecular dynamics; drug design

1. Introduction

Intrinsically disordered proteins (IDPs) have emerged as an important class of biomolecules that are involved in a variety of cellular functions, ranging from signaling to gene expression, chaperoning, and cellular transport [1]. These proteins lack a definite folded structure and adopt an ensemble of conformations in their physiological environment. Their disordered nature is essential for their biological function, as has been discussed in many recent reviews [1–4]. The IDP function is regulated through a fine balance of alternative splicing, post-translational modifications, expression level, and duration of presence in the cell [2]. Due to their dynamic nature, many IDPs can interact with multiple proteins with low affinity but high specificity, enabling them to act as hubs in signaling networks, or adapters for multi-protein scaffolds [1]. The low affinity of certain IDPs facilitates fast disengagement from signaling partners, which could be advantageous for rapid shutdown and switching of signaling, allowing better control over the cellular machinery [5]. Conversely, IDPs have also been found to interact with their partner proteins with ultra-high affinity, while maintaining structural disorder and flexibility in the bound state. [6] Dysregulation of IDP function has been linked to multiple cancers, as well as diabetes, cardiovascular, and neurodegenerative diseases [4]. IDP conformational dynamics has been proposed to facilitate phenotypic switching in stem cells and malignancy, without involving mutagenesis [7]. Therefore, IDPs form an important class of therapeutic targets, whose novel mechanisms and dynamic properties open new ways of regulating cellular function through clinical intervention [8].

In past decades, the emergence of IDPs has changed the traditional structure-function paradigm of folded proteins, which posits that sequence dictates the native state (an ensemble of closely related structures), which in turn dictates function. In contrast, the sequence of an IDP encodes an ensemble of structurally diverse conformations, which exchange in the picosecond to millisecond timescale under physiological conditions [9]. The biological function of the IDP is governed by the nature of this ensemble as well as the associated dynamics of conformational exchange. Experimentally, the IDPs are studied using a combination of techniques, including nuclear magnetic resonance (NMR), small angle X-ray scattering (SAXS), circular dichroism (CD), and single molecule spectroscopy [3]. These methods provide information about local residue contacts and side chain orientations, secondary structure content, as well as the dynamics and lifetime of such contacts. Such information, however, comes as statistical averages of entire ensembles, and do not give information about individual conformations in the ensemble. The structural heterogeneities of IDPs require further development of analytical/computational tools for an accurate description of their statistical properties. Previous major efforts include using modified polymer models that are more relevant for the dynamics of IDPs [10–12], testing and improving on the solvent model [13,14], and the development of new tools for analyses of experimental data [15,16]. An alternative approach would be to combine experimental data with statistical structural models and physics-based simulations of protein dynamics to generate the molecular models that account for the heterogeneous IDP ensemble [17]. Besides this, coarse grain and enhanced sampling simulations can give valuable insights into the oligomerization and interaction of IDPs with partner proteins. However, the sheer time and length scales associated with IDP dynamics pose serious challenges to the application of computational methods, as is evident from the recent literature [18,19]. Needless to say, there is an acute demand in the scientific community for precise atomistic models of IDPs for gaining functional insights as well as designing therapeutic agents inhibiting their functions. In this review, we discuss the various computational protocols that are relevant to IDP research. Such protocols range from structure prediction of IDPs, studying their dynamic behavior and mechanisms of partner protein interaction, to small molecule inhibitor design. In the end, we summarize the challenges involved in applying these methods and possible future directions in this field.

2. Energy Landscape of Intrinsically Disordered Proteins

All proteins exhibit complex dynamic behavior, ranging from high frequency vibrations to slower local perturbations (picoseconds to microseconds), to even slower domain motions (microseconds to seconds). In a landmark paper, Wolynes and coworkers connected the dynamics, conformational sampling, and folding of proteins to the concept of free energy landscape [20]. Well folded proteins that adopt a definite three-dimensional (3D) structure show a funnel like landscape, where the initially formed secondary structure elements cooperatively fold into a tertiary structure stabilized by native contacts. The sequence of such a protein contains strategically placed hydrophobic residues, which in the folded state come together and form a hydrophobic core by efficient expulsion of water. An energy landscape describing such a process is relatively smooth with less frustration (as shown in the schematic in Figure 1A), although misfolded states and intermediate stable states could be populated in the landscape. In protein folding, frustration refers to the hindrance in progressing down the folding funnel, due to a lack of cooperativity in forming increasingly stable contacts. In contrast with a folded protein, the energy landscape of an IDP is proposed to be rugged (Figure 1B), where multiple states are separated by shallow energy barriers to facilitate exchange between the states [21–23]. Secondary structure elements may be present in free solution, but they do not cooperatively contact each other to fold into a stable structure as in the case of folded proteins. A reasonable explanation for the IDPs' resistance to folding is the relative absence of hydrophobic amino acids in their sequences compared to folded proteins [3]. These amino acids are critical for forming the protein core and their absence stabilizes the unfolded states. In some IDPs, the abundance of disorder promoting residues, such as glycine and proline, inhibit the formation of stable helices and prevent folding tertiary structures. IDPs thus exist as an ensemble of extended or partially folded states in free solution with frequent exchange between these states. This rapid exchange prevents the detection of any single state in NMR or circular dichroism experiments [21]. Each of the IDP conformations could be functionally relevant in recognizing specific partner proteins for signaling or arranging a scaffold. In this regard, IDPs are distinct from random polypeptide sequences [21] because, although disordered, the IDP conformations could strategically orient specific recognition motifs such as phosphorylation sites to facilitate interaction with partner proteins. Post-translational modifications such as phosphorylation play a critical role in reshaping the conformational landscape of IDPs, preparing them for specific binding and signaling events [24,25]. Although IDPs mostly remain disordered in free solution, one or multiple intermediate states with ordered motifs may still be present in the energy landscape [26,27], albeit at a higher (worse) free energy than the disordered conformations [28]. In certain IDPs, such as the Aβ40 peptide, these partially ordered states become more predominant at a higher temperature, indicating their presence in the free energy landscape at a higher free energy than the unfolded states [28]. The presence of such partially ordered states in the IDP energy landscapes has been shown using NMR and circular dichroism, as well as enhanced sampling molecular dynamics (MD) methods [28–30]. The partially ordered states may be lowered in energy and stabilized upon binding to partner proteins or aggregation (e.g., amyloid fibrils), as shown in Figure 1B [28,31]. Also, the presence of diverse partially ordered states in the free energy landscape may facilitate interaction with multiple partner proteins, which is a hallmark of IDPs.

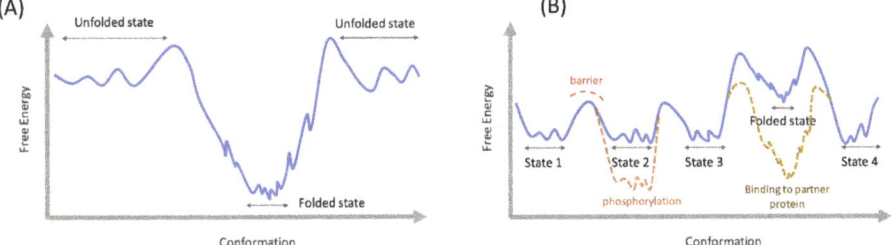

Figure 1. (**A**) Schematic free energy landscape of a folded protein; the folded state is comprised of an ensemble of structurally related states; (**B**) hypothetical intrinsically disordered protein (IDP) landscape showing four disordered (unfolded) states populated in free solution, separated by shallow energy barriers for rapid exchange; the multiple shallow minima in the disordered state free energy landscape indicate high structural flexibility; post translational modifications such as phosphorylation can stabilize one of the states over the others; a folded state is also present in the energy landscape, but only stabilized upon binding to a partner protein.

3. Structure Prediction and Conformational Dynamics

3.1. Conformational Selection Based Methods

Computational structure prediction for folded proteins suffers from the challenges of conformational sampling, due to the numerous degrees of freedom of the polypeptide chain, and the difficulty for a protein to run across thermodynamic barriers among a set of structurally close decoys within limited simulation time to identify the correct native ensemble. In contrast, IDPs have a larger set of "correct answers" with regard to structure—an ensemble of highly diverse conformations ranging from random coil to partially folded structures [32]. The challenge is in exhaustively sampling the set of thermodynamically relevant conformations under physiological conditions, that explain the available experimental structural data (e.g., NMR, SAXS). So far, several computational methods have been proposed that utilize experimental structural information to derive conformational ensembles of IDPs. These methods can be categorized into two groups: a) one that uses NMR, SAXS, or Förster resonance energy transfer (FRET) data to select the relevant conformations from a pool of previously generated structural ensemble, and b) one that uses structural restraints derived from experimental data to drive MD or Monte Carlo (MC) based sampling methods to generate the conformational ensembles [19,22]. The former category includes methods such as TraDES [33,34], flexible-meccano [35], ASTEROIDS [36], and ENSEMBLE [37]. Both TraDES and flexible-meccano use probability distributions of amino acid orientations from crystal structures to sample the IDP conformations. While flexible-meccano generates chain conformations by randomly selecting the Φ/ψ dihedral angles of the residues from the distributions derived from the crystal structure database, TraDES grows the chain one residue at a time, using a Markov process. Both methods use specialized algorithms to accelerate the conformational sampling, by using fast detection of steric clashes between atoms and avoiding slow force field-based energy calculations. The conformational sampling can also be further guided by utilizing secondary structure prediction or other user-defined criteria. Such a conformational search is by no means exhaustive and becomes more challenging for larger proteins. Moreover, electrostatics and solvent-protein interactions are ignored, which may lead to unrealistic protein conformations in the ensemble, for example with water exposed hydrophobic segments. Conformation generation programs like TraDES and flexible-meccano are often used in conjunction with conformation selection programs such as ASTEROIDS and ENSEMBLE to generate a subset of conformers that fit available experimental data, such as chemical shifts, NOE (nuclear overhauser effect), RDC (residual dipolar coupling), PRE (paramagnetic relaxation enhancement), SAXS, and hydrodynamic radius (Figure 2A). Starting from an initial pool of over 100,000 chain conformations, ENSEMBLE selects a random subset of 5000 or less conformers and calculates the experimental properties, such as RDC, by averaging over the ensemble [37]. It then tests the agreement of the calculated properties to the observed experimental data. The program then adds more conformations to the set and eliminates existing conformations using a Monte Carlo scheme, coupled with simulated annealing. The process converges when further iterations do not improve the agreement with the observed data. ASTEROIDS uses a genetic algorithm to evolve an initial pool of conformations to minimize a fitness function based on the difference between calculated and observed experimental parameters. Such an ensemble filtering approach, when combined with maximum likelihood algorithms, can mitigate the problem of overfitting [38,39].

3.2. Molecular Dynamics Based Methods

In contrast to the above methods that attempt to reproduce the experimentally observed IDP ensemble by random sampling of polypeptide conformations, MD based methods perform the conformational sampling using molecular dynamics algorithms, which simulate the dynamic behavior of IDPs under physiological conditions in a solvent environment. Due to the computationally intensive energy functions and the difficulty to cross over energy barriers, most MD based methods are orders of magnitude slower than random sampling based algorithms. However, the benefit of MD based methods is in the insights gained into the protein dynamics, such as exchange rates between different conformations, persistence of specific inter-residue contacts, or the interactions of solvent and ions with the protein. To facilitate sampling of the rugged conformational landscapes of IDPs, MD algorithms are usually coupled with enhanced sampling methods (also known as generalized-ensemble algorithms [29,40]), such as replica exchange (REMD) [41], bias exchange metadynamics (BEMD) [42], and temperature cool walking (TCW) [29,43]. In REMD, multiple MD simulations (replicas) of the same system are performed in parallel at different temperatures, with frequent exchange of operating temperatures between the replicas [41]. In TCW, the simulations are performed at two different temperatures, the target temperature and a higher temperature with transitions between the two temperatures facilitated by simulated annealing. In both methods, by temporarily raising the temperature of a replica, the system is able to overcome energy barriers that would have restricted sampling, had the MD been performed at a single temperature. The exchange probabilities are selected such that a thermodynamically consistent structural ensemble is obtained at the target temperature. The advantage of TWC over REMD is the lower computational resource requirement. While in REMD, 30 or more separate simulations are often required to cover the desired temperature range, but only two simulations are necessary in TWC, although the transition between the two temperatures is computationally demanding due to the use of simulated annealing (for a comparison between the two methods, please see [29]). In BEMD [42], multiple simulations (replicas) are performed at the same temperature, but with time-dependent biasing potentials along different sets of collective variables for each replica, with frequent exchanges of the biasing potentials between the replicas. Bias exchange metadynamics can be computationally efficient, since fewer replicas are required as compared to REMD. However, as with standard metadynamics simulations, the choice of the collective variables is crucial for proper sampling of the conformational space. Using REMD, Patel et al. compared the disordered conformational ensembles of two heat shock proteins, explaining their difference in efficiency for binding to unfolding proteins at higher temperatures [44]. The BEMD has been used to map the conformational landscapes of several IDPs, such as the Aβ40 peptide involved in Alzheimer's disease and the islet amyloid polypeptide involved in type 2 diabetes [28,45]. Temperature cool walking was used to study the effect of paramagnetic spin labels on the conformational ensembles of IDPs [46]. In relation to the IDP ensemble, the structures themselves and the rates of transition between these structures, which govern the kinetics, are of equal importance. A change in environment, such as pH and temperature and post translation modifications, can affect these rates and hence the biological function of the IDPs. With the advent of fast GPU (graphical processing unit) powered computing networks, it is now possible to map transition rates among various equilibrium states in the protein landscape, using methods such as Markov state model (MSM) analysis [47]. The MSM uses numerous independent MD trajectories to calculate the equilibrium states and the rates of transition between these states. However, due to the numerous degrees of freedom in the IDP landscape, it is still challenging to apply MSM to calculate transition rates in IDPs. Using the distributed computing network GPUGRID.net [48], Stanley et al. developed a MSM for the kinase-inducible domain (KID) of the transcription factor CREB (cAMP response element-binding protein), and showed that phosphorylation slows down the conformational kinetics and facilitates binding with partner proteins [49]. Markov state model was also used to map the conformational landscape of the hIAPP peptide involved in fibril formation in type II diabetes [30]. Alternatively, exhaustive simulations of protein dynamics using ASIC hardwares such as Anton [50,51] have proved successful in folding proteins and studying protein dynamics over recent years [52]. The applications of Anton in studying IDPs provide another avenue for generating and understanding their heterogeneous structural ensembles [32].

One method which is promising for simulating IDP dynamics is generalized Newton–Euler inverse mass operator (GNEIMO) torsional dynamics [53–55]. By performing protein dynamics in the low frequency torsional degrees of freedom (DOF) while freezing the high frequency bond and angle vibrations via constraints, GNEIMO is able to simulate long timescale transitions that are difficult to achieve in all-atom Cartesian MD [56]. Besides the bonds and angles, selective torsional DOFs can be constrained as well, depending on the system of interest. Thus, given a protein with both disordered and folded regions, for instance, GNEIMO can simulate the conformational dynamics of the disordered domain in the environment of the relatively static folded domain, while keeping the backbone (and core sidechains) of the folded domain frozen. Constraining the uninteresting DOFs will lead to accelerated sampling and a higher chance of simulating long timescale transitions in the disordered region [55,56]. The GNEIMO employs specialized algorithms that are designed to preserve accurate dynamics with constrained DOFs, without introducing artifacts [55,57]. The GNEIMO, combined with temperature replica exchange, was used to simulate the dynamics of the flexible regions of fasciculin and calmodulin [56]. During dynamics, two of the experimentally verified conformational states of fasciculin were sampled by GNEIMO. For calmodulin, GNEIMO achieved the transition between the calcium bound and unbound conformations. Such conformational transitions were achieved in all-atom Cartesian MD by using biasing potentials [58], or using an united atom Gō model [59].

The above examples demonstrate that the MD based methods, including both the enhanced sampling and brute force techniques, can give valuable insight into the conformational equilibria and the associated kinetics of IDPs. Intrinsically disordered proteins typically show a wide range of motion, from pico- to microseconds and longer. The rates/correlation times in these different temporal regimes, along with the flexibility of the protein domains (represented by the order parameters), can be obtained by deconvoluting the experimental data from NMR relaxation and fluorescence correlation spectroscopy (FRET-FCS) [60]. The question remains whether MD simulations can accurately reproduce the dynamic behavior of IDPs as reported by these experimental methods. In recent years, several works have compared the quantitative dynamics information of IDPs obtained from the experiments to those from the simulations. Tryptophan fluorescence quenching rates obtained with several model (disordered) peptides were found to be in agreement with microsecond scale MD simulations [61]. This work also addressed the effect of force field and solvent viscosity on the rate of inter-residue contact formation and diffusivity, which govern dynamic behavior. Using FRET-FCS, Soranno et al. [62] measured the relaxation time for inter-termini distance in the unfolded protein L, which agreed with the quantity calculated from microsecond long MD simulations on the ANTON supercomputer by Piana et al. [14]. The MD simulations were performed using an improved water model (TIP4P-D) to better reproduce the extended ensembles of IDPs. Using three different techniques (high-field ^{15}N spin relaxation, low-field ^{1}H relaxometry, nanosecond fluorescence correlation spectroscopy), Rezaei-Ghaleh et al. monitored the conformational dynamics of α-synuclein at different timescales (picoseconds to nanoseconds to 10s of nanoseconds) [63]. These timescales were compared to the equivalent parameters calculated from a 16 µs MD trajectory of α-synuclein in explicit water [14]. While the relaxation rates obtained from the low field ^{1}H relaxometry and nanosecond fluorescence correlation spectroscopy were in agreement with the values obtained from MD, the relaxation times obtained from ^{15}N spin relaxation were over-predicted. Also, compared to the order parameters from NMR, MD showed relatively restrictive backbone motion. To match the order parameter values from MD to those from NMR, the authors had to apply a scaling factor to the MD time axis. The results from these studies indicate that the MD simulations, with the appropriate force field and simulation length, can provide quantitative insights into IDP dynamics. Nevertheless, the discrepancies with experiments depending on the timescale of motion highlights the complex scenario with applying MD methods in studying IDP dynamics. This also impresses upon the need for developing accurate protein and solvent force fields that capture realistic dynamics as well as ensemble properties.

3.3. Force-Field Development for Intrisically Disordered Proteins

For MD based methods, accuracy of the underlying force field is a key determinant of the reliability of the obtained results. From the time when protein crystallography was first introduced in the 1950s, the general paradigm of protein function has rested with its folded structure, and most efforts were originally spent in understanding and predicting the native state of globular proteins. Early force field development focused on stabilizing the protein crystal structures, with less attention being payed to the unfolded state. As a result, these force fields generated conformations with overpopulated secondary structure elements (i.e., alpha helices and beta sheets) [18]. However, such inaccuracies have been largely corrected in the recent versions of these force fields by modifying the protein backbone dihedral parameters, and validating against experimental NMR and SAXS data [64–67]. The other issue with many general-purpose force fields is the over-stabilization of collapsed, molten globule like states compared to extended states. Both these issues are especially relevant while studying IDP structural ensembles, which lack extensive secondary structures and are less compact than folded proteins. The accuracy of various force fields has been widely discussed in the literature [18,68]. Rauscher et al. did a detailed comparison of CHARMM, AMBER, and OPLS force fields in conjunction with several water models (TIP3P, TIP4P, and implicit solvent) [69] (Figure 2B,C). This study highlighted the inherent bias of all-atom force fields towards certain secondary structures, for example, the propensity of CHARMM36 to overpopulate left-handed α-helices in disordered peptides. Also evident was the stabilization of over-compact structures by CHARMM36 and FF99SB*-ILDN (Figure 2C). Corrections to such biases or deficiencies have been partially addressed in revisions to the existing force fields that are targeted specifically towards simulating IDPs. Examples include force fields from the AMBER family, such as FF03* and FF99SB* [65], and CHARMM family force fields CHARMM36m [67] and CHARMM22* [70]. Since solvent–protein interactions play an important role in the structural propensity of IDPs, it is desirable, alongside the protein backbone parameters, to optimize the protein–water interaction parameters as well. Such modifications produced the AMBER FF03ws [71] and, recently, the A99SB-disp [32] force fields. The latter was developed through a combined optimization of protein dihedral parameters, hydrogen-bonding potentials and partial charges alongside water van der Waals parameters to reproduce the structural properties of both folded and disordered proteins. Other efforts in the development of force fields for IDPs include RSFF [72,73], KBFF [74], CUFIX [75], and ff14idp [76].

3.4. Coarse Grain and Multiscale Methods

Due to the computational expense of all-atom MD simulations in explicit water, coarse-grain protein and solvent models are viable alternatives to study the conformational ensemble of IDPs. In the coarse grain description of the polypeptide chain, several atoms are combined into one moiety, with a similar treatment applied to the solvent atoms. A special force field function is developed to model the interaction between the different coarse grain moieties in a way that reproduces protein-specific behavior. An alternative approach to coarse-graining is the implicit solvation model, where the explicit solvent molecules are replaced by a mean field approximation, while the protein is kept fully atomistic. Implicit solvation models can reproduce aspects of the protein–solvent interaction, such as cavity penalty, electrostatic screening, and nonpolar burial. However, the detailed behavior of individual solvent molecules at the protein/bulk water interface, including water mediated hydrogen bonds, are not retrieved in such models. The use of coarse grain models reduces the number of particles in the simulation box, leading to a significant gain in computational performance and enhanced sampling of the conformational space. These models can be potentially used to simulate long timescale processes, such as crowding and self-assembly of IDPs, which are normally beyond the reach of all-atom MD based methods. Implicit solvation methods such as Generalized Born [77] have been widely used to predict structures of folded proteins [78,79]. However, their application to IDPs [23,80] is limited by 1) the computational cost involved in frequently calculating the effective Born radii in a rapidly changing protein environment (more so than in folded proteins) [81], and 2) over-stabilization of secondary structural elements and compact ensembles [31,82]. The latter problem was addressed by Lee et al. by optimizing the GBMV2 (Generalized Born using molecular volume) implicit solvation model [83], in conjunction with the CHARMM36 protein force field. The improved GBMV2 model predicted fewer compact ensembles, in agreement with the experimental structural properties of several IDPs [82]. One of the implicit solvation models that has shown success in the IDP field is the ABSINTH model (self-assembly of biomolecules studied by an implicit, novel, and tunable Hamiltonian) by Vitalis and Pappu [81,84]. The ABSINTH builds and improves upon the EEF1 (effective energy function) solvent model [85] that calculates the solvation free energy of the protein as a sum of individual backbone and sidechain components. The solvation energies of the individual components are obtained from experimental solvation free energies of small molecules that resemble the protein components and are weighted by their solvent exposure during simulation. The ABSINTH has been used to explore the effect of temperature and charged amino acid distribution in the protein sequence on the ensemble properties of IDPs [86,87].

Alongside the implicit solvation models that approximate the electrostatic contribution of the solvent environment towards fully atomistic protein structures, advancements have been made towards modeling the polypeptide chain in a coarse grain form. The associative-memory, water-mediated, structure, and energy model (AWSEM) [88,89], which was originally developed to study globular protein folding, has been successfully modified for application to IDPs [90]. The AWSEM incorporates a coarse grain potential function comprising of terms that model hydrophobic, hydrogen bond, and water mediated interactions, as well as terms to control secondary structure formation and local tertiary interactions, both of which can be obtained from database or experimental/computational studies. A recent computational study applied AWSEM to study a cancer-related IDP, prostate-associated gene 4 (PAGE4), and successfully reproduced the structural switch of this molecule induced by different levels of phosphorylation [91]. Using the modified coarse grain protein model PLUM [92], Rutter et al. reproduced the secondary structures and disorder propensities of amino acids in the N terminus of the n16 peptide involved in biomineralization [93]. The predicted conformations showed agreement with all-atom MD simulations. These coarse grain simulations also successfully distinguished the dimerization propensity of the n16 peptide with its mutant which fails to dimerize, and in a later paper, the aggregation behavior of multiple peptides [94]. Such developments give hope for increasing the scope of MD simulations beyond the conformational sampling of single protein chains and enable simulation of complex processes such as aggregation, self-assembly, and vesicle formation involving IDPs.

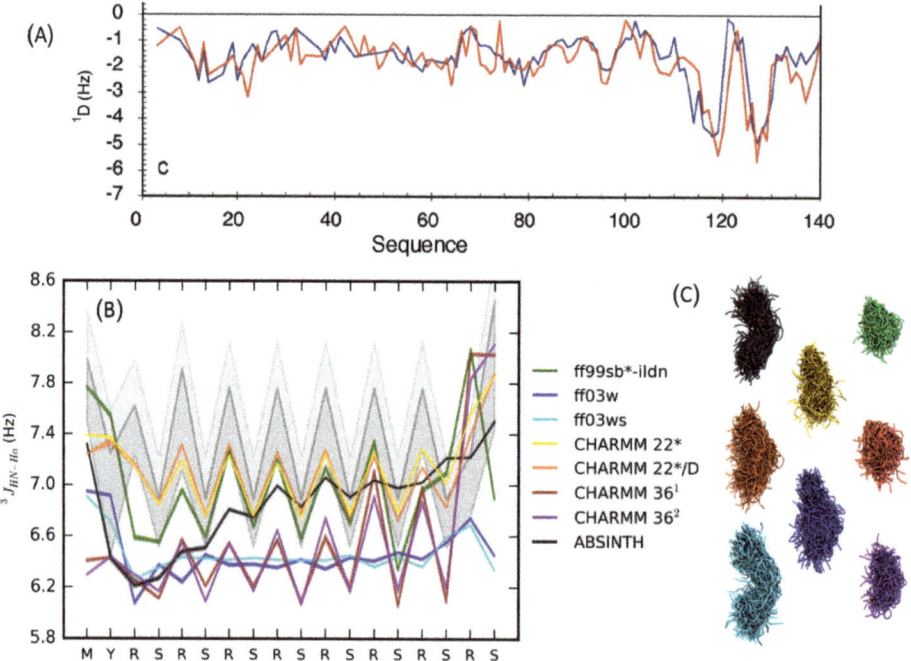

Figure 2. (**A**) Comparison between experimental (blue) and simulated $^1D_{NH}$ residual dipolar coupling (RDCs, red) from ensemble of α-synuclein generated by flexible-meccano and ASTEROIDS (a selection tool for ensemble representations of intrinsically disordered states); reproduced with permission from [95]; (**B**) comparison of experimental J coupling data from a disordered peptide with those calculated from ensembles obtained from replica exchange molecular dynamics (REMD) simulations with various force fields; The experimental $^3J_{HN-H\alpha}$ couplings are shown in gray shading (**C**) ensembles obtained from various force fields in cartoon representation; reproduced with permission from [69].

4. Protein–Protein Interaction Involving Intrinsically Disordered Proteins

Due to their conformational diversity, IDPs interact with multiple partner proteins, DNA, and RNA, leading to signaling, transport, endocytosis, gene expression, and fibril formation. The association of IDPs ranges from homo and hetero-dimerization to aggregation involving hundreds of monomers.

Many IDPs adopt folded structures upon binding to their partners and the same IDP can adopt multiple folded structures depending on its binding partner [5,96]. Alternatively, disorder can be retained upon binding, in the so called fuzzy complexes [97,98]. Besides proteins, IDPs are also involved in interactions with ligands, nucleic acids and membranes, details of which can be found in several reviews [8,99,100].

4.1. Disorder Retained upon Binding: Fuzzy Complexes

Many IDPs are reported to form fuzzy complexes with proteins and nucleic acid polymers, whose importance in the biological processes has become increasingly clear in recent years [97,98]. The IDP involved in a fuzzy complex maintains its structural disorder upon binding to the partner protein. The binding is driven by increase or no loss in entropy and lowering of enthalpy via multiple weak protein–protein interactions [98]. In some cases, both the binding partners remain disordered upon binding, as in the case of histone H1 and prothymosin-α. Here, the binding is driven by long range electrostatic attraction, as opposed to specific inter-residue interactions [6]. As part of a combined theoretical and experimental work, Milles et al. studied the association between nucleoporins and the nuclear transporter importin β using all-atom MD simulations [101]. Out of ten independent simulations, four binding events were observed within 100 ns (Figure 3A), and the predicted binding site interactions agreed with the observed NMR ^{1}H-^{15}N HSQC (heteronuclear single quantum coherence) spectrum. The multiple binding events within a short simulation time is in line with the ultra-fast association rates of fuzzy complexes, which do not have the rate limiting step of structural rearrangement or folding upon binding. Also, fuzzy complex IDPs can bind to their partner proteins through multiple pathways, leading to fast binding.

4.2. Conformational Selection versus Induced Fit

For IDPs that adopt folded structures upon binding to their partner proteins, two types of mechanisms have been proposed: (a) conformational selection and (b) induced fit [1,102]. In conformational selection, one of the preexisting folded monomer conformations binds to the partner protein, whereas in induced fit, the folding happens subsequent to binding (Figure 3B). Most IDPs are thought to follow a combination of the two mechanisms, where one of the partially folded metastable states binds to the partner protein (selection), followed by the rest of the folding (induced fit), which is facilitated by the environment of the other protein [103]. Such complex binding mechanisms often incorporate multiple steps with associated energy barriers and are typically beyond the scope of all-atom unbiased MD simulations in an explicit solvent environment. As a result, coarse grain simulations or all-atom biased simulations are employed where the interaction energy between different parts of the protein are modeled based on experimental structural data and physics-based potentials. Coarse grain models such as the modified Gō-like models have been extensively used in studying the binding of IDPs [104–108]. The coarse-grained Gō model was originally developed to study the folding of globular proteins [109]. It is based on the minimally frustrated energy landscape theory [110,111], which posits that foldable protein sequences have evolved to create a funnel shaped energy landscape, where only the native contacts are energetically favored and non-native contacts are not. Thus, the force field interactions in the Gō model are chosen to stabilize the native state over non-native conformations, in order to approximate the protein free energy landscape. To adapt the Gō model to study IDPs which sample multiple conformations instead of one native state, multiple topology based energy terms (each specific towards one conformation) can be combined together using exponential mixing, as described in [108]. The resulting potential function can describe an energy landscape with multiple local minima, separated by free energy barriers controlled by a mixing temperature. The parameters for modeling the energy function can be derived from the crystal and NMR structures of IDP complexes. Such a model, though simplistic compared to all-atom physics-based models, can be a powerful tool to study kinetics and free energy landscapes of IDP binding. Using a multistate Gō model, Knott et al. studied the binding of the disordered nuclear coactivating binding domain (NCBD) of the CREB binding protein to the ACTR domain of p160 and the interferon regulatory factor IRF-3 (NCBD adopts different folded conformations upon binding to ACTR and IRF-3). The energy parameters of the Gō model were derived from the crystal structures of the two bound complexes and the respective binding affinities. The authors showed that the binding of NCBD to both ACTR and IRF-3 follow an induced fit mechanism. In a separate work, Ganguly and coworkers showed that non-specific electrostatic interactions play a key role in orienting NCBD and ACTR towards the native interaction surface to facilitate fast binding [107]. Wang et al. developed a hybrid potential based on both physics based and native topology-based terms, which they used to study the mechanism of binding between the disordered measles virus nucleoprotein (MeV) and the phosphoprotein X domain (XD) [103]. The resulting binding free energy landscape showed that the initial binding of MeV proceeds via conformational selection of an α-helical monomer conformation, followed by induced fit that results in complete folding of MeV around XD (Figure 3C).

4.3. Liquid–Liquid Phase Separation and Aggregation

Due to their disordered and flexible nature, IDPs can exhibit a variety of complex thermodynamic states, involving multiple proteins, RNA (or DNA), small molecules, and ions [8]. One prominent feature of IDPs is their involvement in the formation of proteinaceous membrane-less organelles (PMLOs) [112]. These organelles, that are abundant in both eukaryotic and plant cells [113], are an essential part of the biological repertoire, being involved in sequestering enzymatic reactions and small molecules or RNA/DNA from the bulk cytoplasm [114]. Such organelles may also be involved in protein aggregation related neurodegenerative diseases [115]. The PMLOs are formed by the localized separation of a protein rich liquid phase (droplet) in equilibrium with a surrounding dilute phase, a phenomenon commonly termed as liquid–liquid phase separation (LLPS). In LLPS, the protein-rich phase shows liquid like properties such as low shear and surface wetting, and is distinct from protein aggregate rich organelles such as inclusion bodies [113]. The flexibility of the IDPs and the abundance of charged amino acids in their sequence are often cited as reasons for facilitating LLPS [112]. The IDP domains that participate in phase separation often consist of charged amino acid repeats (low complexity regions) that create multiple sites of interaction with neighboring proteins, facilitating condensate formation [8,113,116]. However, there are currently unanswered questions regarding the detailed mechanisms of IDPs in undergoing LLPS, and the role of amino acid composition and placement, presence of folded domains, temperature, pH, post translational modification, and concentration of different precursors such as RNA [112,116]. The problem of IDP phase separation is best addressed by coarse grain MD methods [117] and analytical and semi-analytical polymer theory [118], since the timescale of the slow diffusion controlled rearrangement of multiple IDP chains involved in phase separation is beyond the reach of all-atom MD simulations. See [119] for a complete review on coarse grain and multiscale simulations of the phase behavior of IDPs.

Coarse grain models, such as lattice models, are simplistic but highly powerful tools to explore the phase behavior of polymers and surfactants [120,121]. In a lattice model, the simulation box is discretized into a grid, and the protein (and RNA) is modeled as a chain of beads occupying adjacent lattice sites. The beads of neighboring chains interact using a square well potential, where the interaction strength is determined by the knowledge of the individual components. The system is simulated by moving the beads to nearby lattice sites and accepting or rejecting the moves using Monte Carlo. Using both experiments and coarse-grain lattice Monte Carlo simulations, Boeynaems et al. provided insights into the formation of multi-layered PMLOs by IDPs, in the presence of RNA and polyanionic proteins [117]. The authors showed that RNA molecules lacking stable secondary structures facilitate the formation of LLPS droplets, whereas base pairing of RNA leads to (metastable) solid-like gels. In another work using continuum coarse grain models, Dignon et al. simulated the phase properties of two different IDPs (one of which is involved in fibril formation in amyotrophic lateral sclerosis (ALS)) [116]. Their coarse grain model included a single bead for every amino acid, interacting with each other through van der Waals and screened electrostatic interactions, whose parameters were optimized by comparing with experimental radii of gyration of the proteins of interest. The authors simulated the phase behavior of the proteins at different temperatures, thus constructing the complete phase diagram. They also discussed the effect of mutations and the presence of folded domains on the observed phase behavior. Lastly, analytical and semi-analytical polymer theories have been applied for modeling IDP phase behavior. Such theories come with different degrees of approximation and resolution, and they can capture salient features of IDP phase properties, such as the effects of amino acid pattern and chain length. For a recent work in this area, please see [122].

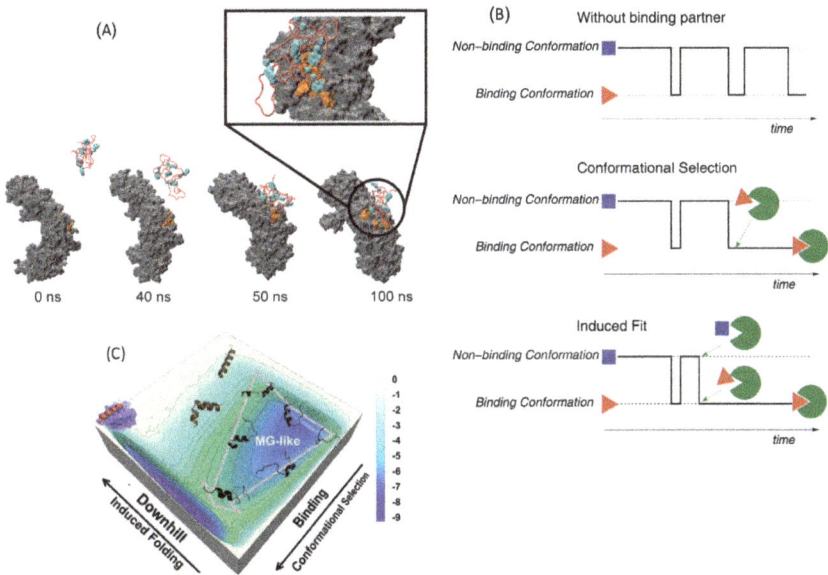

Figure 3. (A) Formation of a fast binding fuzzy complex between nucleoporin (red cartoon) and importinβ (grey surface), simulated using an all-atom molecular dynamics (MD) simulation; the binding sites on importin β and nucleoporin are colored in orange and cyan respectively; reproduced with permission from [101] (https://doi.org/10.1016/j.cell.2015.09.047) under the terms of the Creative Commons Attribution License (CC BY); http://creativecommons.org/licenses/by/4.0/ (B) schematic demonstration of conformational selection and induced fit binding mechanisms; in the absence of binding partner, the IDP switches between the non-binding (blue) and binding (red) conformations; in conformational selection, the IDP binds to the partner protein in the binding conformation without any structural rearrangement; for induced fit binding, the IDP initially encounters the partner using the non-binding conformation, then adopts the binding conformation in presence of the partner; reproduced with permission from ref. [108] (C) coarse-grain free energy landscape showing a combined conformational selection and induced fit binding of a disordered C terminal segment of the measles virus nucleoprotein to the X domain of the measles virus phosphoprotein; reproduced with permission from ref. [103]; Copyright 2013 national Academy of Sciences.

Several IDPs, for example the tau protein, amyloid β peptides, α-synuclein, and hIAPP, show a propensity to form high density, fibril like aggregates that are implicated in diabetes and neurodegenerative diseases like Alzheimer's (AD) and Parkinson's [123]. It has been proposed that transient secondary structure elements naturally present in these IDP ensembles can induce aggregation and fibril formation under overcrowded conditions [31]. Qiao et al. constructed the Markov State Model for the hIAPP peptide involved in amyloid fibril formation in type 2 diabetes through extensive MD simulations [30]. These simulations revealed metastable states in the energy landscape, which were shown to facilitate fibril formation. A well-studied IDP involved in fibril formation is the Aβ peptide. Using REMD simulations, Das et al. studied the conformational landscape of the wild type Aβ peptide and two of its mutants, the disease resistant A2T and A2V, which induces early onset Alzheimer's [124]. While the A2T mutation inhibited the wild type population of β hairpin structures that promote aggregation, the A2V mutation preserved such conformations. Using the MD simulations, the authors were able to provide insights into the mechanisms behind such conformational shifts. In a separate study, REMD simulations were used to explain the binding mechanism of short peptides (based on the A2T and A2V mutants) to wild type Aβ peptide, that were designed to impede fibril formation [125]. The atomistic MD simulations provide insights into the aggregation process by analyzing the conformational propensity of isolated IDP monomers. Simulating the actual aggregation process, however, is beyond the scope of atomistic simulations, and would require coarse grain protein models. Examples of works in this area include [126,127].

5. Intrinsically Disordered Proteins as Therapeutic Targets

Due to the increasing evidence of IDPs being involved in various diseases and their abundance in the human genome [4,128], these proteins have emerged as promising drug targets. Many IDPs act as signaling hubs (central points in cellular signaling networks) and dysregulation of these hubs often has a significant effect on the cellular function. In diabetes and neurodegenerative diseases, aggregation of IDPs, such as hIAPP and tau-protein, lead to β cell death and amyloid fibril formation [123,129]. Thus, designing small molecules or peptides to bind to IDPs is a viable strategy to modulate signaling networks or prevent aggregation and reverse disease phenotypes. To date, the discovery of several drug candidates that bind to disordered regions of proteins reinforces this possibility [130–135]. However, some of the challenges involved in targeting IDPs for drug discovery are: 1) lack of stable binding pockets due to high inherent flexibility [135–137], 2) weak affinity of the binders due to transient interaction with the protein [128], and 3) potential lack of selectivity to the target IDP [128]. The suggested strategies for targeting IDPs with small molecules include stabilizing IDPs in their native disordered ensemble (to prevent aggregation), inhibiting interaction with specific binding partners, and allosteric modulation of protein conformation [136].

Experimental drug discovery relies on high throughput screening assays (HTS), which can be expensive and are limited by the number of compounds that can be screened (up to 100,000 compounds a day). Computational drug screening (high throughput virtual screening, HTVS) [138] can filter small molecule databases with more than a million compounds and significantly reduce the number of candidates to be tested in experimental assays, saving time and effort. However, most of the existing methods for computational drug discovery are designed to identify compounds that bind to deep, well-formed pockets in conventional folded proteins. The principles that help to distinguish binders from non-binders in these proteins are shape fitting, stable, energetically feasible protein–ligand interactions and effective shielding from the solvent upon binding. In contrast, IDPs adopt multiple conformations in free solution (instead of a single dominant one that can be targeted for designing a drug) and lack stable hydrophobic cores that would facilitate the formation of deep pockets. In fuzzy complexes, the protein–protein interface is comprised of many weak and dynamic inter-protein interactions, as opposed to a few stable hotspots. This makes it highly challenging to design small molecules using the established drug design principles to disrupt such interactions. However, IDPs can have relatively rigid hydrophobic pockets, while the rest of the structure remains flexible, as shown in the case of nuclear protein 1 (NUPR1). [132] Such pockets can be targeted for binding small molecules. Several small molecules have been successfully identified and confirmed to bind to disordered regions of proteins, for example the oncogenic transcription factor c-Myc, that disrupts its association with its partner protein Max [130,131]. The NMR nuclear Overhauser effect spectroscopy (NOESY) data showed that two separate binding sites exist in c-Myc, that bind two different small molecules. Multiple small molecule inhibitors have been identified for the IDP α-synuclein, which is a major target for Parkinson's disease [133,134]. An analysis of 51 IDP structures from public databases showed that IDPs contain on average 50% more druggable pockets than folded proteins [139]. This evidence suggests that it is feasible to design small molecules to bind to IDPs and modulate their functions, potentially with high specificity [128]. However, new design principles are needed for identifying small molecule binders to IDPs, which have to be formulated based on mechanistic insights gained from studying existing examples.

The binding sites and interactions between small molecules and their cognate IDP partners have been studied using NMR and molecular simulations. Using NMR guided docking and MD simulations, Neira et al. studied the binding of several small molecules to the IDP NUPR1 involved in pancreatic duct adenocarcinoma [132]. These compounds were found to bind to a hydrophobic region in the NUPR1 monomer that was relatively rigid compared to the rest of the structure. Thus, binding of the compounds didn't significantly reduce the flexibility of the protein and minimized entropy loss. Additionally, they shielded hydrophobic residues such as Phe, Tyr, and Leu from water exposure, leading to favorable binding. A similar binding of small molecules to a hydrophobic/aromatic rich region in c-Myc was reported by Michel et al. [140]. Using BEMD simulations in explicit water, the authors compared the conformational ensemble of c-Myc in the presence and absence of the small molecule 10058-F4, followed by validation with NMR chemical shift data. 10058-F4 was shown to preferentially bind to several protein conformations that were less populated in the free solution. Upon the binding of 10058-F4, the equilibrium shifted towards the increased population of the ligand specific conformations. The preexistence of small molecule binding conformations in free monomer ensemble (although in fringe proportion) was shown in the flexible fusion peptide of HIV-1 using collective MD simulations [141]. These studies give some useful pointers towards targeting IDPs with small molecules: 1) the conformational ensemble of the ligand free IDP may already have conformations that are conducive to binding small molecules, 2) extensive conformational sampling using computational methods is capable of sampling these conformations, and 3) relatively rigid or hydrophobic domains on IDP surfaces could be potential hotspots for drug interaction, and this could serve as a signature for selecting the small molecule specific conformations from an ensemble. However, it may be advantageous to give priority to those conformations that are already highly populated in the ligand free ensemble. As mentioned in [141], targeting less populated IDP conformations for drug design could elicit a higher dose requirement of the resulting drug.

Intrinsically disordered proteins are also promising targets for developing allosteric modulators, since conformational flexibility has been shown to enhance allostery in IDPs and bacterial flagellar switch [142–145]. Methods like ALLOSTEER, which can identify pockets that are both druggable and allosterically active, can immensely benefit IDP drug discovery [146]. Using ALLOSTEER, it is possible to identify allosterically active pockets that are distant from the protein–protein interface and the binding site residues that are critical for allostery [147]. Drugs binding to such pockets can modulate the binding of the IDP to the partner protein, while not having to compete directly with the partner protein by binding at the interface. A computational protocol for designing small molecules for an IDP therefore could start with a protein structural ensemble obtained from experimental data and computational sampling, followed by clustering of conformations and identification of druggable pockets in each cluster representative, using methods such as FindBindSite [148] and FPOCKET [149], and narrowed down using design principles such as structural rigidity, hydrophobicity, and allostery. Then, conventional HTVS methods can be used to screen small molecule libraries in each pocket, and compounds which show low binding energies in multiple conformations can be selected as potential drug candidates (Figure 4). Such protocols are likely to improve with future insights gained in the interaction between IDPs and small molecules.

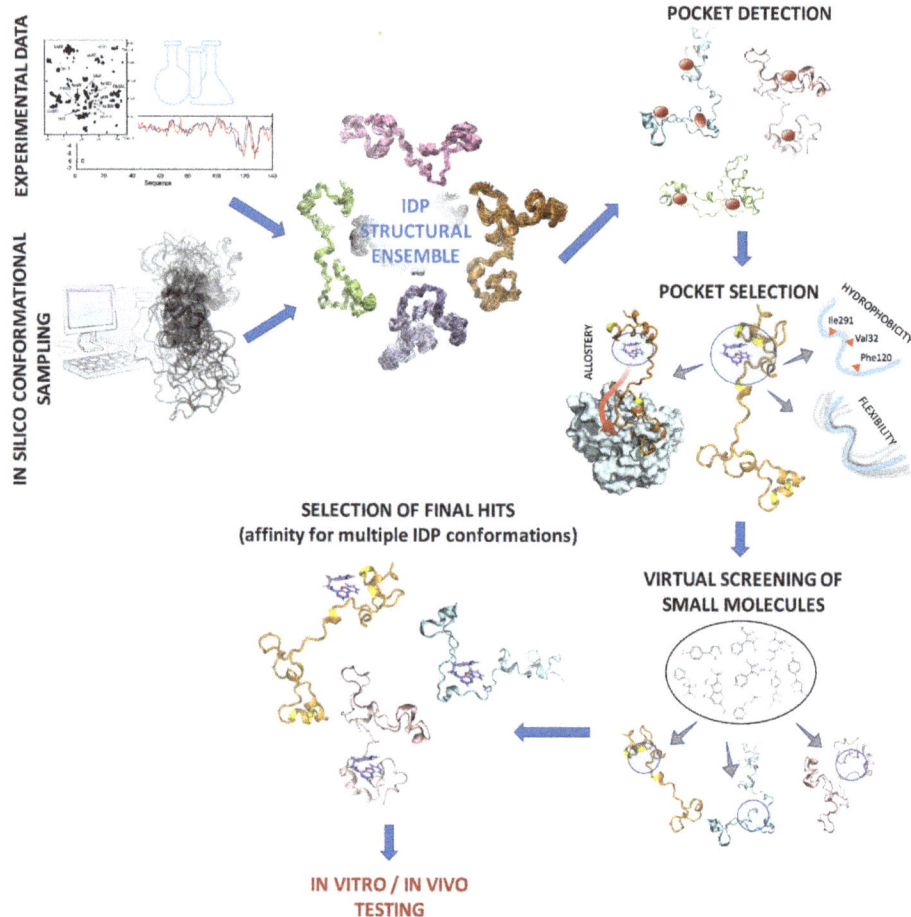

Figure 4. Example computational protocol for identifying drug candidates for IDPs; the IDP structural ensemble is clustered into representative conformations and druggable pockets are identified in each conformation; these pockets are further filtered by criteria such as hydrophobicity, backbone flexibility, and allosteric communication with functional sites. Virtual screening is performed in each pocket and final hits are selected based on high affinity in multiple IDP conformations.

6. Concluding Remarks

Compared to folded proteins, the energy landscape of an IDP is seemingly more complex with multiple populated basins at physiological conditions. With folded proteins, the challenges in computationally exploring the energy landscape come from the free-energy barriers separating the intermediate states along the folding pathway and the difficulty in energetically distinguishing the native ensemble from decoys. In addition to this, the challenges with IDPs are the vast degrees of freedom and the intricate balance between the inter-protein and solvent interactions that govern structural equilibrium. Methods that use experimental data to select a subset of conformations from a statistical coil ensemble do not cover all possible conformations of an IDP, which can be stellar even for a short polypeptide chain. A major concern is that transient or sparsely populated structures that do not significantly contribute to the statistical average properties may be missed. These transient conformations could be nevertheless critical for partner protein recognition or inhibitor binding. The other question is regarding the uniqueness of the structural ensemble that is obtained by fitting to the experimental NMR data, the so called degeneracy issue [22,150]. Normally, a large number of experimental restraints are needed to uniquely reproduce an IDP ensemble using computational sampling. Such experimental data are rarely available, leading to potentially ambiguous results from the fitting [151]. Thus, careful cross-validation of the predicted ensembles is needed, possibly using alternative experimental methods such as site-directed mutagenesis. The relevance and accuracy of the experimental data itself is also a matter of concern, since experimental measurements often require modification of the protein by attaching probes and labels. Given the fact that, for many IDPs, the conformational equilibrium is highly sensitive to post-translational modifications such as phosphorylation, it is debatable to what extent NMR probes affect the IDP ensembles [46]. De novo methods like MD and enhanced sampling algorithms, that model protein dynamics using physics-based approaches, can solve some of the aforementioned issues, but these methods have their own challenges due to limited computational power and inaccurate force fields. Analyzing recent literature, it is clear that more improvement is needed to accurately describe the energetics of IDPs, including the balance between secondary structure formation and solvent interaction. The heterogeneous solvent environment of IDPs makes it harder to model the chemical nature of the polypeptide chain during dynamics simulations, such as polarization effects and protonation states of charged residues and histidines, which can change more rapidly compared to the folded protein environment. Moreover, the expanded structures of IDPs require larger simulation boxes than folded proteins, which is a hindrance towards fully sampling the IDP dynamics using atomistic simulations. Thus, a multiscale approach is better suited for conformational sampling of IDPs, where an initial ensemble of backbone conformations obtained through coarse grain methods can be further refined using finer resolution algorithms, giving detailed information such as the orientation of residue sidechains or transition barriers. These ensembles must be validated against available experimental data and compared with the ensembles obtained through random coil algorithms. The available public databases of IDP ensembles can largely aid in the development and improvement of computational techniques for exploring IDPs [152,153].

In recent years, multiple experimental and computational studies have given insight into the binding mechanisms of IDPs, such as conformational transitions upon binding and the associated kinetics. However, more research is needed in this field, especially since protein–protein binding is a complex topic that is not fully understood, even for folded proteins. It is not clear, for example, how IDPs recognize their partner proteins with such high specificity, despite a lack of specific inter-residue interactions at the binding interface, and how dynamics plays its role in the binding specificity. Molecular modeling and simulation studies can be complemented by co-evolutionary analysis of IDPs and their partners. Co-evolutionary analysis has been heavily explored for folded proteins [154,155], and is just now being studied for IDPs [156]. Such insights will be invaluable in the rational design of therapy targeting IDPs, i.e., small molecules and peptides to disrupt binding and aggregation.

Author Contributions: Conceptualization, S.B.; investigation, S.B. and X.L.; writing—original draft preparation, S.B.; writing—review and editing, S.B. and X.L.; funding acquisition, S.B. and X.L.

Funding: Research reported in this publication included work performed in the Computational Therapeutics Core supported by the National Cancer Institute of the National Institutes of Health under award number P30CA033572. The content is solely the responsibility of the authors and does not necessarily represent the official views of the National Institutes of Health. X.L. was supported by National Science Foundation (NSF) through the Center for Theoretical Biological Physics (NSF-PHY-1427654, NSF MCB-1241332, and NSF-CHE-1614101)

Conflicts of Interest: The authors declare no conflict of interest. The funders had no role in the design of the study; in the collection, analyses, or interpretation of data; in the writing of the manuscript, or in the decision to publish the results.

References

1. Wright, P.E.; Dyson, H.J. Intrinsically disordered proteins in cellular signalling and regulation. *Nat. Rev. Mol. Cell. Biol.* **2015**, *16*, 18–29. [CrossRef]

2. Babu, M.M. The contribution of intrinsically disordered regions to protein function, cellular complexity, and human disease. *Biochem. Soc. Trans.* **2016**, *44*, 1185–1200. [CrossRef] [PubMed]
3. Oldfield, C.J.; Dunker, A.K. Intrinsically disordered proteins and intrinsically disordered protein regions. *Annu. Rev. Biochem.* **2014**, *83*, 553–584. [CrossRef] [PubMed]
4. Uversky, V.N.; Oldfield, C.J.; Dunker, A.K. Intrinsically disordered proteins in human diseases: introducing the D2 concept. *Annu. Rev. Biophys.* **2008**, *37*, 215–246. [CrossRef]
5. Mollica, L.; Bessa, L.M.; Hanoulle, X.; Jensen, M.R.; Blackledge, M.; Schneider, R. Binding Mechanisms of Intrinsically Disordered Proteins: Theory, Simulation, and Experiment. *Front. Mol. Biosci.* **2016**, *3*, 52. [CrossRef] [PubMed]
6. Borgia, A.; Borgia, M.B.; Bugge, K.; Kissling, V.M.; Heidarsson, P.O.; Fernandes, C.B.; Sottini, A.; Soranno, A.; Buholzer, K.J.; Nettels, D.; et al. Extreme disorder in an ultrahigh-affinity protein complex. *Nature* **2018**, *555*, 61–66. [CrossRef]
7. Jia, D.; Jolly, M.K.; Kulkarni, P.; Levine, H. Phenotypic Plasticity and Cell Fate Decisions in Cancer: Insights from Dynamical Systems Theory. *Cancers (Basel)* **2017**, *9*, 70. [CrossRef] [PubMed]
8. Uversky, V.N. Intrinsically Disordered Proteins and Their "Mysterious" (Meta)Physics. *Front. Phys-Lausanne* **2019**, *7*, 10. [CrossRef]
9. Dunker, A.K.; Babu, M.M.; Barbar, E.; Blackledge, M.; Bondos, S.E.; Dosztanyi, Z.; Dyson, H.J.; Forman-Kay, J.; Fuxreiter, M.; Gsponer, J.; et al. What's in a name? Why these proteins are intrinsically disordered: Why these proteins are intrinsically disordered. *Intrinsically Disord. Proteins* **2013**, *1*, e24157. [CrossRef]
10. O'Brien, E.P.; Morrison, G.; Brooks, B.R.; Thirumalai, D. How accurate are polymer models in the analysis of Forster resonance energy transfer experiments on proteins? *J. Chem. Phys.* **2009**, *130*, 124903. [CrossRef]
11. Zheng, W.W.; Zerze, G.H.; Borgia, A.; Mittal, J.; Schuler, B.; Best, R.B. Inferring properties of disordered chains from FRET transfer efficiencies. *J. Chem. Phys.* **2018**, *148*, 123329. [CrossRef]
12. Zheng, W.W.; Best, R.B. An Extended Guinier Analysis for Intrinsically Disordered Proteins. *J. Mol. Biol.* **2018**, *430*, 2540–2553. [CrossRef]
13. Vitalis, A.; Wang, X.L.; Pappu, R.V. Quantitative characterization of intrinsic disorder in polyglutamine: Insights from analysis based on polymer theories. *Biophys. J.* **2007**, *93*, 1923–1937. [CrossRef]
14. Piana, S.; Donchev, A.G.; Robustelli, P.; Shaw, D.E. Water Dispersion Interactions Strongly Influence Simulated Structural Properties of Disordered Protein States. *J. Phys. Chem. B.* **2015**, *119*, 5113–5123. [CrossRef]
15. Song, J.H.; Gomes, G.N.; Shi, T.F.; Gradinaru, C.C.; Chan, H.S. Conformational Heterogeneity and FRET Data Interpretation for Dimensions of Unfolded Proteins. *Biophys. J.* **2017**, *113*, 1012–1024. [CrossRef] [PubMed]
16. Riback, J.A.; Bowman, M.A.; Zmyslowski, A.M.; Knoverek, C.R.; Jumper, J.M.; Hinshaw, J.R.; Kaye, E.B.; Freed, K.F.; Clark, P.L.; Sosnick, T.R. Innovative scattering analysis shows that hydrophobic disordered proteins are expanded in water. *Science* **2017**, *358*, 238–241. [CrossRef] [PubMed]
17. Schuler, B.; Soranno, A.; Hofmann, H.; Nettels, D. Single-Molecule FRET Spectroscopy and the Polymer Physics of Unfolded and Intrinsically Disordered Proteins. *Annu. Rev. Biophys.* **2016**, *45*, 207–231. [CrossRef] [PubMed]
18. Best, R.B. Computational and theoretical advances in studies of intrinsically disordered proteins. *Curr. Opin. Struct. Biol.* **2017**, *42*, 147–154. [CrossRef] [PubMed]
19. Varadi, M.; Vranken, W.; Guharoy, M.; Tompa, P. Computational approaches for inferring the functions of intrinsically disordered proteins. *Front Mol. Biosci.* **2015**, *2*, 45. [CrossRef]
20. Frauenfelder, H.; Sligar, S.G.; Wolynes, P.G. The energy landscapes and motions of proteins. *Science* **1991**, *254*, 1598–1603. [CrossRef] [PubMed]
21. Wei, G.; Xi, W.; Nussinov, R.; Ma, B. Protein Ensembles: How Does Nature Harness Thermodynamic Fluctuations for Life? The Diverse Functional Roles of Conformational Ensembles in the Cell. *Chem. Rev.* **2016**, *116*, 6516–6551. [CrossRef] [PubMed]
22. Fisher, C.K.; Stultz, C.M. Constructing ensembles for intrinsically disordered proteins. *Curr. Opin. Struct. Biol.* **2011**, *21*, 426–431. [CrossRef] [PubMed]
23. Chebaro, Y.; Ballard, A.J.; Chakraborty, D.; Wales, D.J. Intrinsically disordered energy landscapes. *Sci. Rep.* **2015**, *5*, 10386. [CrossRef]
24. He, Y.; Chen, Y.; Mooney, S.M.; Rajagopalan, K.; Bhargava, A.; Sacho, E.; Weninger, K.; Bryan, P.N.; Kulkarni, P.; Orban, J. Phosphorylation-induced Conformational Ensemble Switching in an Intrinsically Disordered Cancer/Testis Antigen. *J. Biol. Chem.* **2015**, *290*, 25090–25102. [CrossRef] [PubMed]

25. Bah, A.; Vernon, R.M.; Siddiqui, Z.; Krzeminski, M.; Muhandiram, R.; Zhao, C.; Sonenberg, N.; Kay, L.E.; Forman-Kay, J.D. Folding of an intrinsically disordered protein by phosphorylation as a regulatory switch. *Nature* **2015**, *519*, 106–109. [CrossRef]
26. Ma, B.Y.; Nussinov, R. Simulations as analytical tools to understand protein aggregation and predict amyloid conformation. *Curr. Opin. Chem. Biol.* **2006**, *10*, 445–452. [CrossRef]
27. Tycko, R. Solid-State NMR Studies of Amyloid Fibril Structure. *Annu. Rev. Phys. Chem.* **2011**, *62*, 279–299. [CrossRef] [PubMed]
28. Granata, D.; Baftizadeh, F.; Habchi, J.; Galvagnion, C.; De Simone, A.; Camilloni, C.; Laio, A.; Vendruscolo, M. The inverted free energy landscape of an intrinsically disordered peptide by simulations and experiments. *Sci. Rep.* **2015**, *5*, 15449. [CrossRef]
29. Lincoff, J.; Sasmal, S.; Head-Gordon, T. Comparing generalized ensemble methods for sampling of systems with many degrees of freedom. *J. Chem. Phys.* **2016**, *145*, 174107. [CrossRef]
30. Qiao, Q.; Bowman, G.R.; Huang, X.H. Dynamics of an Intrinsically Disordered Protein Reveal Metastable Conformations That Potentially Seed Aggregation. *J. Am. Chem. Soc.* **2013**, *135*, 16092–16101. [CrossRef] [PubMed]
31. Das, P.; Matysiak, S.; Mittal, J. Looking at the Disordered Proteins through the Computational Microscope. *ACS Central Sci.* **2018**, *4*, 534–542. [CrossRef]
32. Robustelli, P.; Piana, S.; Shaw, D.E. Developing a molecular dynamics force field for both folded and disordered protein states. *Proc. Natl. Acad. Sci. USA* **2018**, *115*, E4758–E4766. [CrossRef] [PubMed]
33. Feldman, H.J.; Hogue, C.W. A fast method to sample real protein conformational space. *Proteins* **2000**, *39*, 112–131. [CrossRef]
34. Feldman, H.J.; Hogue, C.W. Probabilistic sampling of protein conformations: new hope for brute force? *Proteins* **2002**, *46*, 8–23. [CrossRef] [PubMed]
35. Ozenne, V.; Bauer, F.; Salmon, L.; Huang, J.R.; Jensen, M.R.; Segard, S.; Bernado, P.; Charavay, C.; Blackledge, M. Flexible-meccano: a tool for the generation of explicit ensemble descriptions of intrinsically disordered proteins and their associated experimental observables. *Bioinformatics* **2012**, *28*, 1463–1470. [CrossRef]
36. Nodet, G.; Salmon, L.; Ozenne, V.; Meier, S.; Jensen, M.R.; Blackledge, M. Quantitative description of backbone conformational sampling of unfolded proteins at amino acid resolution from NMR residual dipolar couplings. *J. Am. Chem. Soc.* **2009**, *131*, 17908–17918. [CrossRef] [PubMed]
37. Krzeminski, M.; Marsh, J.A.; Neale, C.; Choy, W.Y.; Forman-Kay, J.D. Characterization of disordered proteins with ENSEMBLE. *Bioinformatics* **2013**, *29*, 398–399. [CrossRef] [PubMed]
38. Theobald, D.L.; Wuttke, D.S. Accurate structural correlations from maximum likelihood superpositions. *PLoS Comput. Biol.* **2008**, *4*, e4310. [CrossRef]
39. Marchetti, J.; Monzon, A.M.; Tosatto, S.C.E.; Parisi, G.; Fornasari, M.S. Ensembles from Ordered and Disordered Proteins Reveal Similar Structural Constraints during Evolution. *J. Mol. Biol.* **2019**, *431*, 1298–1307. [CrossRef]
40. Mitsutake, A.; Sugita, Y.; Okamoto, Y. Generalized-ensemble algorithms for molecular simulations of biopolymers. *Biopolymers* **2001**, *60*, 96–123. [CrossRef]
41. Sugita, Y.; Okamoto, Y. Replica-exchange molecular dynamics method for protein folding. *Chem. Phys. Lett.* **1999**, *314*, 141–151. [CrossRef]
42. Piana, S.; Laio, A. A bias-exchange approach to protein folding. *J. Phys. Chem. B* **2007**, *111*, 4553–4559. [CrossRef]
43. Brown, S.; Head-Gordon, T. Cool walking: a new Markov chain Monte Carlo sampling method. *J. Comput. Chem.* **2003**, *24*, 68–76. [CrossRef]
44. Patel, S.; Vierling, E.; Tama, F. Replica exchange molecular dynamics simulations provide insight into substrate recognition by small heat shock proteins. *Biophys. J.* **2014**, *106*, 2644–2655. [CrossRef]
45. Zerze, G.H.; Miller, C.M.; Granata, D.; Mittal, J. Free energy surface of an intrinsically disordered protein: comparison between temperature replica exchange molecular dynamics and bias-exchange metadynamics. *J. Chem. Theory. Comput.* **2015**, *11*, 2776–2782. [CrossRef]
46. Sasmal, S.; Lincoff, J.; Head-Gordon, T. Effect of a Paramagnetic Spin Label on the Intrinsically Disordered Peptide Ensemble of Amyloid-β. *Biophys. J.* **2017**, *113*, 1002–1011. [CrossRef]
47. Pande, V.S.; Beauchamp, K.; Bowman, G.R. Everything you wanted to know about Markov State Models but were afraid to ask. *Methods* **2010**, *52*, 99–105. [CrossRef]

48. Buch, I.; Harvey, M.J.; Giorgino, T.; Anderson, D.P.; De Fabritiis, G. High-throughput all-atom molecular dynamics simulations using distributed computing. *J. Chem. Inf. Model* **2010**, *50*, 397–403. [CrossRef] [PubMed]
49. Stanley, N.; Esteban-Martin, S.; De Fabritiis, G. Kinetic modulation of a disordered protein domain by phosphorylation. *Nat. Commun.* **2014**, *5*, 5272. [CrossRef] [PubMed]
50. Deneroff, M.M.; Shaw, D.E.; Dror, R.O.; Kuskin, J.S.; Larson, R.H.; Salmon, J.K.; Young, C. Anton: A specialized ASIC for molecular dynamics. In Proceedings of the 2008 IEEE Hot Chips 20 Symposium (HCS), Stanford, CA, USA, 24–26 August 2008; pp. 1–34.
51. Shaw, D.E.; Grossman, J.P.; Bank, J.A.; Batson, B.; Butts, J.A.; Chao, J.C.; Deneroff, M.M.; Dror, R.O.; Even, A.; Fenton, C.H.; et al. Anton 2: Raising the Bar for Performance and Programmability in a Special-Purpose Molecular Dynamics Supercomputer. In Proceedings of the SC 14: Proceedings of the International Conference for High Performance Computing, Networking, Storage and Analysis, New Orleans, LA, USA, 16–21 November 2014; pp. 41–53.
52. Lindorff-Larsen, K.; Piana, S.; Dror, R.O.; Shaw, D.E. How Fast-Folding Proteins Fold. *Science* **2011**, *334*, 517–520. [CrossRef] [PubMed]
53. Jain, A.; Vaidehi, N.; Rodriguez, G. A Fast Recursive Algorithm for Molecular-Dynamics Simulation. *J. Comput. Phys.* **1993**, *106*, 258–268. [CrossRef]
54. Vaidehi, N.; Jain, A.; Goddard, W.A. Constant temperature constrained molecular dynamics: The Newton-Euler inverse mass operator method. *J. Phys. Chem.* **1996**, *100*, 10508–10517. [CrossRef]
55. Vaidehi, N.; Jain, A. Internal Coordinate Molecular Dynamics: A Foundation for Multiscale Dynamics. *J. Phys. Chem. B* **2015**, *119*, 1233–1242. [CrossRef] [PubMed]
56. Gangupomu, V.K.; Wagner, J.R.; Park, I.H.; Jain, A.; Vaidehi, N. Mapping Conformational Dynamics of Proteins Using Torsional Dynamics Simulations. *Biophys. J.* **2013**, *104*, 1999–2008. [CrossRef]
57. Kandel, S.; Salomon-Ferrer, R.; Larsen, A.B.; Jain, A.; Vaidehi, N. Overcoming potential energy distortions in constrained internal coordinate molecular dynamics simulations. *J. Chem. Phys.* **2016**, *144*, 044112. [CrossRef]
58. Bui, J.M.; McCammon, J.A. Protein complex formation by acetylcholinesterase and the neurotoxin fasciculin-2 appears to involve an induced-fit mechanism. *Proc. Natl. Acad. Sci. USA* **2006**, *103*, 15451–15456. [CrossRef] [PubMed]
59. Zhang, B.W.; Jasnow, D.; Zuckerman, D.M. Efficient and verified simulation of a path ensemble for conformational change in a united-residue model of calmodulin. *Proc. Natl. Acad. Sci. USA* **2007**, *104*, 18043–18048. [CrossRef]
60. Elson, E.L. Fluorescence Correlation Spectroscopy: Past, Present, Future. *Biophys. J.* **2011**, *101*, 2855–2870. [CrossRef] [PubMed]
61. Zerze, G.H.; Mittal, J.; Best, R.B. Diffusive Dynamics of Contact Formation in Disordered Polypeptides. *Phys. Rev. Lett.* **2016**, *116*, 068102. [CrossRef]
62. Soranno, A.; Holla, A.; Dingfelder, F.; Nettels, D.; Makarov, D.E.; Schuler, B. Integrated view of internal friction in unfolded proteins from single-molecule FRET, contact quenching, theory, and simulations. *Proc. Natl. Acad. Sci. USA* **2017**, *114*, E1833–E1839. [CrossRef]
63. Rezaei-Ghaleh, N.; Parigi, G.; Soranno, A.; Holla, A.; Becker, S.; Schuler, B.; Luchinat, C.; Zweckstetter, M. Local and Global Dynamics in Intrinsically Disordered Synuclein. *Angew. Chem. Int. Edit.* **2018**, *57*, 15262–15266. [CrossRef]
64. Maier, J.A.; Martinez, C.; Kasavajhala, K.; Wickstrom, L.; Hauser, K.E.; Simmerling, C. ff14SB: Improving the Accuracy of Protein Side Chain and Backbone Parameters from ff99SB. *J. Chem. Theory Comput.* **2015**, *11*, 3696–3713. [CrossRef]
65. Best, R.B.; Hummer, G. Optimized molecular dynamics force fields applied to the helix-coil transition of polypeptides. *J. Phys. Chem. B* **2009**, *113*, 9004–9015. [CrossRef]
66. Lindorff-Larsen, K.; Piana, S.; Palmo, K.; Maragakis, P.; Klepeis, J.L.; Dror, R.O.; Shaw, D.E. Improved side-chain torsion potentials for the Amber ff99SB protein force field. *Proteins* **2010**, *78*, 1950–1958. [CrossRef]
67. Huang, J.; Rauscher, S.; Nawrocki, G.; Ran, T.; Feig, M.; de Groot, B.L.; Grubmuller, H.; MacKerell, A.D., Jr. CHARMM36m: an improved force field for folded and intrinsically disordered proteins. *Nat. Methods* **2017**, *14*, 71–73. [CrossRef]
68. Palazzesi, F.; Prakash, M.K.; Bonomi, M.; Barducci, A. Accuracy of current all-atom force-fields in modeling protein disordered states. *J. Chem. Theory Comput.* **2015**, *11*, 2–7. [CrossRef]

69. Rauscher, S.; Gapsys, V.; Gajda, M.J.; Zweckstetter, M.; de Groot, B.L.; Grubmuller, H. Structural Ensembles of Intrinsically Disordered Proteins Depend Strongly on Force Field: A Comparison to Experiment. *J. Chem. Theory Comput.* **2015**, *11*, 5513–5524. [CrossRef]
70. Piana, S.; Lindorff-Larsen, K.; Shaw, D.E. How robust are protein folding simulations with respect to force field parameterization? *Biophys. J.* **2011**, *100*, L47–L49. [CrossRef] [PubMed]
71. Best, R.B.; Zheng, W.; Mittal, J. Balanced Protein-Water Interactions Improve Properties of Disordered Proteins and Non-Specific Protein Association. *J. Chem. Theory. Comput.* **2014**, *10*, 5113–5124. [CrossRef]
72. Jiang, F.; Zhou, C.Y.; Wu, Y.D. Residue-specific force field based on the protein coil library. RSFF1: modification of OPLS-AA/L. *J. Phys. Chem. B* **2014**, *118*, 6983–6998. [CrossRef]
73. Zhou, C.Y.; Jiang, F.; Wu, Y.D. Residue-specific force field based on protein coil library. RSFF2: modification of AMBER ff99SB. *J. Phys. Chem. B* **2015**, *119*, 1035–1047. [CrossRef]
74. Mercadante, D.; Milles, S.; Fuertes, G.; Svergun, D.I.; Lemke, E.A.; Grater, F. Kirkwood-Buff Approach Rescues Overcollapse of a Disordered Protein in Canonical Protein Force Fields. *J. Phys. Chem. B* **2015**, *119*, 7975–7984. [CrossRef]
75. Yoo, J.; Aksimentiev, A. New tricks for old dogs: improving the accuracy of biomolecular force fields by pair-specific corrections to non-bonded interactions. *Phys. Chem. Chem. Phys.* **2018**, *20*, 8432–8449. [CrossRef]
76. Song, D.; Wang, W.; Ye, W.; Ji, D.; Luo, R.; Chen, H.F. ff14IDPs force field improving the conformation sampling of intrinsically disordered proteins. *Chem. Biol. Drug. Des.* **2017**, *89*, 5–15. [CrossRef]
77. Still, W.C.; Tempczyk, A.; Hawley, R.C.; Hendrickson, T. Semianalytical Treatment of Solvation for Molecular Mechanics and Dynamics. *J. Am. Chem. Soc.* **1990**, *112*, 6127–6129. [CrossRef]
78. Kleinjung, J.; Fraternali, F. Design and application of implicit solvent models in biomolecular simulations. *Curr. Opin. Struc. Biol.* **2014**, *25*, 126–134. [CrossRef]
79. Zhou, R.H. Free energy landscape of protein folding in water: Explicit vs. implicit solvent. *Proteins-Structure Function Genetics* **2003**, *53*, 148–161. [CrossRef]
80. Awile, O.; Krisko, A.; Sbalzarini, I.F.; Zagrovic, B. Intrinsically Disordered Regions May Lower the Hydration Free Energy in Proteins: A Case Study of Nudix Hydrolase in the *Bacterium Deinococcus* radiodurans. *PLoS Comput. Biol.* **2010**, *6*, e1000854. [CrossRef]
81. Vitalis, A.; Pappu, R.V. ABSINTH: A New Continuum Solvation Model for Simulations of Polypeptides in Aqueous Solutions. *J. Comput. Chem.* **2009**, *30*, 673–699. [CrossRef]
82. Lee, K.H.; Chen, J.H. Optimization of the GBMV2 implicit solvent force field for accurate simulation of protein conformational equilibria. *J. Comput. Chem.* **2017**, *38*, 1332–1341. [CrossRef]
83. Lee, M.S.; Feig, M.; Salsbury, F.R.; Brooks, C.L. New analytic approximation to the standard molecular volume definition and its application to generalized born calculations. *J. Comput. Chem.* **2003**, *24*, 1348–1356. [CrossRef]
84. Choi, J.M.; Pappu, R.V. Improvements to the ABSINTH Force Field for Proteins Based on Experimentally Derived Amino Acid Specific Backbone Conformational Statistics. *J. Chem. Theory Comput.* **2019**, *15*, 1367–1382. [CrossRef]
85. Lazaridis, T.; Karplus, M. Effective energy function for proteins in solution. *Proteins* **1999**, *35*, 133–152. [CrossRef]
86. Das, R.K.; Pappu, R.V. Conformations of intrinsically disordered proteins are influenced by linear sequence distributions of oppositely charged residues. *Proc. Natl. Acad. Sci. USA* **2013**, *110*, 13392–13397. [CrossRef]
87. Wuttke, R.; Hofmann, H.; Nettels, D.; Borgia, M.B.; Mittal, J.; Best, R.B.; Schuler, B. Temperature-dependent solvation modulates the dimensions of disordered proteins. *Proc. Natl. Acad. Sci. USA* **2014**, *111*, 5213–5218. [CrossRef]
88. Davtyan, A.; Schafer, N.P.; Zheng, W.H.; Clementi, C.; Wolynes, P.G.; Papoian, G.A. AWSEM-MD: Protein Structure Prediction Using Coarse-Grained Physical Potentials and Bioinformatically Based Local Structure Biasing. *J. Phys. Chem. B* **2012**, *116*, 8494–8503. [CrossRef]
89. Davtyan, A.; Zheng, W.H.; Schafer, N.; Wolynes, P.; Papoian, G. AWSEM-MD: Coarse-Grained Protein Structure Prediction using Physical Potentials and Bioinformatically Based Local Structure Biasing. *Biophys. J.* **2012**, *102*, 619a. [CrossRef]
90. Wu, H.; Wolynes, P.G.; Papoian, G.A. AWSEM-IDP: A Coarse-Grained Force Field for Intrinsically Disordered Proteins. *J. Phys. Chem. B* **2018**, *122*, 11115–11125. [CrossRef]

91. Lin, X.C.; Roy, S.; Jolly, M.K.; Bocci, F.; Schafer, N.P.; Tsai, M.Y.; Chen, Y.H.; He, Y.N.; Grishaev, A.; Weninger, K.; et al. PAGE4 and Conformational Switching: Insights from Molecular Dynamics Simulations and Implications for Prostate Cancer. *J. Mol. Biol.* **2018**, *430*, 2422–2438. [CrossRef]
92. Bereau, T.; Deserno, M. Generic coarse-grained model for protein folding and aggregation. *J. Chem. Phys.* **2009**, *130*, 235106. [CrossRef]
93. Rutter, G.O.; Brown, A.H.; Quigley, D.; Walsh, T.R.; Allen, M.P. Testing the transferability of a coarse-grained model to intrinsically disordered proteins. *Phys. Chem. Chem. Phys.* **2015**, *17*, 31741–31749. [CrossRef]
94. Rutter, G.O.; Brown, A.H.; Quigley, D.; Walsh, T.R.; Allen, M.P. Emergence of order in self-assembly of the intrinsically disordered biomineralisation peptide n16N. *Mol. Simulat.* **2018**, *44*, 463–469. [CrossRef]
95. Salmon, L.; Nodet, G.; Ozenne, V.; Yin, G.W.; Jensen, M.R.; Zweckstetter, M.; Blackledge, M. NMR Characterization of Long-Range Order in Intrinsically Disordered Proteins. *J. Am. Chem. Soc.* **2010**, *132*, 8407–8418. [CrossRef]
96. Hsu, W.L.; Oldfield, C.J.; Xue, B.; Meng, J.; Huang, F.; Romero, P.; Uversky, V.N.; Dunker, A.K. Exploring the binding diversity of intrinsically disordered proteins involved in one-to-many binding. *Protein Sci.* **2013**, *22*, 258–273. [CrossRef]
97. Sharma, R.; Raduly, Z.; Miskei, M.; Fuxreiter, M. Fuzzy complexes: Specific binding without complete folding. *Febs. Lett.* **2015**, *589*, 2533–2542. [CrossRef]
98. Arbesu, M.; Iruela, G.; Fuentes, H.; Teixeira, J.M.C.; Pons, M. Intramolecular Fuzzy Interactions Involving Intrinsically Disordered Domains. *Front. Mol. Biosci.* **2018**, *5*. [CrossRef]
99. Jakob, U.; Kriwacki, R.; Uversky, V.N. Conditionally and Transiently Disordered Proteins: Awakening Cryptic Disorder to Regulate Protein Function. *Chem. Rev.* **2014**, *114*, 6779–6805. [CrossRef]
100. Sigalov, A.B. Membrane binding of intrinsically disordered proteins: Critical importance of an appropriate membrane model. *Self. Nonself.* **2010**, *1*, 129–132. [CrossRef]
101. Milles, S.; Mercadante, D.; Aramburu, I.V.; Jensen, M.R.; Banterle, N.; Koehler, C.; Tyagi, S.; Clarke, J.; Shammas, S.L.; Blackledge, M.; et al. Plasticity of an Ultrafast Interaction between Nucleoporins and Nuclear Transport Receptors. *Cell* **2015**, *163*, 734–745. [CrossRef]
102. Arai, M.; Sugase, K.; Dyson, H.J.; Wright, P.E. Conformational propensities of intrinsically disordered proteins influence the mechanism of binding and folding. *Proc. Natl. Acad. Sci. USA* **2015**, *112*, 9614–9619. [CrossRef]
103. Wang, Y.; Chu, X.K.; Longhi, S.; Roche, P.; Han, W.; Wang, E.K.; Wang, J. Multiscaled exploration of coupled folding and binding of an intrinsically disordered molecular recognition element in measles virus nucleoprotein. *Proc. Natl. Acad. Sci. USA* **2013**, *110*, E3743–E3752. [CrossRef]
104. Ganguly, D.; Chen, J.H. Topology-based modeling of intrinsically disordered proteins: Balancing intrinsic folding and intermolecular interactions. *Proteins* **2011**, *79*, 1251–1266. [CrossRef]
105. Turjanski, A.G.; Gutkind, J.S.; Best, R.B.; Hummer, G. Binding-induced folding of a natively unstructured transcription factor. *PLoS Comput. Biol.* **2008**, *4*, e1000060. [CrossRef]
106. Lu, Q.; Lu, H.P.; Wang, J. Exploring the mechanism of flexible biomolecular recognition with single molecule dynamics. *Phys. Rev. Lett.* **2007**, *98*, 263602. [CrossRef]
107. Ganguly, D.; Zhang, W.H.; Chen, J.H. Electrostatically Accelerated Encounter and Folding for Facile Recognition of Intrinsically Disordered Proteins. *PLoS Comput. Biol.* **2013**, *9*, e1003363. [CrossRef]
108. Knott, M.; Best, R.B. Discriminating binding mechanisms of an intrinsically disordered protein via a multi-state coarse-grained model. *J. Chem. Phys.* **2014**, *140*, 175102. [CrossRef] [PubMed]
109. Clementi, C.; Nymeyer, H.; Onuchic, J.N. Topological and energetic factors: What determines the structural details of the transition state ensemble and "en-route" intermediates for protein folding? An investigation for small globular proteins. *J. Mol. Biol.* **2000**, *298*, 937–953. [CrossRef]
110. Bryngelson, J.D.; Wolynes, P.G. Spin-Glasses and the Statistical-Mechanics of Protein Folding. *Proc. Natl. Acad. Sci. USA* **1987**, *84*, 7524–7528. [CrossRef]
111. Bryngelson, J.D.; Onuchic, J.N.; Socci, N.D.; Wolynes, P.G. Funnels, Pathways, and the Energy Landscape of Protein-Folding - a Synthesis. *Proteins* **1995**, *21*, 167–195. [CrossRef]
112. Uversky, V.N. Intrinsically disordered proteins in overcrowded milieu: Membrane-less organelles, phase separation, and intrinsic disorder. *Curr. Opin. Struc. Biol.* **2017**, *44*, 18–30. [CrossRef] [PubMed]
113. Cuevas-Velazquez, C.L.; Dinneny, J.R. Organization out of disorder: liquid-liquid phase separation in plants. *Curr. Opin. Plant. Biol.* **2018**, *45*, 68–74. [CrossRef]

114. Darling, A.L.; Liu, Y.; Oldfield, C.J.; Uversky, V.N. Intrinsically Disordered Proteome of Human Membrane-Less Organelles. *Proteomics* **2018**, *18*, 1700193. [CrossRef]
115. Ambadipudi, S.; Biernat, J.; Riedel, D.; Mandelkow, E.; Zweckstetter, M. Liquid-liquid phase separation of the microtubule-binding repeats of the Alzheimer-related protein Tau. *Nat. Commun.* **2017**, *8*, 275. [CrossRef]
116. Dignon, G.L.; Zheng, W.W.; Kim, Y.C.; Best, R.B.; Mittal, J. Sequence determinants of protein phase behavior from a coarse-grained model. *PLoS Comput. Biol.* **2018**, *14*, e1005941. [CrossRef]
117. Boeynaems, S.; Holehouse, A.S.; Weinhardt, V.; Kovacs, D.; Van Lindt, J.; Larabell, C.; Van Den Bosch, L.; Das, R.; Tompa, P.S.; Pappu, R.V.; et al. Spontaneous driving forces give rise to protein-RNA condensates with coexisting phases and complex material properties. *Proc. Natl. Acad. Sci. USA* **2019**. [CrossRef]
118. Lin, Y.H.; Forman-Kay, J.D.; Chan, H.S. Theories for Sequence-Dependent Phase Behaviors of Biomolecular Condensates. *Biochemistry* **2018**, *57*, 2499–2508. [CrossRef]
119. Ruff, K.M.; Pappu, R.V.; Holehouse, A.S. Conformational preferences and phase behavior of intrinsically disordered low complexity sequences: insights from multiscale simulations. *Curr. Opin. Struct. Biol.* **2018**, *56*, 1–10. [CrossRef]
120. Kremer, K.; Binder, K. Monte-Carlo Simulations of Lattice Models for Macromolecules. *Comput. Phys. Rep.* **1988**, *7*, 259–310. [CrossRef]
121. Bhattacharya, S.; Coasne, B.; Hung, F.R.; Gubbins, K.E. Modeling Micelle-Templated Mesoporous Material SBA-15: Atomistic Model and Gas Adsorption Studies. *Langmuir* **2009**, *25*, 5802–5813. [CrossRef]
122. McCarty, J.; Delaney, K.T.; Danielsen, S.P.O.; Fredrickson, G.H.; Shea, J.E. Complete Phase Diagram for Liquid-Liquid Phase Separation of Intrinsically Disordered Proteins. *J. Phys. Chem. Lett.* **2019**, *10*, 1644–1652. [CrossRef]
123. Levine, Z.A.; Larini, L.; LaPointe, N.E.; Feinstein, S.C.; Shea, J.E. Regulation and aggregation of intrinsically disordered peptides. *Proc. Natl. Acad. Sci. USA* **2015**, *112*, 2758–2763. [CrossRef]
124. Das, P.; Murray, B.; Belfort, G. Alzheimer's protective A2T mutation changes the conformational landscape of the Aβ_{1-42} monomer differently than does the A2V mutation. *Biophys. J.* **2015**, *108*, 738–747. [CrossRef]
125. Chakraborty, S.; Das, P. Emergence of Alternative Structures in Amyloid Beta 1-42 Monomeric Landscape by N-terminal Hexapeptide Amyloid Inhibitors. *Sci. Rep.-UK* **2017**, *7*, 9941. [CrossRef]
126. Mondal, B.; Reddy, G. Cosolvent Effects on the Growth of Protein Aggregates Formed by a Single Domain Globular Protein and an Intrinsically Disordered Protein. *J. Phys. Chem. B* **2019**, *123*, 1950–1960. [CrossRef]
127. Zheng, W.H.; Schafer, N.P.; Wolynes, P.G. Free energy landscapes for initiation and branching of protein aggregation. *Proc. Natl. Acad. Sci. USA* **2013**, *110*, 20515–20520. [CrossRef] [PubMed]
128. Metallo, S.J. Intrinsically disordered proteins are potential drug targets. *Curr. Opin. Chem. Biol.* **2010**, *14*, 481–488. [CrossRef] [PubMed]
129. Camargo, D.C.R.; Tripsianes, K.; Buday, K.; Franko, A.; Gobl, C.; Hartlmuller, C.; Sarkar, R.; Aichler, M.; Mettenleiter, G.; Schulz, M.; et al. The redox environment triggers conformational changes and aggregation of hIAPP in Type II Diabetes. *Sci. Rep.-UK* **2017**, *7*, 44041. [CrossRef]
130. Follis, A.V.; Hammoudeh, D.I.; Wang, H.B.; Prochownik, E.V.; Metallo, S.J. Structural Rationale for the Coupled Binding and Unfolding of the c-Myc Oncoprotein by Small Molecules. *Chem. Biol.* **2008**, *15*, 1149–1155. [CrossRef]
131. Hammoudeh, D.I.; Follis, A.V.; Prochownik, E.V.; Metallo, S.J. Multiple Independent Binding Sites for Small-Molecule Inhibitors on the Oncoprotein c-Myc. *J. Am. Chem. Soc.* **2009**, *131*, 7390–7401. [CrossRef]
132. Neira, J.L.; Bintz, J.; Arruebo, M.; Rizzuti, B.; Bonacci, T.; Vega, S.; Lanas, A.; Velazquez-Campoy, A.; Iovanna, J.L.; Abian, O. Identification of a Drug Targeting an Intrinsically Disordered Protein Involved in Pancreatic Adenocarcinoma. *Sci. Rep.-UK* **2017**, *7*, 39732. [CrossRef] [PubMed]
133. Price, D.L.; Koike, M.A.; Khan, A.; Wrasidlo, W.; Rockenstein, E.; Masliah, E.; Bonhaus, D. The small molecule alpha-synuclein misfolding inhibitor, NPT200-11, produces multiple benefits in an animal model of Parkinson's disease. *Sci. Rep.-UK* **2018**, *8*, 16165. [CrossRef]
134. Pujols, J.; Pena-Diaz, S.; Lazaro, D.F.; Peccati, F.; Pinheiro, F.; Gonzalez, D.; Carija, A.; Navarro, S.; Conde-Gimenez, M.; Garcia, J.; et al. Small molecule inhibits alpha-synuclein aggregation, disrupts amyloid fibrils, and prevents degeneration of dopaminergic neurons. *Proc. Natl. Acad. Sci. USA* **2018**, *115*, 10481–10486. [CrossRef]
135. Ruan, H.; Sun, Q.; Zhang, W.L.; Liu, Y.; Lai, L.H. Targeting intrinsically disordered proteins at the edge of chaos. *Drug Discov. Today* **2019**, *24*, 217–227. [CrossRef]

136. Joshi, P.; Vendruscolo, M. Druggability of Intrinsically Disordered Proteins. *Adv. Exp. Med. Biol.* **2015**, *870*, 383–400. [CrossRef] [PubMed]
137. Cheng, Y.; LeGall, T.; Oldfield, C.J.; Mueller, J.P.; Van, Y.Y.J.; Romero, P.; Cortese, M.S.; Uversky, V.N.; Dunker, A.K. Rational drug design via intrinsically disordered protein. *Trends Biotechnol.* **2006**, *24*, 435–442. [CrossRef]
138. Subramaniam, S.; Mehrotra, M.; Gupta, D. Virtual high throughput screening (vHTS)—A perspective. *Bioinformation* **2008**, *3*, 14–17. [CrossRef]
139. Zhang, Y.; Cao, H.; Liu, Z. Binding cavities and druggability of intrinsically disordered proteins. *Protein Sci.* **2015**, *24*, 688–705. [CrossRef]
140. Michel, J.; Cuchillo, R. The Impact of Small Molecule Binding on the Energy Landscape of the Intrinsically Disordered Protein C-Myc. *PLoS ONE* **2012**, *7*. [CrossRef]
141. Venken, T.; Voet, A.; De Maeyer, M.; De Fabritiis, G.; Sadiq, S.K. Rapid Conformational Fluctuations of Disordered HIV-1 Fusion Peptide in Solution. *J. Chem. Theory Comput.* **2013**, *9*, 2870–2874. [CrossRef]
142. Motlagh, H.N.; Wrabl, J.O.; Li, J.; Hilser, V.J. The ensemble nature of allostery. *Nature* **2014**, *508*, 331–339. [CrossRef]
143. Motlagh, H.N.; Li, J.; Thompson, E.B.; Hilser, V.J. Interplay between allostery and intrinsic disorder in an ensemble. *Biochem. Soc. T.* **2012**, *40*, 975–980. [CrossRef] [PubMed]
144. Ferreon, A.C.M.; Ferreon, J.C.; Wright, P.E.; Deniz, A.A. Modulation of allostery by protein intrinsic disorder. *Nature* **2013**, *498*, 390–394. [CrossRef] [PubMed]
145. Bai, F.; Branch, R.W.; Nicolau, D.V.; Pilizota, T.; Steel, B.C.; Maini, P.K.; Berry, R.M. Conformational Spread as a Mechanism for Cooperativity in the Bacterial Flagellar Switch. *Science* **2010**, *327*, 685–689. [CrossRef] [PubMed]
146. Bhattacharya, S.; Vaidehi, N. Differences in Allosteric Communication Pipelines in the Inactive and Active States of a GPCR. *Biophys. J.* **2014**, *107*, 422–434. [CrossRef]
147. Tautermann, C.S.; Binder, F.; Buttner, F.H.; Eickmeier, C.; Fiegen, D.; Gross, U.; Grundl, M.A.; Heilker, R.; Hobson, S.; Hoerer, S.; et al. Allosteric Activation of Striatal-Enriched Protein Tyrosine Phosphatase (STEP, PTPN5) by a Fragment-like Molecule. *J. Med. Chem.* **2019**, *62*, 306–316. [CrossRef] [PubMed]
148. Li, H.; Kasam, V.; Tautermann, C.S.; Seeliger, D.; Vaidehi, N. Computational Method to Identify Druggable Binding Sites That Target Protein-Protein Interactions. *J. Chem. Infor. Model.* **2014**, *54*, 1391–1400. [CrossRef]
149. Le Guilloux, V.; Schmidtke, P.; Tuffery, P. Fpocket: An open source platform for ligand pocket detection. *BMC Bioinformatics* **2009**, *10*. [CrossRef] [PubMed]
150. Fisher, C.K.; Huang, A.; Stultz, C.M. Modeling Intrinsically Disordered Proteins with Bayesian Statistics. *J. Am. Chem. Soc.* **2010**, *132*, 14919–14927. [CrossRef] [PubMed]
151. Gong, H.C.; Zhang, S.; Wang, J.D.; Gong, H.P.; Zeng, J.Y. Constructing Structure Ensembles of Intrinsically Disordered Proteins from Chemical Shift Data. *J. Comput. Biol.* **2016**, *23*, 300–310. [CrossRef] [PubMed]
152. Sickmeier, M.; Hamilton, J.A.; LeGall, T.; Vacic, V.; Cortese, M.S.; Tantos, A.; Szabo, B.; Tompa, P.; Chen, J.; Uversky, V.N.; et al. DisProt: the database of disordered proteins. *Nucleic Acids Res.* **2007**, *35*, D786–D793. [CrossRef] [PubMed]
153. Varadi, M.; Kosol, S.; Lebrun, P.; Valentini, E.; Blackledge, M.; Dunker, A.K.; Felli, I.C.; Forman-Kay, J.D.; Kriwacki, R.W.; Pierattelli, R.; et al. pE-DB: a database of structural ensembles of intrinsically disordered and of unfolded proteins. *Nucleic Acids Res.* **2014**, *42*, D326–D335. [CrossRef]
154. Morcos, F.; Pagnani, A.; Lunt, B.; Bertolino, A.; Marks, D.S.; Sander, C.; Zecchina, R.; Onuchic, J.N.; Hwa, T.; Weigt, M. Direct-coupling analysis of residue coevolution captures native contacts across many protein families. *Proc. Natl. Acad. Sci. USA* **2011**, *108*, E1293–E1301. [CrossRef] [PubMed]
155. Bai, F.; Morcos, F.; Cheng, R.R.; Jiang, H.L.; Onuchic, J.N. Elucidating the druggable interface of protein-protein interactions using fragment docking and coevolutionary analysis. *Proc. Natl. Acad. Sci. USA* **2016**, *113*, E8051–E8058. [CrossRef]
156. Pancsa, R.; Zsolyomi, F.; Tompa, P. Co-Evolution of Intrinsically Disordered Proteins with Folded Partners Witnessed by Evolutionary Couplings. *Int. J. Mol. Sci.* **2018**, *19*, 3315. [CrossRef] [PubMed]

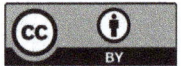

© 2019 by the authors. Licensee MDPI, Basel, Switzerland. This article is an open access article distributed under the terms and conditions of the Creative Commons Attribution (CC BY) license (http://creativecommons.org/licenses/by/4.0/).

MDPI
St. Alban-Anlage 66
4052 Basel
Switzerland
Tel. +41 61 683 77 34
Fax +41 61 302 89 18
www.mdpi.com

Biomolecules Editorial Office
E-mail: biomolecules@mdpi.com
www.mdpi.com/journal/biomolecules

www.ingramcontent.com/pod-product-compliance
Lightning Source LLC
LaVergne TN
LVHW070407100526
838202LV00014B/1406